Burn Care: Rescue, Resuscitation, and Resurfacing

Editors

CHARLES SCOTT HULTMAN
MICHAEL W. NEUMEISTER

CLINICS IN PLASTIC SURGERY

www.plasticsurgery.theclinics.com

July 2017 • Volume 44 • Number 3

ELSEVIER

1600 John F. Kennedy Boulevard • Suite 1800 • Philadelphia, Pennsylvania, 19103-2899

http://www.theclinics.com

CLINICS IN PLASTIC SURGERY Volume 44, Number 3
July 2017 ISSN 0094-1298, ISBN-13: 978-0-323-53148-1

Editor: Jessica McCool
Developmental Editor: Donald Mumford

Clinics in Plastic Surgery (ISSN 0094-1298) is published quarterly by Elsevier Inc., 360 Park Avenue South, New York, NY 10010-1710. Months of issue are January, April, July, and October. Business and Editorial Offices: 1600 John F. Kennedy Blvd., Suite 1800, Philadelphia, PA 19103-2899. Periodicals postage paid at New York, NY and additional mailing offices. Subscription prices are $495.00 per year for US individuals, $825.00 per year for US institutions, $100.00 per year for US students and residents, $561.00 per year for Canadian individuals, $982.00 per year for Canadian institutions, $636.00 per year for international individuals, $982.00 per year for international institutions, and $305.00 per year for Canadian and foreign students/residents. To receive student/resident rate, orders must be accompanied by name of affiliated institution, date of term, and the *signature* of program/residency coordinator on institution letterhead. Orders will be billed at individual rate until proof of status is received. Foreign air speed delivery is included in all *Clinics* subscription prices. All prices are subject to change without notice. **POSTMASTER:** Send address changes to *Clinics in Plastic Surgery*, Elsevier Health Sciences Division, Subscription Customer Service, 3251 Riverport Lane, Maryland Heights, MO 63043. **Customer Service: 1-800-654-2452 (US and Canada). From outside of the United States and Canada, call 314-447-8871. Fax: 314-447-8029. E-mail: JournalsCustomerService-usa@elsevier.com (for print support); JournalsOnlineSupport-usa@ elsevier.com (for online support).**

Reprints. For copies of 100 or more of articles in this publication, please contact the Commercial Reprints Department, Elsevier Inc., 360 Park Avenue South, New York, New York 10010-1710. Tel.: +1-212-633-3874; Fax: +1-212-633-3820; E-mail: reprints@elsevier.com.

Clinics in Plastic Surgery is covered in *Current Contents, EMBASE/Excerpta Medica, Science Citation Index, MEDLINE/ PubMed (Index Medicus), ASCA, and ISI/BIOMED.*

Contributors

EDITORS

CHARLES SCOTT HULTMAN, MD, MBA, FACS
Ethel F. and James A. Valone Distinguished Professor of Surgery, Chief, Division of Plastic Surgery, Founder and Medical Director, University of North Carolina Aesthetic, Laser, and Burn Reconstruction Center, Department of Surgery, University of North Carolina School of Medicine, Chapel Hill, North Carolina

MICHAEL W. NEUMEISTER, MD, FRCSC, FACS
Professor and Chair, Department of Surgery, The Elvin G. Zook Endowed Chair in Plastic Surgery, Institute for Plastic Surgery, Southern Illinois University School of Medicine, Springfield, Illinois

AUTHORS

WONE BANDA, MD, FCS(plast)-ECSA, MSc
Consultant Plastic Surgeon, Queen Elizabeth Central Hospital, Blantyre, Malawi

NORAN BARRY, MD
Assistant Professor of Surgery, Acute Care Surgery, Department of Surgery, Duke University Medical Center, Durham, North Carolina

EDWARD A. BITTNER, MD, PhD
Associate Professor, Department of Anesthesia, Critical Care and Pain Medicine, Massachusetts General Hospital, Boston, Massachusetts

DAVID A. BROWN, MD, PhD
Plastic and Reconstructive Surgery Resident, Duke University School of Medicine, Durham, North Carolina

BRUCE A. CAIRNS, MD, FACS
Professor, Department of Surgery, North Carolina Jaycee Burn Center, University of North Carolina School of Medicine, University of North Carolina at Chapel Hill, Chapel Hill, North Carolina

ROBERT CARTOTTO, MD, FRCS(C)
Associate Professor, Division of Plastic Surgery, Department of Surgery, Ross Tiley Burn Centre, Sunnybrook Health Sciences Centre, University of Toronto, Toronto, Ontario, Canada

ANTHONY G. CHARLES, MD, MPH, FACS
Associate Professor, Department of Surgery, North Carolina Jaycee Burn Center, School of Medicine, University of North Carolina at Chapel Hill, Chapel Hill, North Carolina

AMALIA L. COCHRAN, MD, MA
Associate Professor, Department of Surgery, University of Utah Burn Center, University of Utah, Salt Lake City, Utah

ZACHARY J. COLLIER, BA
Biological Sciences Division, Pritzker School of Medicine, University of Chicago, Chicago, Illinois

ELIZABETH L. DALE, MD
Medical Director, Burn Center, Assistant Professor of Surgery, Division of Plastic/Burn Surgery, Shriners Hospital for Children, University of Cincinnati, Cincinnati, Ohio

TIMOTHY H.F. DAUGHERTY, MD, MS
Resident Physician, Institute for Plastic
Surgery, Southern Illinois University School of
Medicine, Springfield, Illinois

PAUL DIEGIDIO, MD
Department of Surgery, University of North
Carolina School of Medicine, Chapel Hill, North
Carolina

STEPHEN TYLER ELKINS-WILLIAMS, MD
Resident, Division of Plastic and
Reconstructive Surgery, Department of
Surgery, University of North Carolina Medical
Center, University of North Carolina at Chapel
Hill, Chapel Hill, North Carolina

JONATHAN FRIEDSTAT, MD
Division of Burns, Massachusetts General
Hospital and Boston Shriners Hospital for
Children, Instructor in Surgery, Harvard
Medical School, Boston, Massachusetts

JARED GALLAHER, MD, MPH
Department of Surgery, North Carolina Jaycee
Burn Center, University of North Carolina at
Chapel Hill, Chapel Hill, North Carolina

ROJA GARIMELLA, BS
Alpert Medical School, Brown University,
Providence, Rhode Island

WARREN GARNER, MD
Professor, Division of Plastic Surgery,
Department of Surgery, Keck School of
Medicine, University of Southern California,
Los Angeles, California

GIORGIO GIATSIDIS, MD
Instructor, Harvard Medical School, Division of
Plastic Surgery, Brigham and Women's
Hospital, Boston, Massachusetts

JUSTIN GILLENWATER, MD, MS
Assistant Professor of Surgery, Division of
Plastic Surgery, Department of Surgery, Keck
School of Medicine, University of Southern
California, Los Angeles, California

AMANDA A. GOSMAN, MD
Professor of Plastic Surgery, Craniofacial
Fellowship Program Director, Director of
Craniofacial and Pediatric Plastic Surgery,
Residency Program Director, School of
Medicine, University of California San Diego,
San Diego, California

LAWRENCE J. GOTTLIEB, MD
Director of Burn and Complex Wound Center,
Section of Plastic and Reconstructive Surgery,
Professor, Department of Surgery, University
of Chicago, Chicago, Illinois

JEREMY GOVERMAN, MD
Assistant Professor, Division of Burn and
Plastic and Reconstructive Surgery,
Department of Surgery, Massachusetts
General Hospital, Boston, Massachusetts

ERNEST J. GRANT, PhD, RN, FAAN
Nursing Education Clinician, Burn Outreach,
North Carolina Jaycee Burn Center, University
of North Carolina Hospitals, Adjunct Assistant
Professor, University of North Carolina School
of Nursing, Chapel Hill, North Carolina

CORNELIA GRIGGS, MD
House Officer, Department of Surgery,
Massachusetts General Hospital, Boston,
Massachusetts

ANTHONY G. HADDAD, MD
Department of Surgery, Brigham and Women's
Hospital, Boston, Massachusetts

ERIC G. HALVORSON, MD
Plastic Surgery Center of Asheville, Asheville,
North Carolina

STEVEN J. HERMIZ, MD
Department of Surgery, University of
South Carolina School of Medicine, Columbia,
South Carolina

DAVID N. HERNDON, MD, FACS
Professor, Department of Surgery, Shriners
Hospital of Children, University of Texas
Medical Branch, Galveston, Texas

WILLIAM L. HICKERSON, MD, FACS
Medical Director, Department of Plastic
Surgery, Firefighters Regional Burn Center,
Regional One Health, Professor, Department of
Plastic Surgery, College of Medicine,
University of Tennessee Health Science
Center, Memphis, Tennessee

DAVID M. HILL, PharmD, BCPS
Clinical Pharmacist, Department of Pharmacy,
Firefighters Regional Burn Center, Regional
One Health, Department of Clinical Pharmacy,
College of Pharmacy, University of Tennessee
Health Science Center, Memphis, Tennessee

FRANZISKA HUETTNER, MD, PhD, FACS
Assistant Professor, Department of Surgery, Institute for Plastic Surgery, Southern Illinois University School of Medicine, Springfield, Illinois

CHARLES SCOTT HULTMAN, MD, MBA, FACS
Ethel F. and James A. Valone Distinguished Professor of Surgery, Chief, Division of Plastic Surgery, Founder and Medical Director, University of North Carolina Aesthetic, Laser, and Burn Reconstruction Center, Department of Surgery, University of North Carolina School of Medicine, Chapel Hill, North Carolina

ARI ISAACSON, MD
Department of Radiology, University of North Carolina School of Medicine, Chapel Hill, North Carolina

SAMUEL W. JONES, MD, FACS
Associate Professor, Department of Surgery, North Carolina Jaycee Burn Center, University of North Carolina School of Medicine, University of North Carolina at Chapel Hill, Chapel Hill, North Carolina

NEEL A. KANTAK, MD
Plastic and Reconstructive Surgeon, Mid-Atlantic Permanente Medical Group, Largo Medical Center, Upper Marlboro, Maryland

RANDY D. KEARNS, DHA, MSA, CEM
Assistant Professor and Chair, Management Services Division, Tillman School of Business, University of Mount Olive, Mount Olive, North Carolina; Retired Clinical Assistant Professor, University of North Carolina School of Medicine, Chapel Hill, North Carolina

BENJAMIN LEVI, MD
Burn Wound and Regenerative Medicine Laboratory, Assistant Professor, Division of Plastic Surgery, Department of Surgery, University of Michigan School of Medicine, University of Michigan, Ann Arbor, Michigan

LILLIAN F. LIAO, MD, MPH
Assistant Professor, Division of Trauma and Emergency Medicine, University of Texas Health Science Center at San Antonio, San Antonio, Texas

DAVID E. MARCOZZI, MD, MHS-CL, FACEP
Associate Professor of Emergency Medicine, Director of Population Health, The University of Maryland School of Medicine, Baltimore, Maryland; LT COL, USAR, Deputy Surgeon, US Army Special Operations Command, Ft. Bragg, North Carolina

WILLIAM A. MARSTON, MD
Chief, Division of Vascular Surgery, Department of Surgery, University of North Carolina Medical Center, University of North Carolina at Chapel Hill, Chapel Hill, North Carolina

MATTHEW A. MAURO, MD
Department of Radiology, University of North Carolina School of Medicine, Chapel Hill, North Carolina

RIYAM MISTRY, MBChB, BSc (Hons)
Junior Doctor, Department of Plastic Surgery, Royal Devon and Exeter Hospital NHS Foundation Trust, Exeter, United Kingdom

APOORVE NAYYAR, MBBS
Department of Surgery, University of North Carolina School of Medicine, Chapel Hill, North Carolina

MICHAEL W. NEUMEISTER, MD, FRCSC, FACS
Professor and Chair, Department of Surgery, The Elvin G. Zook Endowed Chair in Plastic Surgery, Institute for Plastic Surgery, Southern Illinois University School of Medicine, Springfield, Illinois

ANDREA T. OBI, MD
Vascular Surgery Fellow, Department of Surgery, University of Michigan, Ann Arbor, Michigan

DENNIS P. ORGILL, MD, PhD
Professor, Harvard Medical School, Division of Plastic Surgery, Brigham and Women's Hospital, Boston, Massachusetts

SHIARA ORTIZ-PUJOLS, MD
Department of Surgery, University of North Carolina School of Medicine, Chapel Hill, North Carolina

CHRISTOPHER J. PANNUCCI, MD, MS
Assistant Professor, Division of Plastic Surgery, University of Utah, Salt Lake City, Utah

PRESTON B. RICH, MD, MBA, FACS
Regional Deputy Chief Medical Officer, NDMS,
US Department of Health and Human Services,
Professor of Surgery, Acute Care Surgery,
Department of Surgery, University of
North Carolina School of Medicine, Chapel Hill,
North Carolina

CHRISTINA ROLLINS, RD, CNSC
Director, Food and Nutrition Services,
Memorial Medical Center, Springfield,
Illinois

AMANDA ROSS, MD
Resident Physician, Institute for Plastic
Surgery, Southern Illinois University School of
Medicine, Springfield, Illinois

MICHELLE C. ROUGHTON, MD
Assistant Professor, Division of Plastic and
Reconstructive Surgery, Department of
Surgery, University of North Carolina at
Chapel Hill, Chapel Hill, North Carolina

LEWIS RUBINSON, MD, PhD
Director, Critical Care Resuscitation Unit,
R. Adams Cowley Shock Trauma Center,
Associate Professor, University of Maryland
School of Medicine, Baltimore,
Maryland

ANNA SCHOENBRUNNER, MAS
School of Medicine, University of California
San Diego, San Diego, California

AMITA R. SHAH, MD, PhD
Division of Plastic and Reconstructive Surgery,
University of North Carolina at Chapel Hill,
Chapel Hill, North Carolina; Assistant Professor,
Division of Plastic and Reconstructive Surgery,
University of Texas Health Science Center
at San Antonio, San Antonio, Texas

ROBERT L. SHERIDAN, MD, FAAP, FACS
Burn Service Medical Director, Boston Shriners
Hospital for Children, Division of Burns,
Massachusetts General Hospital, Professor of
Surgery, Harvard Medical School, Boston,
Massachusetts

SCOTT E. SINCLAIR, MD, FCCP
Director of Pulmonary and Critical Care
Services, Department of Medicine,
Firefighters Regional Burn Center, Regional
One Health, Associate Professor, Department
of Medicine, College of Medicine, University of
Tennessee Health Science Center, Memphis,
Tennessee

AMY L. STRONG, MD, PhD, MPH
Plastic Surgery Resident, Division of Plastic
Surgery, Department of Surgery, University of
Michigan, Ann Arbor, Michigan

BENJAMIN H. TIMMINS, MD
Resident Surgeon, Division of Plastic Surgery,
Oregon Health Sciences University, Portland,
Oregon

DAVID VAN DUIN, MD, PhD
Department of Medicine, University of North
Carolina School of Medicine, Chapel Hill, North
Carolina

DAVID E. VARON, BA
Research Assistant, Division of Plastic Surgery,
Brigham and Women's Hospital, Boston,
Massachusetts

KAITLYN VOTTA, BA
Boston Shriners Hospital for Children, Boston,
Massachusetts; Georgetown University
Medical School, Washington, DC

DAVID J. WEBER, MD, MPH
Department of Medicine, University of
North Carolina School of Medicine, Chapel Hill,
North Carolina

FELICIA N. WILLIAMS, MD
Assistant Professor, Department of Surgery,
North Carolina Jaycee Burn Center, University
of North Carolina at Chapel Hill, Chapel Hill,
North Carolina

HYEON YU, MD
Department of Radiology, University of
North Carolina School of Medicine, Chapel Hill,
North Carolina

Contents

Rescue

and illicit substances, characteristics of the burn wound, and concomitant injury are all red flags for inflicted and negligent burns.

This article examines the societal impact of thermal injury in low- and middle-income countries. The authors describe the unique challenges of these health care systems in providing care for burned patients, focusing on resuscitation, excision and grafting, rehabilitation, and reconstruction.

Burns are an often-overlooked health indicator in global health literature, but account for a significant global health burden in lower middle income countries. This article provides an overview of burn injury from the global health perspective. It focuses on education and research, emphasizing the appropriate role of volunteerism.

Resuscitation

This article reviews the pathophysiology of large burn injury and the extreme fluid shifts that occur in the hours and days after this event. The authors focus on acute fluid management, monitoring of hemodynamic status, and end points of resuscitation. Understanding the need and causes for fluid resuscitation after burn injury helps the clinician develop an effective plan to balance the competing goals of normalized tissue perfusion and limited tissue edema. Thoughtful, individualized treatment is the best answer and the most effective compromise.

The classic determinants of mortality from severe burn injury are age, size of injury, delays of resuscitation, and the presence of inhalation injury. Of the major determinants of mortality, inhalation injury remains one of the most challenging injuries for burn care providers. Patients with inhalation injury are at increased risk for pneumonia (the leading cause of death) and multisystem organ failure. There is no consensus among leading burn care centers in the management of inhalation injury. This article outlines the current treatment algorithms and the evidence of their efficacy.

This article highlights the challenges in managing pulmonary failure after burn injury. The authors review several different ventilator techniques, provide weaning parameters, and discuss complications.

Caring for patients with burn injuries is challenging secondary to the acute disease process, chronic comorbidities, and underrepresentation in evidence-based literature. Much current practice relies on extrapolation of guidance from different patient populations and wide variations in universal practices. Identifying infections or sepsis in this hypermetabolic population is imperfect and often leads to overprescribing of antimicrobials, suboptimal dosing, and multidrug resistance. An understanding of pharmacokinetics and pharmacodynamics may aid optimization of dosing regimens to better attain treatment targets. This article provides an overview of the current status of burn infection and attempts recommendations for consideration to improve universally accepted care.

Although pain management is a major challenge for clinicians, appropriate pain control is the foundation of efficacious burn care from initial injury to long-term recovery. The very treatments designed to treat burn wounds may inflict more pain than the initial injury itself, making it the clinician's duty to embrace a multimodal treatment approach to burn pain. Vigilant pain assessment, meaningful understanding of the pathophysiology and pharmacologic considerations across different phases of burn injury, and compassionate attention to anxiety and other psychosocial contributors to pain will enhance the clinician's ability to provide excellent pain management.

Severe burn injury is followed by a profound hypermetabolic response that persists up to 2 years after injury. It is mediated by up to 50-fold elevations in plasma catecholamines, cortisol, and glucagon that lead to whole-body catabolism, elevated resting energy expenditures, and multiorgan dysfunction. Modulation of the response by early excision and grafting of burn wounds, thermoregulation, control of infection, early and continuous enteral nutrition, and pharmacologic treatments aimed at mitigating physiologic derangements have markedly decreased morbidity.

This article provides a clinician's guide to nutritional support of the burn patient. The authors review the assessment and management of the needs of the thermally injured patient and provide recommendations on replacement and supplementation with calories, protein, carbohydrates, lipids, fluids, and minerals. Furthermore, the authors compare and contrast enteral versus parenteral delivery of nutrition.

Although acute acalculous cholecystitis is uncommon in burn patients, this condition can be rapidly fatal due to delays in diagnosis and treatment and should always be considered in the differential diagnosis when burn patients become septic, develop abdominal pain, or have hemodynamic instability. This article reviews the use of percutaneous cholecystostomy in burn patients as both a diagnostic and therapeutic intervention.

Venous thromboembolism (VTE) can be a life-threatening or limb-threatening complication of thermal injury. The severity of burn injury can be used to predict VTE risk among patients with thermal injury, and a weighted risk-stratification tool has been developed. This article reviews the incidence, diagnosis, and management of thromboembolic events in patients with burns. The article particularly focuses on identifying those patients who are at highest risk for VTE and provides recommendations on mechanical and chemical prophylaxis.

Stevens-Johnson syndrome and toxic epidermal necrolysis are rare, life-threatening, cutaneous drug reactions. Medications are the most common cause, although an infection may be responsible. A link between genetics and certain medications has been established. Clinical diagnosis should be confirmed with biopsy. When the area of epidermal detachment approaches 30%, burn center care is advisable. An ophthalmologist should be consulted to optimize ocular care. Pharmacologic interruption has been sought but there is little consensus on the most appropriate agent and no high-quality studies have been conducted to demonstrate if any of these agents lead to improved survival.

This article reviews a single burn center experience with life-threatening skin disorders, over a 10-year period. It explores the incidence of health care–associated infections and the impact on length of stay, hospital charges, and mortality.

Severe pediatric burns require a multidisciplinary team approach at a specialized pediatric burn center. Special attention must be paid to estimations of total body surface area, fluid resuscitation and metabolic demands, and adequate analgesia and sedation. Long-term effects involve scar management and psychosocial support to the child and their family. Compassionate comprehensive burn care is accomplished by a multidisciplinary team offering healing in the acute setting and preparing the child and family for long-term treatment and care.

Resurfacing

Negative pressure wound therapy (NPWT) has become a widely used treatment for acute and chronic wounds. NPWT is indicated for a variety of complex wounds, and some studies validate its use for certain aspects of burn care. Although further research is needed to explore the benefits for burns, NPWT has proven beneficial in its use as a dressing that bolsters skin grafts, promotes integration of bilaminate dermal substitutes, promotes re-epithelialization of skin graft donor sites, and potentially reduces the zone of stasis. This article reviews the literature on NPWT in burns, based on indication/application, and describes our experience with the use of modified NPWT for large burns.

This article reviews the current evidence in using hyperbaric oxygen therapy (HBOT) in burn wounds. There is also separate consideration of diabetic foot burns and a protocol for use of HBOT in a specific case. The challenges of using HBOT in an acute burn care setting are reviewed. Next the pathophysiology of Marjolin ulcers is reviewed. The current thinking in diagnosis, treatment, and prevention of Marjolin ulcers is discussed. Finally, a background in using topical growth factors (tGF) is provided, followed by a summary of the current evidence of tGF in burn wounds.

CLINICS IN PLASTIC SURGERY

FORTHCOMING ISSUES

October 2017
Burn Care: Reconstruction, Rehabilitation, and Recovery
Charles Scott Hultman and
Michael W. Neumeister, *Editors*

January 2018
Contemporary Indications in Breast Reconstruction
Stefan O.P. Hofer, Jian Farhadi, and
Jaume Masià, *Editors*

April 2018
Gluteal Augmentation
Robert F. Centeno and Constantino G. Mendieta,
Editors

RECENT ISSUES

April 2017
Microsurgery: Global Perspectives
Jin Bo Tang and Michel Saint-Cyr, *Editors*

January 2017
Pre-expanded Perforator Flaps
Lee L.Q. Pu and Chunmei Wang, *Editors*

October 2016
Free Tissue Transfer to Head and Neck: Lessons Learned from Unfavorable Results
Fu-Chan Wei and Nidal Farhan AL Deek, *Editors*

ISSUE OF RELATED INTEREST

Surgical Clinics of North America, Volume 94, Issue 4 (August 2014)
Management of Burns
Robert L. Sheridan, *Editor*
Available at: http://www.surgical.theclinics.com/

THE CLINICS ARE AVAILABLE ONLINE!
Access your subscription at:
www.theclinics.com

CLINICS IN PLASTIC SURGERY

Preface

Volume 1: Rescue, Resuscitation, and Resurfacing

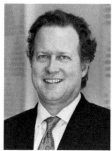

Charles Scott Hultman, MD, MBA, FACS   Michael W. Neumeister, MD, FRCSC, FACS

Editors

Advances in burn care over the last 10 to 15 years have resulted in new innovations, better treatment, and improved outcomes. Patient care is championed by the collaboration of many disciplines focused on the team management of each burn victim. Communication and a comprehension of each discipline's approach to each individual are, therefore, paramount for optimized care.

Our early discussions about running regional burn units identified a mutual passion for managing the acute and chronic care of burn patients. This led to the genesis of the management of burn care in the *Clinics of Plastic Surgery*. Although textbooks may be comprehensive, the material may be outdated soon after publication. The purpose, then, of this two-volume set was to offer the most comprehensive, up-to-date, published communication of knowledge, strategies, and treatment of all aspects of managing the burned patient. Surgeons and other health care providers may find this information useful in the daily care of burn victims. Contributions were solicited from a variety of disciplines, including surgeons, physicians, nurses, therapists, nutritionists, pharmacists, and researchers, each providing their perspective and evidence on issues that arise in the management of the acutely sick, recovering, or chronically debilitated burn patient.

Burn trauma remains one of the most devastating injuries we address as plastic surgeons. The resilience and strength of the burn victims must be respected if not admired as they endure pain, infection, organ failure, scarring, and functional compromise. Their families, social network, and employment can be thrust into turmoil. The complexity of treating burn patients from the moment they enter the burn unit to the conclusion of their reconstructive procedures, and through all of their therapy, mandates dedication and passion of the caregivers involved.

We would therefore like to acknowledge and thank all burn care providers for their commitment and reverence for their role in caring for burn victims. We are especially motivated by the patients themselves, who demonstrate a level of fortitude, conviction, and faith that serves to inspire all of us.

Charles Scott Hultman, MD, MBA, FACS
Department of Surgery
University of North Carolina School of Medicine
7040 Burnett-Womack
Chapel Hill, NC 27599-7195, USA

Michael W. Neumeister, MD, FRCSC, FACS
Department of Surgery
Institute for Plastic Surgery
Southern Illinois University School of Medicine
Baylis Medical Building
747 North Rutledge Street
3rd Floor, Suite 357
Springfield, IL 62702, USA

E-mail addresses:
scott_hultman@med.unc.edu (C.S. Hultman)
mneumeister@siumed.edu (M.W. Neumeister)

Clin Plastic Surg 44 (2017) xv
http://dx.doi.org/10.1016/j.cps.2017.05.001
0094-1298/17/© 2017 Published by Elsevier Inc.

Rescue

Lessons Learned from Burn Disasters in the Post-9/11 Era

 CrossMark

Robert L. Sheridan, MD*, Jonathan Friedstat, MD,
Kaitlyn Votta, BA

KEYWORDS

- Burns • Disasters • Mass casualty

KEY POINTS

- Burns units will be called upon to respond to a variety of disaster scenarios. Although every event is unique, several lessons have been learned in recent years by programs responding to industrial accidents, terrorist incidents, and natural disasters. The burn program should fit within the existing disaster command structure and scene security should precede patient processing.
- On-scene triage by experienced personnel is more effective than moving patients to a central area for triage. Minor injuries should be managed outside the hospital environment. Enteral resuscitation can be effective for many moderate injuries.
- A variety of injures can be expected. Patient categories are delayed, expectant, and immediate, but patients can move between categories as individual status and available resources change.
- Simple protocols, just-in-time training, and real-time expert consultation can effectively expand the number of capable initial burn care providers.
- Less seriously injured patients can consume significant resources later. Secondary long-distance triage is an important strategy for these patients.

INTRODUCTION

Providing care for unexpected, large numbers of burn patients is never easy or neat. Unfortunately, it is sometimes necessary. As burn care has become a defined surgical specialty, practitioners have had to work alongside their emergency and trauma colleagues in addressing these situations. Although every scenario is unique, certain themes have emerged repeatedly and are the foundations of lessons that can be useful to those faced with future burn disasters. These lessons, detailed in later discussion, are loosely organized to follow the flow of a major burn event (**Box 1**).

LESSON: THE BURN PROGRAM SHOULD FIT WITHIN THE EXISTING DISASTER COMMAND STRUCTURE

One of the most essential components of disaster planning is clear delineation of responsibility and communication. Without these essentials, rescue and recovery operations become ineffective and dangerous. Actions at the disaster site and triage stations must be orchestrated with those of transportation vehicles and treatment centers. Examples abound in which disaster responses were impeded by poor coordination and enhanced by strong command and control operations.

Boston Shriners Hospital for Children, 51 Blossom Street, Boston, MA 02114, USA
* Corresponding author.
E-mail address: rsheridan@mgh.harvard.edu

Clin Plastic Surg 44 (2017) 435–440
http://dx.doi.org/10.1016/j.cps.2017.02.003

plasticsurgery.theclinics.com

During the response to the 1970 natural gas pipeline explosion in Osaka, Japan, the response team lacked a chain of command; the lack of central command and control made triage and transfer exceedingly difficult.[1,2] During the response to the 1980 fire in the MGM Grand Hotel in Las Vegas, Nevada, the initial triage post was overrun with patients. Good communication spurred the quick establishment of 2 more stations whose activity was coordinated by a central command post. This prompt response allowed 3000 people to be triaged in 3.5 hours after the fire initially broke out.[3] After the 2002 Bali bombings, where 3 separate bombs were detonated in popular tourist locations, better communication might have allowed available resources to have been delegated much more effectively.[4] In the first hours after the 2003 Station Nightclub fire in Rhode Island, limited communication between the triage sites and local and regional burn centers was a major

issue.[5] Hospitals did not know when or where emergency vehicles were arriving, complicating preparation.[6]

All disaster responders, but especially specialist programs such as burn units, must ensure that they are embedded within a larger response program if they wish to provide the right services to the right patients. With burn patients, who have long and complex aftercare needs, this respect for the overarching response organization remains important long after the initial event.

LESSON: SCENE SECURITY SHOULD PRECEDE PATIENT PROCESSING

Scene safety and security must be reasonably established before care is provided. Safety and security will be provided by the larger command structure and includes such things as reasonable protection from secondary terosit attack and structural integrity of buildings. During the early hours of the response to the 1998 discotheque fire in Gothenburg, Sweden, first responders had trouble with triage due to a lack of crowd control. One provider was physically attacked, while family members of the injured took medical supplies for their own use, impairing triage efforts by the rescuers.[1,7]

LESSON: ON-SCENE TRIAGE BY EXPERIENCED PERSONNEL IS ESSENTIAL AND MUCH PREFERABLE TO MOVING PATIENTS TO A CENTRAL AREA FOR TRIAGE

Focusing the limited skilled personnel and equipment on patients who both need the care and are salvageable is essential. Efficient care is greatly facilitated by triaging as far forward as can be safely done. Given the subtleties of burn wound interpretation and the frequent presence of concomitant nonburn trauma in disaster scenarios, forward triage is ideally assigned to very experienced providers. The goal of triage is to sort patients into 3 rough categories: (1) Patients likely to survive with minimal or delayed care ("delayed patients"); (2) Patients unlikely to live regardless of care ("expectant patients"); and (3) Patients in whom immediate care is likely to improve their probability of survival ("immediate patients"). Individual patient categorization will vary with a host of factors, including burn injury severity, concomitant injury, patient age and preexisting conditions, disaster scene location, scene security, transport and regional resources, and available medical resources. Individual patient categorization will also change with time, as more resources are brought to bear on the situation. Initial patient categorization requires mature judgment to best integrate all of these factors. Triaging as close to the scene as possible will minimize overtaxing limited care available for immediate patients. For example, in the 1970 Osaka natural gas line explosion, many nearby pedestrians and inhabitants sustained relatively minor injuries, but the lack of field triage required hospital-based providers to do the initial sorting, which was thought to compromise their ability to provide immediate care to those most in need.[1,2]

LESSON: MINOR INJURIES SHOULD BE MANAGED OUTSIDE THE HOSPITAL ENVIRONMENT

To optimize urgent care of patients who are truly in need of such care (immediate patients), those with minor injuries who can wait for care (delayed patients) are ideally removed from both the scene of injury and the sites of immediate care. In most scenarios, this group forms the large majority of patients. If they are not efficiently processed, they can make it virtually impossible for providers to address the needs of the immediate patients. There are examples of incidents where this was done well. In the 1980 MGM Grand fire, those with less severe injuries were bused to burn centers further away, while the closer hospitals were reserved for people with more severe injuries.[3] In the Gothenburg discotheque fire in Sweden, they used buses to transport the minimally injured quickly away from the scene.[7] This use of mass transportation clears out the burn centers and hospitals nearby to handle the influx of more critical patients. Ideally, expectant patients are similarly cohorted and managed outside the areas of immediate care.

LESSON: THERE WILL BE A VARIETY AND COMPLEXITY OF MIXED INJURIES

Pure burn injury disasters are rare, and the burn program skill set is useful for a host of nonburn trauma. Depending on the disaster mechanism, providers must expect to deal with concomitant blast and crush injury, penetrating and blunt visceral injury, and neurologic and orthopedic injury.[8] In addition, depending on the scenario details and extrication delay, environmental injury such as frostbite may complicate the initial burn.[9] Burn programs may also be brought in as primary responders or to provide secondary care for disaster victims involved in scenarios that cause extensive nonburn soft tissue injury. Examples include blast injury, such as seen in terrorist activities (**Fig. 1**), or crush injury, as seen in earthquake-associated building collapses (**Fig. 2**). In the days following the initial event, soft tissue infections

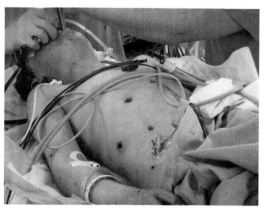

Fig. 1. Blast and fragmentation injury caused by suicide terrorist bombing in Afghanistan.

are common (**Fig. 3**). Burn care providers tasked to respond to incidents at which mixed trauma can be expected must be prepared with appropriate training and experience to manage these patients, whose needs often present conflicts requiring mature judgment.[10]

LESSON: MAJOR PATIENT CATEGORIES ARE DELAYED, EXPECTANT, AND IMMEDIATE; PATIENTS CAN MOVE BETWEEN CATEGORIES AS INDIVIDUAL STATUS AND AVAILABLE RESOURCES CHANGE

Every disaster scenario is different.[11] Resources available for immediate response are frequently very limited. However, in the hours and days following the events, available resources for patient transportation and care often surge. In light of the additional resources, patient categories can change. For example, immediately after the 2010 Haiti earthquake, available resources were very limited for survivors with severe orthopedic injuries. However, as the days and weeks passed,

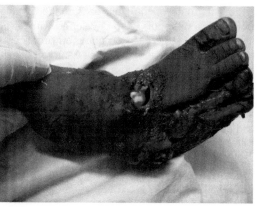

Fig. 2. Crush injury seen in earthquake-associated building collapse in Haiti.

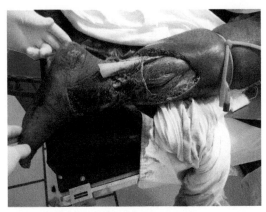

Fig. 3. Invasive soft tissue infections are common in the days following soft tissue injury such as occur in large numbers in earthquakes or blasts.

a massive international response brought significant resources to bear, resulting in patients moving from the delayed to immediate care categories.[12] The international response also resulted in available dialysis for patients with crush injuries, and transportation to alternative sites of care, such as aboard the hospital ship *Comfort*. In the immediate aftermath of the disaster, patients may be appropriately sorted into the expectant category, but as resources for care increase, may be appropriately recategorized as immediate. Providers should be prepared for continual reassessment of patients for changing physiology and in light of changing available resources.

LESSON: USE SIMPLE PROTOCOLS

In the early response to disasters, many providers will be working together who have never worked before in the same program. Furthermore, many nonburn providers will be expected to provide burn care with limited direction. The use of extremely simple protocols will greatly facilitate patient care in these circumstances. For example, in the aftermath of the Haiti earthquake, simple wound care protocols were developed with ketamine analgesia, modeled on common practice in burn programs.[13] In long-distance transport of military burn casualties, long-acting silver dressings can be applied without need for wound care en route.[14] Keeping care strategies as simple as possible facilitates quick "just-in-time" training and communication between providers unfamiliar with burn care and with each other.

LESSON: HAVE REAL-TIME EXPERT CONSULTATION AVAILABLE

In a mass disaster involving burns, most burn care will need to be provided by nonburn

specialists. Expert burn providers will be more valuable advising than caring directly for patients in many circumstances. Local sharing of specialty knowledge is common when mass casualty events are managed within a single institution. Medical professionals coached by local expert burn providers are able to provide excellent care to larger numbers of patients than the local experts could care. This concept can be extended to regions. For example, traveling "B-teams" were formed in response to the 2001 Volendam café disaster in the Netherlands. "B-teams" comprised experienced burn care experts and traveled around to regional hospitals to provide advice and help with transfer decisions.[15] Ideally, in a large area disaster, such consultation could be provided in real time using electronic communication means. Such advice can be invaluable to guide resuscitation, wound evaluation, patient sorting, and initial procedures such as escharotomy and fasciotomy.[16,17]

LESSON: PUSH FORWARD JUST-IN-TIME TRAINING

Providers who do not provide burn care on a regular basis will not be able to maintain competency in the early needs of such patients. The concept of "just-in-time training" is important and should be further developed. The American Burn Association has developed the "ABLS–Now" (Advanced Burn Life Support Now) program, which can provide immediate access to online training modules relevant to the early care of burn patients.[18] The Open Pediatrics project at Boston's Children's Hospital contains on-line burn content that is also useful for providers faced with the need to care for burn patients in the absence of experience.[19] This concept of Internet-based just-in-time training has the potential to immediately expand the knowledge base of experienced providers in facing mass burn disasters.

LESSON: CONSIDER ENTERAL RESUSCITATION

Although traditionally performed intravenously, there is significant experience with enteral resuscitation in the developing world[20] and in disaster scenarios.[21] Enteral resuscitation can be accomplished via spontaneous consumption or nasogastric administration of electrolyte-containing formulas, such as the World Health Organization rehydration formula. Simple saline-based formulas can also be made using usually available kitchen supplies.[22] Monitoring proceeds as in intravenous resuscitation.[23]

LESSON: LESS SERIOUSLY INJURED PATIENTS CAN CONSUME SIGNIFICANT RESOURCES LATER

In a mass burn disaster, delayed patients are likely to have full-thickness wounds of limited extent (**Fig. 4**). Although reasonably delayed in a disaster scenario, these patients will later require significant surgery and rehabilitation services. Plans for care of this potentially large cohort of patients must be made and may include regional transfer as transport becomes available.

LESSON: LONG-TERM PATIENT NEEDS ARE VERY SIGNIFICANT, LONG TRANSCENDING THE ACUTE EVENT

In the aftermath of the Rhode Island nightclub fire, providers at the Massachusetts General Hospital burn unit who cared for some of the most seriously injured victims found that the late acute and reconstructive needs of this cohort of patients consumed enormous staff time and resources. Early post-acute phase patients have very significant needs for hospital care, surgery, rehabilitation, and emotional support. These needs must be included in the disaster planning process. In some cases, patients should be transferred to distant burn programs for this phase of care or they may exhaust local resources. At this point, typically between bulk wound closure and discharge, a very useful transfer window exists.

LESSON: USE SECONDARY REGIONAL AND LONG-DISTANCE TRANSFER WINDOWS CREATIVELY

During the care of burn patients, there are several windows available during which long-distance

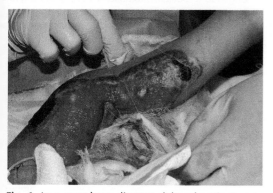

Fig. 4. In a mass burn disaster, delayed patients may be likely to have full-thickness wounds of limited extent. Although reasonably delayed in a disaster scenario, these patients will later require significant surgery and rehabilitation services. Plans for care of this potentially large cohort of patients must be made.

transfer is reasonably safe. If the individual patient will receive better care after transfer, it is appropriate to accept the small risk incurred with transportation. Commonly, there exist transfer windows between fluid resuscitation and initial excision, between initial excision and definitive closure, and between definitive closure and rehabilitation. Even long-distance international transfer is possible during these windows,[24] with en route care needs decreasing with each window.[25] When patient numbers are large, and regional or national resources suffice, these windows should be taken advantage of to optimize patient care.

LESSON: MAINTAIN RELATIONSHIPS WITH REGIONAL AND NATIONAL UNITS TO FACILITATE DISTRIBUTION OF PATIENTS

Finally, maintenance of close collegial relationships between regional and national burn programs is very useful.[26] These relationships may include documentation of burn bed availability. Most importantly, they can facilitate optimal use of transfer windows to broadly distribute patients to ensure that individual patient care is not compromised by excessive demand on the staff of a small number of burn units. In some circumstances, these relationships can be used to increase staffing of individual units near the site of disaster with experienced personnel from regional and national burn programs, but credentialing and other logistic issues usually make patient transfer more practical than staff transfer.

SUMMARY

Burns are a common component of disaster scenarios. Although every event is unique, several lessons have been repeatedly emphasized by providers who have successfully weathered mass casualty events involving burns. Flexibility and communication are at the core of most of these lessons. By analyzing and learning from past events, it is hoped that future events will be less traumatic for victims and responders alike.

REFERENCES

1. Cancio LC, Pruitt BA. Management of mass casualty burn disasters. Intl J Disaster Med 2005;1–16. http://dx.doi.org/10.1080/15031430510034640.
2. Ishida T, Ohta M, Sugimoto T. The breakdown of an emergency system following a gas explosion in Osaka and the subsequent resolution of problems. J Emerg Med 1985;2:183–9.

3. Buerk CA, Batdorf JW, Cammack KV, et al. The MGM grand hotel fire: lessons learned from a major disaster. Arch Surg 1982;117:641–4.

4. Tran MD, Garner AA, Morrison I, et al. The Bali bombing: civilian aeromedical evacuation. Med J Aust 2003;179:353–6.

5. Mahoney EJ, Harrington DT, Biffl WL, et al. Lessons learned from a nightclub fire: institutional disaster preparedness. J Trauma 2005;58(3):487–91.

6. Harrington DT, Biffl WL, Cioffi WG. The station nightclub fire. J Burn Care Rehabil 2005;26:141–3.

7. Cassuto J, Tarnow P. The discotheque fire in Gothenburg 1998. A tragedy among teenagers. Burns 2003;29:405–16.

8. Chipman M, Hackley BE, Spencer TS. Triage of mass casualties: concepts for coping with mixed battlefield injuries. Mil Med 1980;145(2):99–100.

9. Cancio LC, Lundy JB, Sheridan RL. Evolving changes in the management of burns and environmental injuries. Surg Clin North Am 2012;92(4):959–86, ix.

10. Rosenkranz KM, Sheridan R. Management of the burned trauma patient: balancing conflicting priorities. Burns 2002;28(7):665–9.

11. Cancio LC, Sheridan RL, Dent R, et al. Guidelines for burn care under austere conditions: special etiologies: blast, radiation, and chemical injuries. J Burn Care Res 2017;38(1):e482–96.

12. van Berlaer G, Staes T, Danschutter D, et al. Disaster preparedness and response improvement: comparison of the 2010 Haiti earthquake-related diagnoses with baseline medical data. Eur J Emerg Med 2016. [Epub ahead of print].

13. Rice MJ, Gwertzman A, Finley T, et al. Anesthetic practice in Haiti after the 2010 earthquake. Anesth Analg 2010;111(6):1445–9.

14. Barillo DJ, Pozza M, Margaret-Brandt M. A literature review of the military uses of silver-nylon dressings with emphasis on wartime operations. Burns 2014;40(Suppl 1):S24–9.

15. Kuijper EC. The 2003 Everett Idris Evans memorial lecture: every cloud has a silver lining. J Burn Care Rehabil 2004;25:45–53.

16. Bell RC, Yager PH, Clark ME, et al. Telemedicine versus face-to-face evaluations by respiratory therapists of mechanically ventilated neonates and children: a pilot study. Respir Care 2016;61(2):149–54.

17. Yager PH, Cummings BM, Whalen MJ, et al. Nighttime telecommunication between remote staff intensivists and bedside personnel in a pediatric intensive care unit: a retrospective study. Crit Care Med 2012;40(9):2700–3.

18. Cochran A, Edelman LS, Morris SE, et al. Learner satisfaction with Web-based learning as an adjunct to clinical experience in burn surgery. J Burn Care Res 2008;29(1):222–6.

19. Wolbrink TA, Kissoon N, Burns JP. The development of an internet-based knowledge exchange platform for pediatric critical care clinicians worldwide*. Pediatr Crit Care Med 2014;15(3):197–205.

20. Rode H, Rogers AD, Cox SG, et al. Burn resuscitation on the African continent. Burns 2014;40(7):1283–91.

21. Kramer GC, Michell MW, Oliveira H, et al. Oral and enteral resuscitation of burn shock the historical record and implications for mass casualty care. Eplasty 2010;10:e56.

22. Young AW, Graves C, Kowalske KJ, et al. Guideline for burn care under austere conditions: special care topics. J Burn Care Res 2017;38(2):e497–509.

23. Kearns RD, Conlon KM, Matherly AF, et al. Guidelines for burn care under austere conditions: introduction to burn disaster, airway and ventilator management, and fluid resuscitation. J Burn Care Res 2016;37(5):e427–39.

24. Sheridan RL, Schaefer PW, Whalen M, et al. Case records of the Massachusetts General Hospital. Case 36-2012. Recovery of a 16-year-old girl from trauma and burns after a car accident. N Engl J Med 2012;367(21):2027–37.

25. Schmidt PM, Sheridan RL, Moore CL, et al. From Baghdad to Boston: international transfer of burned children in time of war. J Burn Care Res 2014;35(5):369–73.

26. Kearns RD, Conlon KM, Valenta AL, et al. Disaster planning: the basics of creating a burn mass casualty disaster plan for a burn center. J Burn Care Res 2014;35(1):e1–13.

Disaster Preparedness and Response for the Burn Mass Casualty Incident in the Twenty-first Century

Randy D. Kearns, DHA, MSA, CEM[a],*,
David E. Marcozzi, MD, MHS-CL[b,c], Noran Barry, MD[d],
Lewis Rubinson, MD, PhD[e],
Charles Scott Hultman, MD, MBA[f],
Preston B. Rich, MD, MBA[g]

KEYWORDS

• Burn injury • Mass casualty incident • Disaster preparedness • Surge capacity

KEY POINTS

- Managing the Burn Mass Casualty Incident requires planning and a unique knowledge of where the resources are located.
- More resources are available (trauma services) when the disaster includes only burn injured patients (nightclub fire versus industrial plant explosion).
- If the disaster includes infrastructure damage such as an earthquake or a terrorist explosion, it may hinder patients coming to you or being able to transfer them to other facilities.
- The first line of defense is what you have at your facility to include what you can create by adapted spaces and reverse triage in the hospital with the aim of discharging those who can go home.
- Housekeeping staff play a vital role getting rooms cleaned if rapid discharge decisions need to be made to create more space. Involve them in the planning process.

INTRODUCTION

Due to their unpredictability and indiscriminate impact on either unprepared and seemingly risk-free populations or military populations, disasters of even local magnitude tend to be large-scale media events, and the associated responses to them are subject to intense media scrutiny. As a result, society's exposure to mass casualty incidents (MCIs) and their associated management are commonly measured through a sensational and incomplete lens of media outlets. This skewed, remote, and occasionally distanced perspective can often lead to harsh unproductive critiques of observed actions viewed out of context, focused praise of certain isolated high-profile efforts, or harsh judgment of perceived failures with little science to judge operations, outcomes, or perspectives offered.

In contrast, the perspective of health care responders who become engulfed in the actual

[a] Management Services Division, Tillman School of Business, University of Mount Olive, Mount Olive, NC, USA; [b] The University of Maryland School of Medicine, 620 West Lexington Street, Baltimore, MD 21201, USA; [c] USAR, US Army Special Operations Command, Ft. Bragg, NC, USA; [d] Acute Care Surgery, Department of Surgery, Duke University Medical Center, 2301 Erwin Road, Durham, NC 27710, USA; [e] Critical Care Resuscitation Unit, R. Adams Cowley Shock Trauma Center, University of Maryland School of Medicine, Baltimore, MD, USA; [f] Department of Surgery, University of North Carolina School of Medicine, Chapel Hill, NC, USA; [g] Acute Care Surgery, Department of Surgery, University of North Carolina School of Medicine, Chapel Hill, NC, USA
* Corresponding author.
E-mail address: randy.kearns@earthlink.net

Clin Plastic Surg 44 (2017) 441–449
http://dx.doi.org/10.1016/j.cps.2017.02.004

chaos of an unfolding disaster is real, dynamic, complicated, and inherently linked to emotion. The scope and scale of a given disaster, the quantity or quality of available resources, or the geopolitical implications of a particular event can vary widely. Each disaster response can be universally reduced to the aggregate actions of individuals who are called on to make complex, immediate, and high-stake decisions that ultimately contribute to the outcome. Although the process always begins with first responders, it systematically evolves and expands throughout the entire health care system, inclusive of 9-1-1 call systems, emergency medical systems (EMS), triage centers, initial receiving hospitals, and definitive care and postacute facilities, extending well into available rehabilitation and psychosocial support infrastructure. Disasters are fundamentally local community events that commonly grow to involve regions, nations, and sometimes even manifest global impact.

Disasters are local events. Therefore, sound community MCI planning is critical to effecting excellent patient outcomes. Capacity and capability are inherently resource-based. This requires the development and implementation of thoughtful, carefully crafted, and individually designed emergency plans that match potential needs with a progressive echelon of available or potentially available response assets.[1]

Although first-responder personnel commonly consist of local EMS, fire, hazardous materials (HAZMAT), or rescue assets, training and available equipment often vary significantly between jurisdictions. Furthermore, the initial facilities that receive the first wave of patients may range from major regional referral medical centers to minimally staffed critical access hospitals and may even consist of temporary mobile shelters.

Given these known and anticipated variabilities in available resources, pre-incident planning is crucial. This planning contributes to the provision of consistent care delivered through the rational coordination of integrated system-level care networks.[2–4] When disaster strikes, the first calls for help are funneled to the local 9-1-1 center (although 9-1-1 is the number used primarily in the United States and other countries, this number varies in other countries to include 9-9-9 and 1-1-2 being several of the more common).

Once the call is placed to the emergency communications center, the trigger point for all disasters with a medical component will rest on the shoulders of the local EMS system. Thus, the first wave of patients will be managed by EMS personnel (the *First Responders*) and the emergency department physicians and nurses (the *First Receivers*). It should be noted that casualty evacuation may take on many forms, including the use of privately owned and law enforcement vehicles. Nevertheless, a vast majority of patients are initially managed by first responders and all those with serious injuries are managed by the first receivers.

TYPES OF MEDICAL DISASTERS

Burn injuries are one of the most challenging medical disaster scenarios. Burn MCI (BMCI) typically can be linked to 1 of 3 broad scenarios: a mass gathering, such as a theater, dinner, or nightclub with a sudden fire; natural disaster, such as wildfire or earthquake; or purposeful hostilities, such as terrorism, bomb blast, or an act of war.[5] As an event becomes more complex, the variety of wounds and concomitant injuries will require a more diverse response. If there is concurrent damage to infrastructure that limits hospital care or limits transportation access, the problems and limitations may grow exponentially.

Despite the infrequent nature of medical disasters, their initial management and the subsequent surge in capacity that necessarily follows, quickly becomes the greatest challenge, and potential threat to a given hospital, health care system, or region.[3,6] Learning from these events, whether civilian or military, offers opportunities for improvement in approach to trauma delivery across the nation and around the world.[7] The purpose of this article was to review the basics of disaster planning, preparedness, response, and recovery in the aftermath of a medical disaster. Although the primary focus is BMCI, illustrative examples include natural disaster and infectious disease principles.

CONTENT: WHY BURN INJURIES?

Patients with significant burn injuries represent a small subset of patients; however, due to their complexity and injury severity, they impose a disproportionate impact on health care systems. A recent survey revealed that even seasoned practitioners, including experienced physicians, nurses, and paramedics, stated they were "uncomfortable with their knowledge, skills, and ability to care for a burn-injured patient."[8]

The capability to effectively manage and care for BMCI is a critical determinant of desirable outcomes in the care of patients with burn injuries.[9–12] Given the scarcity of resources and the infrequency of BMCI events, it is reasonable to consider and plan for these events as worst-case scenarios in modern health care systems.

Successful BMCI planning includes thorough examination of existing internal protocols, patient flow parameters, and the engagement of all pertinent stakeholders.[5,13] Geography and lines of political jurisdiction are important planning factors, and close coordination and communication between various burn centers are essential for a successful response.[14,15]

ALL-HAZARDS, CAPABILITY-BASED PLANNING, SURGE CAPACITY, AND THE STANDARD OF CARE

The critical phase of MCI planning involves initial patient assessment and management, individualized triage, and subsequent referral to accepting definitive care centers. Preparations for large-scale events must include plans to address surge resources on local, regional, and national scales.[1,4,16–18] Capacity refers to the quantity of staff, space, and supplies (pharmaceuticals and equipment) available. Capability refers to the types of clinicians available to render appropriate care for the sick and injured, as well as the quality of equipment needed to perform certain procedures.

Key factors that determine capacity include commonly available routinely used resources in addition to key assets that can be flexed to specifically accommodate MCI needs, such as holding areas, outpatient facilities, conference rooms, and often the adaptation of temporary structures to serve this purpose.[19,20] An important measure of scalable capacity is the ability to increase bed availability through flexing by 20% within 4 hours for the highest acuity patients.[19]

Factors to consider in a capability analysis include available equipment and its asset typing, noninventory materials that have the potential for shipping and receiving, and available personnel with detailed credentialing information.[4] In addition, an understanding of transportation assets, multijurisdictional, and multiagency are imperative.[21]

FACILITY PLANNING

Over the past 10 years, clinicians have gained a greater understanding in the assessment and management of MCIs with regard to the fine balance of *staff, space, and supplies.*[22,23] By 2009, the surge planning had evolved to stratify surge capacity into 3 defined categories: *Conventional, Contingency, and Crisis Surge Capacities.*[18,21]

Some mass casualty events can be managed with limited strain on existing health care resources. At times, surging requires only small modifications in staffing, hospital-based equipment, and treatment facility spaces. In these cases, traditional standards of care may remain intact.

In events where needs outstrip resources, traditional standards of care and expectations require modification. *Contingency surge capacity* measures may include such things as provision of medical care in otherwise nontraditional settings and/or by nontraditional practitioners. Staffing will still often include clinicians with traditional credentials but who may be unaccustomed with the specialized care that will need to be delivered. Supplies are commonly limited in these settings, and in some cases substitute medications or fluids may need to be used. The most unpredictable limitation is the availability of and access to supplies and specialty equipment, such as intravenous pumps and ventilators.

Crisis Surge Capacity implies that the practices of care may, by necessity, extend outside of what may be considered traditional standards of care. Although often required under these conditions, mitigation strategies should be enacted to alleviate them as soon as is reasonably possible. The pre-incident planning process provides an ideal opportunity to engage informed policymakers to define community care standards under various potential disaster scenarios, provide guidelines for acceptable care under resource-constrained conditions, and outline reasonable expectations for the infrastructure needed to manage any given disaster event.

SURGE EQUILIBRIUM

As a disaster scenario unfolds, there are trigger points that often mark event stabilization. The achievement of this state of relative balance (known as *surge equilibrium,* represented in **Fig. 1**) can be identified when sufficient numbers of patients have been transferred, discharged, or died. This inflection point creates conditions whereby patients with ongoing needs can be met on a steady and predictable basis by the staff, space, and supplies available for use. Effective and efficient transportation resources are often effective tools to enable relative patient decompression during a disaster by allowing rational triage of acutely injured or ill patients to appropriate receiving facilities and simultaneously shuttling supplies, personnel, and temporary treatment facilities to the disaster site.

IMMEDIATE BED AVAILABILITY, ALTERNATIVE STAFF RESOURCES, JUST-IN-TIME TRAINING, AND FORCE MULTIPLIERS

A core strategy for disaster process planning is implementation of an immediate bed availability

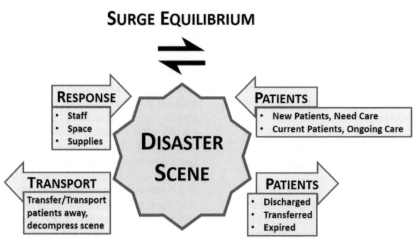

Fig. 1. The target is to reach surge equilibrium and provide care based on traditional standards of care. The 3 time phases may vary slightly based on quantity of available resources and proximity to the site of the BMCI (or burn disaster). Thus, as ranges in other state and regional plans are reviewed, they may not have the same precise 3 blocks of time. Nevertheless, the 3 general periods, immediate, intermediate (loosely defined as 6–120 hours), and extended (the 120 hours post disaster), are general windows for what is identified as a type III burn disaster. These windows of time may grow when the BMCI is competing for resources, such as with an explosion (type II), or there is impact to the infrastructure, such as an earthquake that damages the hospital or limits highway access for patient transport (type I). Surge Equilibrium: all competing influences of the disaster are balanced at the point of where the patients are being managed, disaster scene or at the hospital.

(IBA) approach, which emphasizes the deliberate triage and discharge of affected patients to available medical resources with reliance on existing personnel to receive and treat the initial influx of patients from an MCI. Ideally, IBA tactics should be expected to generate 20% more resources with no more than 4 hours' notice.

Strategies to surge staff include force multipliers through just-in-time (JIT) training by using personnel who have the aptitude to quickly learn, adapt, and assist.[24] Cross-training before a disaster can effectively augment personnel pools in preparation for an MCI event, but for logistic reasons may not be a viable option for smaller organizations. Military surge strategies offer excellent examples of how to systematically leverage medical resources by flexing available manpower that may not be considered traditional clinical complements. JIT training paradigms can augment targeted capabilities over relatively short time frames and can provide large groups of caregivers led by specially trained medical team leaders, allowing systems to manage large numbers of acute care patients.[25,26] Telemedicine platforms may also be used to augment staff and provide expert assistance "virtually" when the necessary technology is available to support the effort.[27]

Effective strategies that are commonly used to expand staffing resources during a crisis surge is the planned incorporation of disaster medical responders from other communities via preexisting

memoranda of understanding or capability expansion through the JIT training and use of nontraditional personnel. Availability of these resources varies widely between jurisdictions, and often includes state or regional teams in addition to federal disaster resources. The federal disaster teams are incorporated into the National Disaster Medical System (NDMS) within the US Department of Health and Human Services. This multifaceted approach facilitates the coordinated surge response, including both specialized equipment and personnel directly into the affected area and provides integrated transportation resources allowing patient movement away from the disaster site.[28]

Historically, the BMCI has also been widely discussed as a burn disaster.[5] For the purpose of using a common language, 3 general BMCI scenarios were identified, relying on National Incident Management System standards,[29] to aid disaster planners with a common language (detailed in **Box 1**). The 3 scenarios established 3 broad groups that escalate in complexity: one that impacts the burn care system, one that impacts the broader health care system, and one that reflects an impact on critical infrastructure.

The inherent complexity of disasters that include both trauma and burn-injured patients creates a scenario of competition for resources placing enormous pressure on the health care system to meet all of the needs within a traditional standard of care.[5] However, when infrastructure is catastrophically

---

Box 1
These are the 3 basic types of burn mass casualty incidents relying on the National Incident Management System order of classification; these classifications were first published in 2014

Burn Mass Casualty Incident (BMCI) (Burn Disaster) Scenarios

Type I BMCI:

- Description and example: catastrophic event, to include multiple casualties with various and combined burn injuries over a wide geographic area, such as earthquakes to include the 1994 Northridge earthquake,[68,69] the 9/11 attacks,[70–72] the Great East Japan earthquake (2011),[51,73] or an improvised nuclear device.[57,60,74,75]

- Impact: critical infrastructure

- Logic: impact to the infrastructure could be devastating. When the infrastructure is damaged, from highways to utilities, the magnitude of the disaster is amplified by the compromised facilities. When the facilities in which care is provided are damaged or essential utilities are disrupted, in addition to the surge of both burn and general traumatic injuries, most likely the management of the disaster will be suboptimal. Radiation-related incidents would include activation of the Radiation Injury Treatment Network, a cooperative effort of the National Marrow Donor Program and the American Society for Blood and Marrow Transplantation.[76]

Type II BMCI:

- Description and example: multiple-aspect burn disaster, such as an explosion, with significant numbers of traumatic as well as burn-injured patients producing multiple casualties with various blunt force and combined thermal injuries. This type of disaster would include the Madrid train bombings (2004)[65,66] and London subway attack (2005).[67]

- Impact: health care system

- Logic: impact to the health care system may be significant; due to the nature of the disaster, there may or may not be ample critical care and trauma care beds that can be adapted to care for those burn-injured patients who need less intensive attention by burn care professionals. Given the competing interests of traumatic injury with burn injury, filling the need without crossing into a crisis surge capacity may be problematic in the immediate geographic area near the site of the disaster.

Type III BMCI:

- Description and example: an isolated burn disaster with mostly thermal injuries, such the Rhode Island Station Night Club fire (2003)[61–63] or the Kiss Nightclub fire in Santa Maria, Brazil (2013).[64]

- Impact: burn care system

- Logic: impact to the burn care system may be significant; but due to the nature of the disaster, critical care and trauma care beds can be adapted to provide care for burn-injured patients who need less intensive attention by burn care professionals.

---

damaged or destroyed (eg, earthquakes), the result will most likely include widespread care being provided outside the typical standards. The downstream effect includes extending the stress into a region well beyond the impacted area. As such, earthquakes or any disaster that creates widespread damage to the infrastructure continues to be a focus for disaster planning.[5]

THREE STAGES OF ACTIVITY DURING A DISASTER PLAN
Activation Point/Trigger(s)

Disaster plans must include an activation point (trigger). Triggers are identified by a combination of data or science and the opinions of the subject matter experts. All disaster plans should offer sufficient latitude to move into the context of the plan early on in the disaster, in an attempt to control the common tendency toward chaos.

Functional Period of Activity

Disaster plans must have a functional period of activity. This functional activity can be tested and assessed through simulation and actual use. Simulation provides an opportunity to simultaneously test numerous inputs and variables in a cost-effective laboratory setting to identify potential plan weaknesses and augment plan strengths.

Three commonly used modeling techniques include Monte Carlo Simulation, Discrete Event Simulation, and Continuous Simulation. Modeling is routinely performed in an academic environment and numerous published surge models exist based on these systems.[30–38]

Methods to test planning efforts can include (virtual) table-top exercises, functional scenarios (in which 1 or more specific components are tested), and full-scale simulation involving the physical participation of many personnel and structures.[39] In the aftermath of any disaster, it is essential to develop an after-action report (AAR) to identify successes and opportunities for improvement in which existing plans can be modified or improved based on actual experiences. Incorporating Lean and Six Sigma tools, such as spaghetti plots and process maps, can significantly enhance the quality of AARs.

Plan Failure

No disaster plan is infinitely scalable. In fact, when plans attempt to capture both the focus and the obscurity of disaster needs, inevitably disaster planning can become less focused and therefore potentially less effective. This can result in a plan that may, under certain conditions, fail to provide the appropriate guidance needed in a given event. In contrast, developing flexible plans that contain key components can serve as an operational framework providing responders with critical guidance in the event of loss of containment.

Any plan must also consider where additional resources can be accessed and facilitate efficient and effective coordination with other hospitals or burn centers within an immediate area (referred to as interfaculty planning). Based on geography and proximity, the closest resources may be located in an adjacent community or across a state line. The immediate resources, along with contact information, should be reflected in the plan.

WORST-CASE SCENARIOS

Aside from the BMCI, pandemic events have produced several of the greatest threats faced by health care systems over the past 100 years. Recently there have been several large-scale global events, such as the 2009 H1N1 influenza outbreak,[40] that reached pandemic proportions based on patient numbers and viral characteristics but not in terms of patient mortality. On the other hand, several outbreaks, including Severe Acute Respiratory Syndrome Coronavirus[41,42] and the Ebola Virus Disease,[43–46] manifested higher mortality rates but never reached pandemic proportions as defined by World Health Organization.

Although infrequent, radiation-related disasters represent novel and challenging threats that can put health care systems at great risk. The use of radiation equipment is common in hospitals. As such, there is ready access to detection equipment as well. Experience shows that large radionuclear events, such as occurred in Chernobyl, Russia (1986),[47,48] and Fukushima, Japan (2011),[49–51] can have devastating and long-term local, regional, national, and global impact.

Nuclear weapons, such as those used in Hiroshima and Nagasaki, Japan, killed more than 100,000 and left an equal number of people with acute radiation illnesses.[52–54] Modern technology allows for highly enriched weapons, with a similar yield to the Hiroshima weapon, that could be concealed in a small container the size of suitcase. The potential use of highly enriched weaponized fissile materials represents the ultimate terrorism threat. If used, this would rapidly overwhelm all traditional resources for an extended period, even in developed countries such as the United States.[55–60]

SUMMARY

The BMCI scenario represents a very challenging and clinically significant event. Successful pre-incident planning can help facilitate the coordinated care of the these severely injured patients. Flexibility in planning must account for initial patient management, the surging of available resources, and the coordinated regional dispersion of patients to definitive care facilities. Plans can be effectively tested through well-recognized simulation techniques, which can help identify opportunities for improvement, and augment existing strengths. The AAR process is an ideal opportunity to reinforce effective practices, and fill in gaps previously unanticipated. During an MCI, speed, repetition, simplicity, and creativity are critical components of success.

REFERENCES

1. Healthcare Preparedness Capabilities, National Guidance for Healthcare System Preparedness. In: Response OotASfPa, ed. US DHHS ASPR. 2012. Available at: http://www.phe.gov/Preparedness/planning/hpp/reports/Documents/capabilities.pdf. p. 72. Accessed April 1, 2017.
2. VandenBerg SL, Davidson SB. Preparation for mass casualty incidents. Crit Care Nurs Clin North Am 2015;27(2):157–66.
3. Hick JL, Hanfling D, Cantrill SV. Allocating scarce resources in disasters: emergency department principles. Ann Emerg Med 2012;59(3):177–87.

4. Kearns RD, Cairns BA, Cairns CB. Surge capacity and capability. A review of the history and where the science is today regarding surge capacity during a mass casualty disaster. Front Public Health 2014;2:29.

5. Kearns RD, Conlon KM, Valenta AL, et al. Disaster planning: the basics of creating a burn mass casualty disaster plan for a burn center. J Burn Care Res 2014;35(1):e1–13.

6. Hick JL, Einav S, Hanfling D, et al. Surge capacity principles: care of the critically ill and injured during pandemics and disasters: CHEST consensus statement. Chest 2014;146(4 Suppl):e1S–16S.

7. National Academies of Sciences E, Medicine. A National Trauma Care System: integrating military and civilian trauma systems to achieve zero preventable deaths after injury. Washington, DC: The National Academies Press; 2016.

8. Kearns RD, Ortiz-Pujols SM, Craig CK, et al. Advanced burn life support for day-to-day burn injury management and disaster preparedness: stakeholder experiences and student perceptions following 56 advanced burn life support courses. J Burn Care Res 2015;36(4):455–64.

9. Barillo DJ. Planning for burn mass casualty incidents. J Trauma 2007;62(6 Suppl):S68.

10. Barillo DJ, Wolf S. Planning for burn disasters: lessons learned from one hundred years of history. J Burn Care Res 2006;27(5):622–34.

11. Conlon KM, Ruhren C, Johansen S, et al. Developing and implementing a plan for large-scale burn disaster response in New Jersey. J Burn Care Res 2014;35(1):e14–20.

12. Conlon KM, Martin S. 'Just send them all to a burn centre': managing burn resources in a mass casualty incident. J Bus Contin Emer Plan 2011;5(2):150–60.

13. Wachtel TL, Cowan ML, Reardon JD. Developing a regional and national burn disaster response. J Burn Care Rehabil 1989;10(6):561–7.

14. Kearns RD, Cairns BA, Hickerson WL, et al. ABA Southern Region Burn disaster plan: the process of creating and experience with the ABA southern region burn disaster plan. J Burn Care Res 2014; 35(1):e43–8.

15. Kearns R, Holmes JT, Cairns B. Burn disaster preparedness and the southern region of the United States. South Med J 2013;106(1):69–73.

16. Hick JL, DeVries AS, Fink-Kocken P, et al. Allocating resources during a crisis: you can't always get what you want. Minn Med 2012;95(4):46–50.

17. Hanfling D, Hick JL, Cantrill SV. Understanding the role for crisis standards of care. Ann Emerg Med 2012;60(5):669–70 [author reply: 670–1].

18. Hick JL, Barbera JA, Kelen GD. Refining surge capacity: conventional, contingency, and crisis capacity. Disaster Med Public Health Prep 2009;3(2 Suppl):S59–67.

19. Emergency PH. Immediate bed availability. 2014. Available at: http://www.phe.gov/Preparedness/planning/sharper/Pages/iba.aspx. Accessed July, 7 2016.

20. Kearns RD, Skarote MB, Peterson J, et al. Deployable, portable, and temporary hospitals; one state's experiences through the years. Am J Disaster Med 2014;9(3):195–210.

21. Kearns RD, Hubble MW, Holmes JH, et al. Disaster planning: transportation resources and considerations for managing a burn disaster. J Burn Care Res 2014;35(1):e21–32.

22. Gerberding JL, Falk H, Arias I, et al. In a moment's notice: surge capacity for terrorist bombings challenges and proposed solutions. US Department of Health and Human Services, Centers for Disease Control. Available at: https://emergency.cdc.gov/masscasualties/pdf/surgecapacity.pdf. Accessed April 7, 2017.

23. Kelen GD, McCarthy ML. The science of surge. Acad Emerg Med 2006;13(11):1089–94.

24. Posner Z, Admi H, Menashe N. Ten-fold expansion of a burn unit in mass casualty: how to recruit the nursing staff. Disaster Manag Response 2003;1(4):100–4.

25. Lennarson P, Boedeker BH, Kuper GM, et al. Utilization of a civilian academic center as a force multiplier in support of NATO special operations medicine—a pilot demonstration. Stud Health Technol Inform 2012;173:260–2.

26. Bryan J, Miyamoto D, Holman V. Medical civil-military operations: the deployed medical brigade's role in counterinsurgency operations. US Army Med Department J 2008;25–8.

27. Simmons S, Alverson D, Poropatich R, et al. Applying telehealth in natural and anthropogenic disasters. Telemed J E health 2008;14(9):968–71.

28. Franco C, Toner E, Waldhorn R, et al. The national disaster medical system: past, present, and suggestions for the future. Biosecurity and bioterrorism: biodefense strategy, practice, and. science 2007; 5(4):319–25.

29. National Incident Management System. 2008. Available at: http://www.fema.gov/pdf/emergency/nims/NIMS_core.pdf. Accessed December 7, 2012.

30. Abir M, Davis MM, Sankar P, et al. Design of a model to predict surge capacity bottlenecks for burn mass casualties at a large academic medical center. Prehosp Disaster Med 2013;28(1):23–32.

31. Albores P, Shaw D. Government preparedness: using simulation to prepare for a terrorist attack. Comput Oper Res 2008;35(6):1924–43.

32. Dallas CE, Bell WC. Prediction modeling to determine the adequacy of medical response to urban nuclear attack. Disaster Med Public Health Prep 2007;1(2):80–9.

33. Franc-Law JM, Bullard M, Della Corte F. Simulation of a hospital disaster plan: a virtual, live exercise. Prehosp Disaster Med 2008;23(4):346–53.

34. Hirshberg A, Scott BG, Granchi T, et al. How does casualty load affect trauma care in urban bombing incidents? A quantitative analysis. J Trauma 2005; 58(4):686–95.

35. Smith SW, Portelli I, Narzisi G, et al. A novel approach to multihazard modeling and simulation. Disaster Med Public Health Prep 2009;3(2):75–87.

36. Steward D, Wan TT. The role of simulation and modeling in disaster management. J Med Syst 2007;31(2):125–30.

37. Kearns R, Zoller J, Hubble M, et al. Using Monte Carlo simulation for modeling surge capacity in the ABA southern region. J Burn Care Res 2012; 33(2):1.

38. Kearns RD. Burn surge capacity in the south: what is the capacity of burn centers within the American Burn Association southern region to absorb significant numbers of burn injured patients during a medical disaster? Medical University of South Carolina. [ProQuest Dissertations and Theses]. 2011.

39. Federal Emergency Management Agency. Homeland Security Exercise and Evaluation program. 2013; Available at: http://www.fema.gov/media-library-data/20130726-1914-25045-8890/hseep_apr13_.pdf. Accessed July 6, 2016.

40. H1N WHOINfMMfPI. Studies needed to address public health challenges of the 2009 H1N1 influenza pandemic: insights from modeling. PLoS Curr 2009; 1:RRN1135.

41. Cheng VC, Chan JF, To KK, et al. Clinical management and infection control of SARS: lessons learned. Antiviral Res 2013;100(2):407–19.

42. Xing W, Hejblum G, Leung GM, et al. Anatomy of the epidemiological literature on the 2003 SARS outbreaks in Hong Kong and Toronto: a time-stratified review. PLoS Med 2010;7(5):e1000272.

43. Kearns RD, Leaming LE. 'An abundance of caution' and Ebola in the US Healthcare System: what is the new normal? J Bus Contin Emer Plan 2015; 8(4):317–25.

44. McCarthy M. Liberian man being treated for Ebola in Texas dies. BMJ 2014;349:g6145.

45. McCarthy M. US issues new guidelines for health workers caring for Ebola patients. BMJ 2014;349: g6418.

46. Ki M. What do we really fear? The epidemiological characteristics of Ebola and our preparedness. Epidemiol Health 2014;36:e2014014.

47. Takada J. Chernobyl nuclear power plant accident and Tokaimura criticality accident. Nihon rinsho. Jpn J Clin Med 2012;70(3):405–9 [in Japanese].

48. Svendsen ER, Runkle JR, Dhara VR, et al. Epidemiologic methods lessons learned from environmental public health disasters: Chernobyl, the World Trade Center, Bhopal, and Graniteville, South Carolina. Int J Environ Res Public Health 2012;9(8):2894–909.

49. Sugimoto A, Krull S, Nomura S, et al. The voice of the most vulnerable: lessons from the nuclear crisis in Fukushima, Japan. Bull World Health Organ 2012; 90(8):629–30.

50. Robertson AG, Pengilley A. Fukushima nuclear incident: the challenges of risk communication. Asia Pac J Public Health 2012;24(4):689–96.

51. Fuse A, Yokota H. Lessons learned from the Japan earthquake and tsunami, 2011. J Nippon Med Sch 2012;79(4):312–5.

52. Matsunari Y, Yoshimoto N. Comparison of rescue and relief activities within 72 hours of the atomic bombings in Hiroshima and Nagasaki. Prehosp Disaster Med 2013;28(6):536–42.

53. Stalpers LJ, van Dullemen S, Franken NA. Medical and biological consequences of nuclear disasters. Ned Tijdschr Geneeskd 2012;156(20):A4394 [in Dutch].

54. Dallas CE. Medical lessons learned from Chernobyl relative to nuclear detonations and failed nuclear reactors. Disaster Med Public Health Prep 2012;6(4):330–4.

55. Knebel AR, Coleman CN, Cliffer KD, et al. Allocation of scarce resources after a nuclear detonation: setting the context. Disaster Med Public Health Prep 2011;5(Suppl 1):S20–31.

56. Hick JL, Weinstock DM, Coleman CN, et al. Health care system planning for and response to a nuclear detonation. Disaster Med Public Health Prep 2011; 5(Suppl 1):S73–88.

57. Goffman TE. Nuclear terrorism and the problem of burns. Am J Emerg Med 2011;29(2):224–8.

58. DiCarlo AL, Maher C, Hick JL, et al. Radiation injury after a nuclear detonation: medical consequences and the need for scarce resources allocation. Disaster Med Public Health Prep 2011;5(Suppl 1):S32–44.

59. Coleman CN, Weinstock DM, Casagrande R, et al. Triage and treatment tools for use in a scarce resources—crisis standards of care setting after a nuclear detonation. Disaster Med Public Health Prep 2011;5(Suppl 1):S111–21.

60. Coleman CN, Knebel AR, Hick JL, et al. Scarce resources for nuclear detonation: project overview and challenges. Disaster Med Public Health Prep 2011;5(Suppl 1):S13–9.

61. Gutman D, Biffl WL, Suner S, et al. The station nightclub fire and disaster preparedness in Rhode Island. Med Health R I 2003;86(11):344–6.

62. Harrington DT, Biffl WL, Cioffi WG. The station nightclub fire. J Burn Care Rehabil 2005;26(2):141–3.

63. Mahoney EJ, Harrington DT, Biffl WL, et al. Lessons learned from a nightclub fire: institutional disaster preparedness. J Trauma 2005;58(3):487–91.

64. Dal Ponte ST, Dornelles CF, Arquilla B, et al. Mass-casualty response to the Kiss nightclub in Santa

Maria, Brazil. Prehosp Disaster Med 2015;30(1): 93–6.

65. Gutierrez de Ceballos JP, Turegano Fuentes F, Perez Diaz D, et al. Casualties treated at the closest hospital in the Madrid, March 11, terrorist bombings. Crit Care Med 2005;33(1 Suppl):S107–12.

66. Turegano-Fuentes F, Caba-Doussoux P, Jover-Navalon JM, et al. Injury patterns from major urban terrorist bombings in trains: the Madrid experience. World J Surg 2008;32(6):1168–75.

67. Chim H, Yew WS, Song C. Managing burn victims of suicide bombing attacks: outcomes, lessons learnt, and changes made from three attacks in Indonesia. Crit Care 2007;11(1):R15.

68. Shoaf KI, Sareen HR, Nguyen LH, et al. Injuries as a result of California earthquakes in the past decade. Disasters 1998;22(3):218–35.

69. Peek-Asa C, Kraus JF, Bourque LB, et al. Fatal and hospitalized injuries resulting from the 1994 Northridge earthquake. Int J Epidemiol 1998;27(3): 459–65.

70. Cushman JG, Pachter HL, Beaton HL. Two New York City hospitals' surgical response to the September 11, 2001, terrorist attack in New York City. J Trauma 2003;54(1):147–54 [discussion: 154–5].

71. Yurt RW, Bessey PQ, Bauer GJ, et al. A regional burn center's response to a disaster: September 11, 2001, and the days beyond. J Burn Care Rehabil 2005;26(2):117–24.

72. Jordan MH, Hollowed KA, Turner DG, et al. The Pentagon attack of September 11, 2001: a burn center's experience. J Burn Care Rehabil 2005;26(2):109–16.

73. Koyama A, Fuse A, Hagiwara J, et al. Medical relief activities, medical resourcing, and inpatient evacuation conducted by Nippon medical school due to the Fukushima Daiichi nuclear power plant accident following the Great East Japan earthquake 2011. J Nippon Med Sch 2011;78(6):393–6.

74. Bargues L, Donat N, Jault P, et al. Burns care following a nuclear incident. Ann Burns Fire Disasters 2010;23(3):160–4 [in French].

75. Caro JJ, DeRenzo EG, Coleman CN, et al. Resource allocation after a nuclear detonation incident: unaltered standards of ethical decision making. Disaster Med Public Health Prep 2011;5(Suppl 1): S46–53.

76. Ross JR, Case C, Confer D, et al. Radiation injury treatment network (RITN): healthcare professionals preparing for a mass casualty radiological or nuclear incident. Int J Radiat Biol 2011;87(8):748–53.

Burn Injuries
Prevention, Advocacy, and Legislation

Ernest J. Grant, PhD, RN

KEYWORDS

- Burn prevention • Advocacy • Legislative process • The Five-Step process • Five E's
- Collaboration

KEY POINTS

- It is crucial that the plastic surgeon, as the head of the prevention team, recognizes the influence such a position may hold in an effort to get the hospital administration to support fire and burn prevention initiatives.
- Every effort should be made to collaborate with community fire and life safety organizations to address the fire and burn issues.
- The goal of public education is to provide information that creates awareness that gets individuals to recognize and reduce their risks of sustaining a burn injury.
- The plastic surgeon should have a working knowledge of the legislative process to influence legislation that could reduce burn injuries.

INTRODUCTION

Each year, more than 486,000 individuals visit emergency departments to seek some form of medical treatment for a burn injury (National Hospital Ambulatory Medical Care Survey, 2011).[1] Additionally, more than 30,000 individuals are burned so significantly that they require admission to the 132 designated burn care facilities in the United States and Canada each year for the treatment of a burn injury (American Burn Association, 2016).[2] Most of these injuries are preventable. The plastic surgeon is in a unique position to help promote prevention initiatives. This article presents an historical perspective related to burn prevention and elements of successful burn prevention programs and explores ways in which the plastic surgeon can promote burn prevention through education, advocacy, and the legislative process. Because the best way to treat a burn is to prevent it from occurring, prevention efforts undertaken by the surgeon can increase awareness, ensure a safe environment, and reduce burn injuries.

THE HISTORY OF BURN PREVENTION

Ever since humans first discovered fire, a burn injury probably occurred shortly thereafter. Numerous records exist that describes the treatment of burns dating from the times of cave dwellers to 1500 to 1600 BC.[3] The first recorded burn injury in the United States occurred in 1609 to Captain John Smith of the Jamestown Colony. Records indicate that Smith was badly injured (burned) from a mysterious gunpowder explosion in October of that year. He returned to England for treatment and never set foot in Virginia again.[4] Technologic advances and changes in cultural mores may have contributed to the increase in burn injuries, as little or no emphasis on safety

Disclosure Statement: The author has nothing to disclose.
Burn Outreach, North Carolina Jaycee Burn Center, University of North Carolina Hospitals, 5th Floor P. S. T., 101 Manning Drive, Chapel Hill, NC 27514, USA
E-mail address: Ernest.Grant@unchealth.unc.edu

Clin Plastic Surg 44 (2017) 451–466
http://dx.doi.org/10.1016/j.cps.2017.02.005

was required for new products. It was not until the late 19th and mid-20th centuries that society began to recognize that most burn injuries could be prevented. It could easily be argued that the recognition for burn prevention came about because of published injury data reports and reaction to local, regional, or national disasters that resulted in injury or the loss of life. As a consequence of these incidents, legislation in the form of laws or codes and standards were enacted to prevent or minimize their reoccurrence. These regulatory measures, when adopted, help ensure the safety of the general public but may not necessarily be applicable to individuals or specific forms of burn injuries such as scalds and flames that may occur in the home environment. It is difficult to determine the success of such methods, but the steady decline in burn-related injures over the ensuing years may be one way to measure its success. **Table 1** shows several major historical fire events in US history, their causes, and the resultant legislative changes enacted to promote public fire safety. Some of the significant fires of note were the following.

A fire at the Triangle Shirtwaist Company of New York was believed to have started in a rag bin on the evening of March 25, 1911. Hazardous working conditions, blocked exits, and poor communication played a role in the death of 147 workers. Codes enacted after this tragedy evolved into the National Fire Protection Association's (NFPA's) Life Safety Code 101. This code addressed the standardization of fire escape (exits) planning for factories, schools, department stores, and theaters.[5]

The Coconut Grove Nightclub fire occurred on November 28, 1942 in Boston, Massachusetts. Because of a lack of sprinklers, blocked and locked exits, and other fire code violations, 492 individuals lost their lives. Significant advancement in the treatment of burns (comprehensive treatment of inhalation injuries, fluid resuscitation, and the use of antibiotics) and public safety initiatives (revolving doors must also have swing doors, disaster planning, and no combustibles in places of assembly) occurred as a result of this fire.[6–9]

Two years later, on July 6, 1944, a fire occurred in the big tent of the Ringling Brother's Circus in Hartford, Connecticut. This fire was thought to have occurred as a result of arson, but waterproofing efforts applied to the tents (coating with a mixture of paraffin and gasoline) may have contributed to the death of 168 individuals (two-thirds were children). Furthermore, blocked exits and a panicked crowd that headed for exits in which they entered (instead of more accessible exits) created congestion and slowed egress

from the burning structure. New codes and standards initiated after this fire addressed the construction, location, protection, and maintenance of grandstands and bleachers. This code also affected seating facilities located in the open air or within enclosed or semienclosed structures such as tents, membrane structures, and stadium complexes.

The middle of the 20th century saw significant progress related to fire and burn prevention. For example, Congress passed the Flammable Fabrics Act in 1953. This act was designed to regulate the manufacture or sale of highly flammable clothing.[10] Technology in the mid-1960s brought about the introduction of residential smoke alarms. Although considered to be expensive at the time of its introduction, smoke alarms served (and continue to present day) as early warning devices that alert consumers of a possible fire and permit early egress. In 1972, the independent federal regulatory agency known as the Consumer Products Safety Commission was founded by the Consumer Product Safety Act. In that law, Congress directed the Commission to "Protect the public against unreasonable risks of injury and deaths associated with consumer products."[11] Since its inception, the Commission has called for and removed many products that have proven to be dangerous to the public. Some products that may cause or have actually been related to a burn injury have been the focus of many such recalls. However, safety is not totally the responsibility of regulatory agencies or technologic advances. As the US and Canada become more culturally diverse, Fire and Life Safety professionals along with medical and public health officials recognize that everyone must work together to educate and ensure the safety of the general public.

FIRE AND BURN PREVENTION TODAY

Fire and burn prevention initiatives of the last half of the 20th century have tended to focus on specific topics or behaviors. Campaigns such as National Fire Prevention Week, National Burn Awareness Week, and The National Scald Prevention Campaign are a few examples of such initiatives. These campaigns have encouraged consumer knowledge and participation in the proper installation and maintenance of smoke alarms and the setting of hot water heater temperatures, creating a safe home environment, and the practice of home escape planning in the event of a fire. A unique feature of these campaigns is the collaboration and inclusion of fire and life safety professionals. For example, fire fighters may canvas a targeted high-risk residential area to

Table 1
Historical fire events and the resultant safety legislation adopted as a result

	Description of the Event	Safety Codes or Standard Enacted
The Great Chicago Fire (1871)	The Chicago Fire of 1871, also called the Great Chicago Fire, burned from October 8 to October 10, 1871 and destroyed thousands of buildings, killed an estimated 300 people and caused an estimated $200 million in damages. It is estimated that one-third of the city was destroyed by this fire.	Fire and building codes in place for new spacing and construction materials required to be used for reconstruction. The week of October 9th is known as National Fire Prevention Week marks the anniversary of this fire.
The Triangle Shirtwaist Fire, New York City, 1911	A fire in the rag bin spread from the rags to cutting tables and then to cloth patterns hanging on wire above the tables. Working conditions, locked doors, and lack of communication caused the deaths of 147 people.	The New York City Fire Prevention Bureau was established. The first in the country, the bureau expanded the powers of the fire commissioner. Publications regarding standardization of fire escape (exits) planning for factories, schools, department stores, and theaters were presented.
Coconut Grove Nightclub Fire - Boston (1942)	More than 491 individuals died because of blocked or locked exits and overcrowding and flammable materials within the building.	Advancement made in burn treatment (better comprehension of the treatment of inhalation injuries, fluid resuscitation, and the use of antibiotics). Public safety (revolving doors required the addition of swing doors), disaster preparedness, no combustibles in places of assembly, battery-operated emergency lighting, and addition of codes to the Life Safety Code.
Ringling Brother's Big Tent Fire (Also known as the Hartford Circus Fire of 1944)	The cause of the fire is listed as "undetermined," but an arsonist who was captured confessed to starting the fire and later recanted his story. A postfire investigation revealed waterproofing efforts (paraffin wax treated with 3 parts gasoline) had been recently applied to the canvas. A total of 168 individuals (two-thirds of them children) perished in the fire and hundreds were severely injured. It was thought the large amount of injuries and life loss was the result of the crowd rushing to the exits they had entered instead of using other exits. Two exits were blocked by animal cages.	The waterproofing method of paraffin and gasoline were prohibited. NFPA Standard 102 was developed (grandstands, folding and telescopic seating, tents, and membrane structures). This code is also reflected in the 2000 International Building Code and 2003 NFPA 5000.
Our Lady of Angles School Fire, December 1958	Combustible interior finish work may have contributed to the fire spread. The investigative report of the fire indicated that inadequate facility exits may have contributed to the high number of deaths. Ninety students and 3 nuns died in this fire.	The 1958 edition of the Building Exits Code provided for sprinklers in schools. Reclassification of schools that may have different safety requirements.

(continued on next page)

Table 1
(continued)

	Description of the Event	Safety Codes or Standard Enacted
The Beverly Hill Supper Club Fire, May 28, 1977	Inadequate training and preparedness of personnel, delayed notification, blocked exits, and noncompliance with codes contributed to this fire. A total of 164 people died.	Sprinkler requirements for buildings having 4 or more stories required for new buildings (some retroactive for existing buildings). Class A and class B buildings are required to be sprinklered throughout (applies only to new construction).
The Rhode Island Nightclub Fire, 2003	Pyrotechnics display ignited expanded foam plastic insulation after the band started to play. A total of 100 occupants perished and more than 200 were injured. It is ranked as the fourth deadliest nightclub fire in US history.	Changes made to fire and life safety codes in an effort to make public assembly occupancies safer. Fire sprinklers must be installed in new nightclubs and similar assembly occupancies regardless of occupant load and in existing facilities that accommodate more than 100. • Building owners must inspect exits to ensure they are free of obstructions and must maintain records of each inspection. • At least 1 trained crowd manager must be present for all gatherings of more than 50, except religious services. (For gatherings of more than 250, additional crowd managers are required at a ratio of 1:250.) • Festival seating is prohibited for crowds of more than 250 unless a life-safety evaluation approved by the authority having jurisdiction has been performed. (Festival seating, according to NFPA 101, is a form of audience/spectator accommodation in which no seating, other than a floor or ground surface, is provided for the audience to gather and observe a performance.)

ensure that smoke alarms are installed properly. Fire safety education and a free home safety inspection may be offered during the installation process. Fire department personnel may also benefit by gathering previously unknown information about the home such as the presence of window bars (which may block a second means of egress in the event of a fire), home oxygen (which could accelerate fire growth or cause an explosion), or the health of the resident(s) (invalid, blind, deaf, or hard of hearing). Such information may assist fire personnel in designing their plan of action when answering an emergency call.

In addition to the aforementioned campaigns, formal fire and burn safety education curriculums have been promoted by national organizations such as the American Burn Association, the NFPA, the Centers for Disease Control and Prevention, the American Red Cross, Safe Kids Worldwide, and the United States Fire Administration. Each of these curriculums provides vital injury prevention education and advocacy to the general public and those considered at highest risk—the very young, older adults, and persons with disabilities. For example, The American Burn Association's National Burn Awareness Week campaign focuses on a variety of fire and scald prevention topics aimed at specific high-risk groups. The NFPA's Learn-Not-To-Burn and Learn-Not-To-Burn Preschool curriculums are designed to enhance preschool and elementary student's knowledge and safety behavior regarding fire and burns. Another program offered by this organization (Remembering When) addresses fall, fire, and burn safety education targeted to the needs of the older adult.[12,13] The Centers for Disease Control and Prevention offer key prevention safety tips and other resources that may be useful for the establishment of community-based safety programs. The American Red Cross and Safe Kids Worldwide offer a variety of fire and burn safety tips specifically aimed at the general public and caregivers for the very young, respectively. The United States Fire Administration encourages fire departments and other life safety organizations to increase community awareness about preventing home fires through the use of its Fire is Everyone's Fight program.[14]

The aforementioned prevention efforts may take many forms in the delivery of their messages. Most of these programs tend to follow the premise of the Injury Control Model (introduced through the public health model of injury prevention), the Five-Step Process (utilized by public health and other federal agencies) or the Five E's of Prevention when creating and establishing safety and prevention programs. These models use tools and concepts that allow educators to thoroughly evaluate the problem, create an intervention strategy, and evaluate the results after implementation. Use of these models also ensures and promotes consistent messages and safety guidelines.

The Injury Control Model

The Injury Control Model has been in use since the 1950s and 1960s and was introduced by William Haddon, Jr, an engineer and public health physician. Haddon theorized that injury prevention depended on controlling the agent. He introduced the Haddon Matrix (**Table 2**), which consisted of a framework that allowed for the identification of factors related to the host, agent, and environment. A guiding principle of injury control that emerged from Haddon's work was that effective injury control (prevention) relied on a combination of intervention strategies.[15] Haddon's work was initially applied to motor vehicle safety and is credited with saving more than 300,000 lives from 1960 to 2002.[16] Because the model provides a compelling framework for understanding the origins of the injury problems and identifying multiple countermeasures to address those problems, it has been adopted and used to develop other safety initiatives such as fire and burn prevention.[17] **Table 3** uses the Haddon matrix to address the problem of residential fires caused by cigarettes igniting upholstered furniture.

The Five-Step Process

Beginning in the mid to late 1970s, injury prevention professionals recognized that the Haddon matrix did not fully address the safety needs faced by a changing society. Fire and burn safety awareness was greatly influenced by the publication of the report America Burning in 1973 and America Burning Recommissioned in 2000. This report laid the foundation that identified, among other things, (1) the need for the establishment of codes and standards, (2) fire protection planning programs, and, most importantly, (3) fire and life-safety education programs.[18,19] Whereas the matrix continued to provide a blueprint for exploring the problem, newer initiatives such as the Five-Step Process and the Three E's provided a step-by-step process approach as called for in the report. The Five-Step Process was created and first introduced by the US Fire Administration to specifically assist with public fire education programs. The process used a systemic step-by-step approach that assisted the educator in designing, implementing, and evaluating their specific community safety education programs. Unique to this process was the encouragement of public educators to collaborate with local community partners (ie, police, churches, senior centers, civic groups) to assist with gaining access to high-risk communities and support the implementation of their programs.[20] The 5 steps consist of the following:

Step 1: Conduction of a community risk assessment

Step 2: Development of community partnerships

Step 3: Creation of an intervention strategy

Step 4: Implementation of strategy

Step 5: Evaluation of results

Fig. 1 lists the step-by-step components of implementation of the Five-Step Process.

Step 1—Conduction of a Community Risk Assessment

A community risk assessment must be performed to help the educator determine whether there is a problem that needs to be addressed. Local, state, and regional data collected over a period (weeks, months, or years) may be assessed when considering data needs. The assessment will also find other important data or exact facts such as the demographic and cultural characteristics of the community, the suspected (or potential) safety risk that needs attention, and what efforts the community may be taking to alleviate the problem. When conducting a community risk assessment, it is

Table 2
Haddon matrix

| | Human | Agent/Vehicle | Environment | |
			Physical	Social
Pre-event	Driver age, gender, experience, drug or alcohol use, vision, fatigue, frequency of travel, risk-taking behavior	Vehicle speed, brakes, tires, road-holding ability, visibility (eg, daytime running lights)	Road design and traffic flow, road conditions, weather, traffic density, traffic control (lights, signals), visibility	Speed restrictions, impaired driving laws, licensing restrictions, road rage, seat belt and child restraint laws
Event	Age, pre-existing conditions (eg, osteoporosis), restraint use	Vehicle speed, size, crash-worthiness, type of seat belts, airbag, interior surface hazards	Guardrails, median dividers, break-away poles, road-side hazards	Enforcement of speed limits
Postevent	Age, comorbidities	Integrity of fuel system	Distance from emergency medical care, obstacles to extrication	Emergency medical services planning and delivery, bystander control, quality of trauma care, rehabilitation

Courtesy of The McGraw-Hill Companies, Inc; with permission; and *From* Western Journal of Emergency Medicine, Orange, CA. Need for injury-prevention education in medical school curriculum. Available at: http://westjem.com/articles/need-for-injury-prevention-education-in-medical-school-curriculum.html. Accessed July 28, 2016; and Runyan C. Using the Haddon Matrix: Introducing the third dimension. Inj Prev 1998;4(4):303; with permission.

essential that the educator recognize that the analysis process is always ongoing, as communities and people are constantly changing.

The risk assessment may serve as a roadmap that will assist the educator in developing a safety program that specifically targets the identified problem facing the community. For example, after looking over a fire department's monthly call report, an educator may have noted that the department was called to a specific high-rise building where seniors reside. Just by looking at the report, the educator may perceive that every person who resides in the building may be causing the fires. The problem may not be revealed until a complete assessment of all the data is completed. It could be that most of the fires may be caused by one individual who resides on a particular floor. Further assessment of that one individual may disclose that the fires may be caused by a new resident that is thought to have little or no literacy skills and cannot read the temperature settings of the electric stove used in the apartment. The resident may be used to cooking on an open flame such as a gas stove rather than an electric range. Now the educator has a little bit more information that will help with the development of an action plan.

The educator should consider the development of a specific education plan for the new resident. However, that does not mean the rest of the building residents should not receive some educational safety tips as well. In addition to tackling the specific problem of teaching the new resident how to safely use the appliances, the educator may also wish to instruct or remind other residents of cooking safety tips, fire escape planning, and how to activate emergency services. The educator should anticipate stumbling blocks as attempts are made to conduct the classes. For example, other residents may feel that the safety program is unnecessary and that the only problem exists with the new resident who needs to learn the temperature settings. They may not see themselves as being vulnerable because of their longevity and familiarity with cooking on electric appliances.

Step 2—Develop Community Partners

There are multiple advantages of developing and collaborating with community partners. First, from an economic perspective, working with community partners may result in cost savings to everyone involved in the project. Rather than one

Table 3
Haddon matrix applied to the problem of residential fires caused by cigarettes igniting upholstered furniture

	Host (Children in Home)	Agent/Vehicle (Cigarette, Matches, and Upholstered Furniture)	Physical Environment (Home)	Social Environment (Community Norms, Policies, Rules)
Pre-event (before fire starts)	Teach children not to play with matches	Redesign cigarettes so they self-extinguish before ignition of upholstery.	Lower flammability of structures.	Improve efforts to curb smoking initiation. Improve smoking cessation efforts.
Event (during fire)	Teach children to stop, drop, and roll. Plan and practice a fire escape route with children. Teach children not to hide during a fire.	Design furniture with materials that are less toxic when burned. Design upholstery that is flame resistant.	Install smoke detectors. Install sprinklers. Increase number of usable exits.	Pass ordinances requiring smoke detectors or sprinkler systems. Fund the fire department adequately to provide enough personnel and equipment for rapid response.
Postevent (after child injured by fire)	Provide first aid and CPR training to all family members.	Design heaters with quick and easy shutoff device.	Build homes with less toxic building materials.	Increase availability of burn treatment facilities.

Abbreviation: CPR, cardiopulmonary resuscitation.
Data from Runyan CW. Using the Haddon matrix: Introducing the third dimension. Inj Prev 1998;4(4):302–7.

organization devoting all of its resources to tackle a particular problem, other organizations may be able to contribute their resources resulting in financial and man power savings. Having one or more partners makes sense in terms of having more minds, bodies, and resources to tackle the problem. Sharing the tasks of targeting the problem, developing a plan, and implementing the solution is more productive in terms of creativity, credibility, and overall effectiveness. The most successful risk reduction efforts are those that involve the community in the planning and solution process.[20] The educator must remember that the term *resources* does not necessarily refer to financial assistance. Resources may take the form of knowledge expertise, in-kind support, political support, or community support, to cite a few examples. It is important for the educator to realize that this teamwork approach also means that everyone has a voice in the development,

implementation, and evaluation of any safety programs that develop from any collaboration.

Step 3—Creation of an Intervention Strategy

An intervention strategy is necessary for the group to begin the detailed work of developing a successful safety program. Some important components that need to be considered when exploring strategies include what will be done, where will it implemented, how the implementation will occur, and who will conduct the program once it is developed.[20] It is important for the committee to remember that any strategy should also include a process for evaluation of the program's effectiveness. Evaluation concepts should be addressed during the strategy phase, as this will also help serve as a foundation guide to determine whether the intent of the program is being met. The formation of an intervention strategy involves the

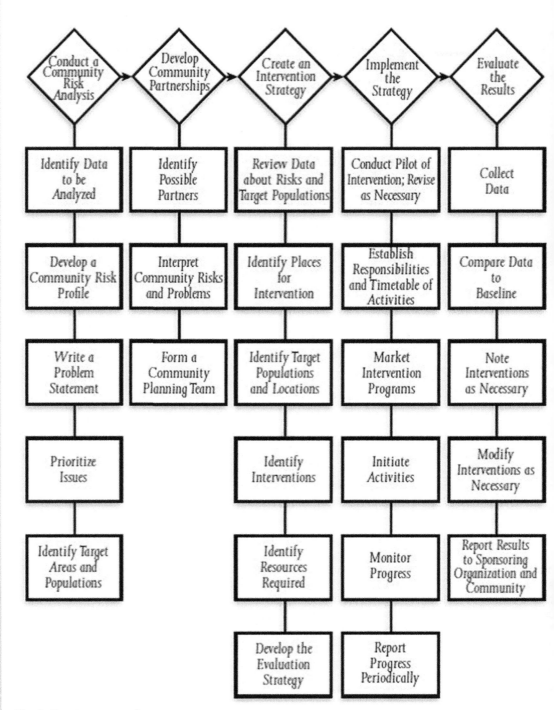

Fig. 1. Five-step-process diagram.

participation of all group members to achieve the intended outcomes.

Step 4—Implementation of Strategy

Before the implementation process, the proposed strategy may involve the need to test and retest the planned interventions. After each test, the process should be evaluated for such things as what worked and what did not, did the intended message remain clear and concise (particularly for individuals from different cultures), and are there any unforeseen barriers? The plan(s) should also include specific steps for implementing the program in the community and include such points as how the program be implemented, the length of time of the program, and, most importantly, the roles and responsibilities of each team member.[20] One of the ways a strategy may be implemented is to use an actual story that reflects the goal of the strategy. For example, if the goal of your strategy is to get seniors who reside in a high-rise building to actually practice a fire escape plan on a regular basis, having a senior who may have actually escaped a fire speak about their experience will provide more credibility that practicing this behavior does save lives and actually works. Listening to the experience of someone in the audience could easily grab the intended audience's attention more than an education program done by professionals. In the end, the result may be the same—the intended audience recognizes the importance of fire escape planning.

Step 5—Evaluating the Results

The primary goal of this process is to determine whether the risk reduction efforts that targeted a specific audience had the intended impact over a short and long period of time. Perhaps the most visible way to view the program's success or failure is to examine data collected over a period after implementation of the program. Validation of the program's goals may be achieved by determining whether stated goals and objectives have been achieved. The success of the program may also be evaluated through the use of tools such as surveys, interviews, reported behavioral change, legislative initiatives, and environmental changes. Because the implementation of the program has been a collaborative effort, it is also essential that information is shared with all members of the planning team. Finally, because of findings discovered during the evaluation process, it may be determine that adjustments are needed if the program is to be implemented again to another group or setting.[20]

THE FIVE E'S

Originally started in 1947 under the orders of President Harry Truman, the concept known as the *Three E's* (**Table 4**) was the result of a national conference on fire prevention. The plan formed at the conclusion of the conference recognized that it was best to prevent fires before they occurred. The prevention effort involved 3 areas, or as it eventually became known as, the *Three E's* (engineering, enforcement, and education) of fire prevention.[21] Two additional components (economic incentive and emergency response) were added by the National Fire Academy in 2000 because of their importance to community risk reduction thus, making this concept known

Table 4
The Five E's of prevention

"E"	Explanation
Engineering/ environment	*Engineering* (*environment*) refers to the use of passive interventions that promote fire and burn safety behaviors. There is no direct action required by the consumer. The use of and installation of a 10-year smoke alarm is a good example of environmental change.
Enforcement	Using legislative codes, standards, or regulations to reduce unsafe behavior. The regulation(s) may govern the actions of manufacturers, consumers, or local government.
Education	Education is used to inform the target group about potential hazards or risks based on their current behavior. Education may not cause the individual to change behavior but does increase injury awareness. An educational example would be informing about the need to change smoke alarm every 10 y.
Emergency response	Emergency responses are initiatives or interventions used by emergency medical services personnel to reduce the potential of a risk. Recognizing potential community dangers or planning for community disasters are example of how emergency response may be used as part of the Five E's of prevention
Economic incentive	Incentives that may be used to influence or persuade individual behaviors either positively or negatively. Positive incentives may be used as a reward (monetary, gifts) for individuals behaving in a certain manner. Negative incentives may be the issuance of tickets, fines or punishment for not behaving in a certain manner. An example of a positive incentive may be a discount on homeowner's insurance if a smoke alarm is present.

as the *Five E's*.[22] The Five E model is unique and can be adapted for promoting prevention initiatives in the primary, secondary, and tertiary settings. Once a potential problem or issue has been assessed and a determination made that a plan of action is necessary, the application of the Five E's is often used.

The engineering component (also referred to as *the environmental approach*) of this model refers to the use of technology and engineered solutions that help reduce or minimize the potential of an injury or hazard from occurring. The unique feature of this concept is that it usually does not depend on the actions of another, but is passive, automatic, or constant in its protective efforts.[22,23] Examples of this component may include the use of fire sprinklers, smoke alarms, and induction engineering technology for stovetops.

The enforcement component relies on the passage of legislation that gives those in authority the right to enforce the intended safety initiative. The intent of enforcement is that it uses the legislative process to promote (or prohibit) individual behavior change, which subsequently is beneficial for the individual or the public. Laws, codes, and standards that govern exits, fire doors, and building codes are examples of such enforcement initiatives.

The education component relies on the dissemination of information to target groups that may be identified as high risk or general public education. The goal of education is to provide information that creates awareness. Once awareness has been achieved, it is hoped that a change in knowledge is realized. Subsequently, the change in knowledge along with the increase in awareness will result in a change in behavior. Without the increase in awareness, there will not be a permanent change in attitude or behavior. When conducting an education campaign, it is important to remember to educate and not lecture to the intended audience. The goal of any educational program is to get individuals to understand their risks rather than be threatened with injury or property damage.[24] Examples of education programs may include safe cooking and heating, grilling, and recreational safety and reducing fire hazards around the home.

The emergency response component of this model describes interventions that may be taken by emergency responders to mitigate risks. This is accomplished by responders having a thorough knowledge of available community resources and capabilities when formulating a community risk reduction assessment plan.[22,23] Responders use their knowledge to identify areas within the community that may be high risk or at an increased risk of hazards that may promote injury or harm. For example, responders may be able to develop and practice a response plan if they know that a local manufacturing plant used extremely hazardous chemicals in its manufacturing process. By preplanning for such an event, responders may be able to determine whether they have all the resources (ie, personnel, tools, protective clothing) available to minimize the effects of such an incident. This process also reduces the possibility of emergency services being overwhelmed by excessive demands.

The last component of this model is economic incentive. *Economic incentive* refers to measures or initiatives executed to influence behaviors in a positive or negative manner. Some examples of a positive influence may include a tax benefit or homeowner's insurance reduction for the installation of residential sprinklers, smoke alarms, or

Table 5
Relationship between the temperature of tap water and time elapse before a scald injury occurs in the adult and infant

Temperature		Degree Burn			
		Adult		Infant	
Degrees Centigrade	Degrees Fahrenheit	Second	Third	Second	Third
70	158	Instant	Instant	Instant	Instant
65	149	Instant	1 s	Instant	Instant
60	140	2 s	5 s	Instant	1 s
55	131	11 s	20 s	2 s	5 s
50	122	2 min	7 min	11 s	20 s
45	113	1 h, 46 min	2 h, 7 min	2 min	7 min
40	104	—	—	1 h, 46 min	2 h, 7 min

Courtesy of N.C. Jaycee Burn Center, UNC Hospitals, Chapel Hill, NC.

other safety equipment. A negative incentive influence may be a fine levied for the violation of a fireworks ordinance or a citation for failing to enact certain safety behaviors such as proper storage of flammables.[22,23]

The combination of these 5 components helps determine whether a program or initiative has been successful. This is achieved through the evaluation process as data and other facts are gathered and examined to determine areas that may need improvement or additional work. Once examined, the decision may be made to continue investing in the programs. Things that may help make that determination may include a reduction in the identified risk and the amount of time, money, and personnel involved to achieve the hopeful outcome. Sometimes, the evaluation process may often be confused with research because they may use some of the same principles. However, the educator must remember the main difference between research and evaluation. According to Michael Q. Patton, the main difference between the 2 is that research seeks to prove and evaluation seeks to improve.[24]

Future Implications

The technology used to make our lives easier changes almost daily. These changes will have an impact on the future of fire and burn safety education. The surgeon must embrace such changes and incorporate them into any program initiatives. Technology, such as the use of global positioning system mapping, data analysis, robotic/interactive play, improved communication techniques (social media) and other resources, such a product improvement and redesign, legislative initiatives, and marketing, are a few examples of how the future of fire and burn safety programs may be influenced by technologic changes. Incorporating these changes will help members of the prevention team ensure a well thought out plan that incorporates every available technology.

The surgeon may serve as the head of the prevention team. In such cases, it is crucial that the surgeon recognizes the influence such a position may hold in an effort to get hospital administration to support fire and burn prevention initiatives. For example, by blending a combination of marketing ingenuity and the identified need for public education, the surgeon should be successful in gaining the full support of hospital administration. The marketing component should stress the branding of the hospital and its burn center as vital community corporate partners that desire to promote a healthy and safe community. Such an approach denotes a sense of comfort to the community and other corporate partners by implying the hospital supports safety first (a cost-effective risk-reduction tool), but if emergency or burn care services are needed, the local hospital can provide the best care available. Another marketing point may also emphasize that the local burn unit or trauma service has undergone a verification process by the American Burn Association, the American Trauma Society, and other agencies that provide their seal of approval of the services offered by the hospital. Prevention initiatives are usually emphasized as a part of such verification programs.

The Role of the Surgeon in Promoting Burn Prevention

It is important that the surgeon recognize the important role they will play in promoting burn prevention initiatives. One of the most important components of that role is the need for the surgeon to consider the available resources within the community and how such resources may affect the culture and socioeconomic makeup of the community. For example, in some communities, the socioeconomic conditions and culture may cause inhabitants to use alternative heating methods such as a wood stove or kerosene heater as the primary source of heating. This method may also be used so that inhabitants may have additional money to pay bills or provide food for the family. The surgeon should realize that poorer homes may be less likely to have a safe heating system, code-compliant electrical services, smoke alarms, or other fire safe security measures. To promote a burn prevention program, the surgeon should recognize that the financial concerns of the community inhabitants may present a challenge. They may not have the resources available to purchase a smoke alarm or safety devices. However, if the surgeon has a working knowledge of available community resources, he or she may be able to connect the individuals with available resources to alleviate a potential injury.[23]

The surgeon should take a proactive stance and use the media to help promote community education and prevention. For example, the perfect opportunity for a teaching/learning moment may present when speaking at a news conference that may involve inquires regarding a local fire or tragedy in which a single or multiple individuals may have been injured. The surgeon should use this opportunity to state the obvious that having an early warning device such as a working smoke or carbon monoxide alarm could have prevented such a tragedy from occurring by giving the occupants an early warning notification to escape. The surgeon should stress that everyone should have a working smoke alarm, that such alarms should be tested frequently and replaced if older than 10 years from the date of manufacture. Local reporters should be encouraged to repeat the safety information when subsequent comments are made regarding the tragedy. The surgeon may also suggest that the local media consider doing a special segment regarding fire and burn safety and post safety tips on their Web site.

Building a community coalition is another important tool the surgeon could use to help promote fire and burn safety initiatives at the local, state, and national levels. As mentioned earlier, such a network of like-minded agencies should have input regarding an initiative and its relevance to the community, costs, and man power. For example, if the local or state government is considering relaxing the age limit for the sale of pyrotechnics within the community or across the state, the lone voice of the surgeon expressing concern that permitting such sales to minors could result in an increase in burn and traumatic injury and possible lifelong disabilities may not be enough to deter the enactment of such legislation. However, by forming and working with members of a coalition composed of local, state, and national organizations with a similar focus, such as the National Fire Protection Association, SafeKid Worldwide, the local fire and life safety educators, Emergency Nurses Association, American Trauma Society, Academy of Family Physicians, may be enough to deter such legislation from going forth.[23] The formation of such a coalition would also present the opportunity for each member to solidify their data and unify the message(s) required for the effort.

AGE-RELATED BURN PREVENTION

Burn injuries may occur to anyone at any given time; however, some individuals tend to be more susceptible to sustaining such an injury than other populations. The infants, toddlers, older adults, and persons with disabilities have been identified as the most susceptible to a burn injury. These individuals may lack the ability to recognize and escape a fire or life-threatening situation. Loss of cognitive ability and sensation may also contribute to that risk. To help the surgeon comprehend the vulnerability of the identified population(s), the next session will provide some suggested strategies and coalition partners associated with each of the identified groups.

Infants and Preschool-Age Children

Infants and young children have little to no ability to recognize, perceive, or escape the dangers that may exist in their environment. This population cannot reason the consequences of their actions that may be brought on by their curiosity or fascination. They depend on adults and caregivers to provide a safe and secure environment. Scald injuries can happen across the age spectrum, but young children are more susceptible to deeper burns because of their thinner skin compared with adults who may be exposed to the same temperature. Because of their total body surface areas, the proportion of a child's body that is exposed to any given amount of a scalding substance is also greater.[25] The most common type of scald injury occurring in children is usually the result of contact with hot liquids or steam and contact by touching hot objects.[23,25]

When planning a fire and burn safety initiative, the American Burn Association and other life safety organizations suggest that educational programs should focus on educating the parents and caregivers. Specific points should include the creation of a safe zone in areas of the house, such as the kitchen and bathroom, where a child's curiosity may be stimulated. In the kitchen, parents should be instructed to always cook on the back burners, turn pot handles away from the edge of the stove, and never hold a child while cooking. Parents may further reduce the possibility of an injury by being instructed to create a "Safe Zone" (a marked off area 3 feet in front of the oven or stove) where children are forbidden to step inside when the stove is operating. Safety consideration should also be given when using appliances such as the microwave, crock pots, and coffee mugs. **Boxes 1** and **2** provide some additional suggestive tips to reduce the possibility of a scald injury in this vulnerable population. Passive safety may be provided through the reduction of the home's hot water heater temperature to 120°F/48°C or just below the medium setting. Installing antiscald devices in the bathroom shower or tub may minimize the possibility of scald injury occurring in the bathroom. These heat-sensitive devices are designed to stop or interrupt water flow when a predetermined temperature is reached (generally 110°–114° degrees) and prevent hot water from coming out of the tap before scalding occurs. **Table 5** provides an example of the time and temperature necessary to produce a full-thickness burn in the older adult and infant.[23,25,26] The surgeon should also remember that children are capable of learning safety behaviors from an early age. Consulting with and forming a coalition with age-appropriate safety-oriented organizations (ie, child safety advocacy groups, daycare associations) will help to ensure that messages are age appropriate and comprehensible for the target audience.

Box 1
Suggested ways to reduce scald injuries caused by hot liquids

- Ensure that the hot water heater is set at temperature of 90°F to 120°F (32.2°C–48.9°C).
- Install tempering valves (antiscald devices) in all faucets and shower heads.
- When preparing a bath, always turn on the cold water first, then, gradually add hot water to the desired temperature.
- Always test the water temperature with your hands before putting children into or stepping into the tub.
- If uncertain about the water temperature, use a commercial thermostat or bath thermometer to check the temperature.
- When using the microwave, always read and follow directions and warnings on microwaveable foods. Open microwave heated containers away from your body as contents may be hot.
- Never cuddle or hold children (or pets) when drinking hot drinks.
- Do not cook with children or pets in the kitchen or cooking area. Create a "No Kids/Pet" zone 3 feet in front of the stove.
- Always turn pot handles in when cooking on the stove.
- When possible, only cook on back burners.
- Keep small appliances (crock pots, toaster ovens) at the back of the counter, with cords out of the way of children.

Box 2
Resources for fire and burn prevention programs

American Burn Association (ABA) www.ameriburn.org

American Association of Retired persons (AARP)

National Center for Injury Prevention and Control (NCIPC/CDC)

National Fire Protection Association (NFPA) www.nfpa.org

US Fire Administration (USFA) www.usfa.fema.org

American Council of the Blind

National Center for Health Statistics (NCHS)

National Fire Incident Reporting System (NFRIS)

The National Institute on Deafness and Other Communication Disorders (NIDOCD)

THE SCHOOL-AGE CHILD

Fire, burn, and life safety information for this age group can be very challenging. Parents want to be supportive of this age group as they begin to express their independence in the kitchen by using the microwave or cooking under parental supervision. However, this age group is still easily distracted and may be prone to unintentional accidents during the cooking process. It is necessary for the parents to provide clear safety instructions (such as opening microwaved foods away from the face, no horse play while cooking, or remaining in the kitchen when cooking) to minimize the potential of a burn injury. Children of this age group may also sustain a burn injury caused by a clothing related fire. Burn-related incidents may occur because of a fascination with or curiosity of fire usually expressed through match and lighter play. Clothing ignition may also occur as a result of performing chores assigned to children as they get older. For example, refueling a lawn mower while the engine is still hot may cause an ignition accident if gasoline comes in contact with a hot engine or if gasoline has spilled onto clothing the child may be wearing.[27] Most school-age children have received some fire and burn safety information at school. During National Fire Prevention Week, local fire departments or fire and life safety educators have instructed them in life safety maneuvers such as the "Stop, Drop, and Roll" technique, " Crawl low under smoke," or knowing 2 ways out in the event of a fire. When considering a burn safety initiative for this age group, the surgeon should collaborate with organizations such as the Boy Scouts or Girls Scouts or local organizations such as the 4-H Club or religious organizations.

OLDER ADULTS

Older adults (age 50 and higher) are 33.5% of the US population, but they accounted for 49.5% of the burn cases admitted to US burn centers from 2004 to 2013. Thus, older adults suffer serious burns at a disproportionately higher rate than younger adults.[28,29] Changes associated with the aging process such as physical and mental abilities and aging/frailty and comorbidities such as diabetes and arthritis make the older adult susceptible to a fire or burn-related injury. A 2008 study[30] found that 50% of the homes of most older adults lacked the appropriate safety equipment (smoke and carbon monoxide alarms) and that 30% of the homes had tap water temperatures in excess of 60°C (140°F). Because of their thinner skin, older adults may suffer a deeper burn injury even with very brief exposure to hot liquids or hot objects. Today's seniors are very concerned about their health, safety, and remaining in their own homes for as long as possible.[31] Seniors also learn new materials in a manner that is different from other populations. They prefer to participate in the discussion of the topic and share their lived experiences. Even though seniors may participate in life safety programs, it does not guarantee that they will adhere to or follow the safety advice that is given. To effectively communicate with this population, the surgeon should have a working knowledge of educational techniques that will ensure better acceptance and adherence to the topic of discussion. Some key elements to consider are:

- Host midmorning educational sessions when seniors are more likely to be at their peak level of performance and alertness.
- Educational setting should be well lit and warm.
- Encourage audience participation during topics of discussion. Invite them to share their lived experiences and incorporate those into the topic of discussion by pointing out successful maneuvers or actions not to take.
- Handouts should have large (12 + point) fonts for easy reading.
- Messages should be kept short and simple.
- Key messages should be repeated at least 3 times during the presentation.
- Provide local examples.

The surgeon should also remember that some older adults may have low or no literacy skills. Appy[32] noted that adults with low literacy skills put themselves in danger of failing to receive and understand basic fire and life safety messages or use essential fire safety devices.[23] One way to minimize or avoid embarrassment and ensure that the message is received is to include simple words, pictures, or videos in the presentation. Organizations such as the local fire department, the Council on Aging, and Social Services may offer some collaborative assistance to the surgeon when planning a program for this vulnerable population. For individuals that may be homebound, the local Meals-on-Wheels program or visiting home health agencies may also be of assistance.

BURN PREVENTION FOR INDIVIDUALS WITH DISABILITIES

The Americans with Disabilities Act became law in 1990 and was amended with a Title I act in 2008. It is the first civil rights law that prohibits discrimination against individuals with disabilities in all areas of public life, including jobs, schools, transportation, and all public and private places that are open to the general public. The purpose of the law is to make sure that people with disabilities have the same rights and opportunities as everyone else.[33] A disability is defined as (1) a physical or mental impairment that substantially limits one or more of the major life activities of an individual, (2) a record of such an impairment, or (3) being regarded as having such an impairment. Major life functioning may be described as thinking and caring for oneself, performing manual tasks, walking, seeing, hearing, and working.[34] Individuals that meet the definition of the Americans with Disabilities Act may have done little or no preparation for emergencies such as a fire or burn injury. Even if such preparation has been made, preventative or rescue actions may depend on a caregiver that may not be present or is distracted when an incident occurs. When planning an educational program, the surgeon should remember that the reinforcement of any skills or activities should be based around the abilities of the individual and should include the individuals and their caregivers. Partnering with local and national organizations that provides specific disability services (ie, the March of Dimes, Deaf and Hard of Hearing services, The United Way) may prove to be beneficial.[23] For example, in preparing a fire and burn safety course for a certain disabled population, the use of alternative formats such as Braille, large print, audio tapes, or assistive communication devices may be considered. The partner organizations may assist with planning, programming (operationalizing), and uploading the educational program into the devices that best suit the needs of the individuals and their learning capabilities.

VISION- HEARING- AND MOBILITY-IMPAIRED PERSONS

Because of their disabilities, vision-, hearing-, and mobility-impaired persons require special sensitivity when considering fire and burn safety initiatives. Even though they may be familiar with their environment, in the event of a fire, confusion and disorientation may arise because of heat, chemicals, and smoke filling the room. When designing a fire and burn prevention program for this population, it is important to remember that the program activities and objectives should be based around the individual's disability and capabilities. For example, a flashing exit sign may prove to be beneficial when the fire alarm has been activated for an individual with partial vision loss. However, an individual with total loss of vision may benefit by recognizing the sound of an alarm designed for the visually impaired and seek safety in an area of refuge or shelter in place.[23,35]

Because of their disabilities, mobility- and thought-impaired individuals may be restricted from taking swift action in the event of a fire. Safety programs designed for this particular group should focus on the individuals' capabilities and their caregivers. If their mental and physical status permits, the individuals should be encouraged to practice techniques that would decrease their chances of sustaining a burn injury in the event of a fire while cooking or performing other activities of daily living. The installation of antiscald devices in the kitchen and bathroom should also be addressed. Any assistive devices used by the individual should also be incorporated in any planned program.

SUMMARY

The plastic surgeon should use every opportunity to promote fire and burn prevention safety initiatives. The unique relationship they develop by caring for individuals who have suffered a devastating burn injury should serve as a driving force to reduce or minimize further harm to others. The plastic surgeon should use their position as head of the burn team to champion the reduction of fire and burn injuries. Whether speaking with the local media, hospital administrators, or community, some form of fire and burn safety should be included in their conversation. The most effective way to achieve a reduction in fire and burn injuries is through their own actions by practicing fire and burn safety in their personal lives.

REFERENCES

1. National Hospital Ambulatory Medical Care Survey: 2100 Emergency Department Summary Tables. Available at: http://www.cdc.gov/nchs/data/ahcd/nhamcs_emergency/2011_ed_web_tables.pdf. Accessed July 10, 2016.
2. American Burn Association 2016 Fact Sheet. Available at: http://ameriburn.org/resources-factsheet.php. Accessed July 10, 2016.
3. Barrow RE, Herndon DN. History of treatment of burns. In: Herndon DN, editor. Total burn care. 3rd edition. New York: Saunders Elsevier; 2007. p. 1–8.
4. Historic Jamestowne fact sheet. 2016. Historic Timeline – Jamestowne Rediscovery. Available at: http://historicjamestowne.org/history/history-timeline/. Accessed July 9, 2016.
5. Teague PE. Case histories: fire influencing the life safety code. Updated by Chief Ronald R. Farr. Supplement 1, life safety code handbook. Quincy (MA): National Fire Protection Association Press; 2009.
6. Esposito JC. Fire in the Grove. Cambridge (MA): Dacapo Press; 2005.
7. Moulton RS. The Cocoanut Grove night club fire, Boston, November 28, 1942. Natl Fire Prot Assoc J 1943;11:1–19.
8. Saffle JR. The 1942 fire at Boston's cocoanut Grove night club. Am J Surg 1993;166(6):581–91.
9. Hall JR Jr, Cote AE. An overview of the fire problems and fire protections. In: Cote AE, Grant CC, Hall JR Jr, et al, editors. Fire protection handbook, vol. 1. Quincy (MA): National Fire Protection Association; 2008. p. 208. Sec. 3.25.
10. U. S. Consumer Product Safety Commission Flammable Fabrics Act: Public Law 88, Chapter 164; 83rd Congress, 1st session, H.R. 5069, U.S> Government Printing Office. 1953. Available at: https://books.google.com/books?id=4vI9AAAAYAAJ&q=Books+about+flammable+Fabrics+act&dq=Books+about+flammable+Fabrics+act&hl=en&sa=X&ved=0ahUKEwj13vbogobTAhVL1CYKHcrWB5kQ6AEIHjAB. Accessed July 17, 2016.
11. U.S. Consumer Product Safety Commission. Who we are-What we do for you. (2106). Available at: http://www.cpsc.gov/en/Safety-Education/Safety-Guides/General-Information/Who-We-Are–What-We-Do-for-You/. Accessed July 17, 2016.
12. National Fire Protection Association. Learn-not-to-burn and learn-not-to- burn Preschool curriculum. Quincy (MA): National Fire Protection Association Press; 2016.
13. National Fire Protection Association. Remembering When: a fire and fall prevention program for the older adult. Quincy (MA): National Fire Protection Association Press; 2016.
14. United States Fire Administration (2016). Fire is Everyone's Fight. Available at: https://www.usfa.fema.gov/prevention/outreach/. Accessed July 10, 2016.
15. Sleet DA, Dahlberg LL, Basavaraju SV, et al. Injury prevention, violence prevention and trauma care: building the scientific base. MMWR Morb Mortal Wkly Rep 2011;60(4):78–85.
16. Kahane CJ. Lives saved by the federal motor vehicle safety standards and other vehicle safety technologies, 1960-2002. Passenger cars and light trucks. With a review of 19 FMVSS and their effectiveness in reducing fatalities, injuries and crashes. Washington, DC: US Department of Transportation, National Highway Traffic Safety Administration; 2004. NHTA Technical report no. DOT HS 809 833. Available at: http://www.nhtsa.gov/cars/rules/regrev/evaluate/809833.html.
17. Runyan CW. Using the Haddon matrix: Introducing the third dimension. Inj Prev 1998;4(4):302–7.
18. National Commission on Fire and Control and the United States Fire Administration. America Burning: The report of the National Commission on Fire Prevention and Control. (Library of Congress Cared

Number 73–600022). 1973. Available at: http://www.usfa.fema.gov/downloads/pdf/publication/fa-264.pdf. Accessed July 10, 2016.

19. United States Fire Administration. American Burning Recommissioned (USFA Publication No. HQ-oo-144). Washington, DC: 2000. Available at: http://www.fema.gov/news-release/2000/12/13/american-burning-recommissioned-issues-final-report. Accessed July 10, 2016.

20. U. S. Fire Administration, Public fire education planning a five step process (FA-219). 2008. Available at: https://www.usfa.fema.gov/dowloads/pdf/publications/fa-219.pdf. Accessed July 10, 2016.

21. Szymanski, TR. Fire Safety Education: The "three E's of "of fire prevention. Firehouse - Prevention and Investigation section. 2013. Available at: http://www.firehouse.com/article/11201116/fire-safety-education-the-three-es-of-fire-prevention. Accessed July 10, 2016.

22. U. S. Department of Homeland Security, Federal Emergency Management Agency. Executive analysis of community risk reduction course. 2012. Available at: https://www.usfa.fema.gov/downloads/pdf/coffee-break/fm/fm_2013_13.pdf. Accessed July 10, 2016.

23. Grant EJ. Burn prevention for the surgeon. In: Greenhalgh DG, editor. Burn care for general surgeons and general practitioners. Switzerland: Springer; 2016. p. 281–93.

24. King MA. Demonstrating your fire prevention program's worth – Part 2. Firehouse – prevention and investigation section. 2011. Available at: http://www.firehouse.com/article/10460617/demonstrating-your-fire-prevention-programs-worth-part-2. Accessed July 17, 2016.

25. American Burn Association: scald injury prevention educator's guide. 2007. Available at: http://www.ameriburn.org/Preven/ScaldInjuryEducator'sGuide.pdf. Accessed July 17, 2016.

26. American Burn Association. Pediatric scalds: a burn issue factsheet. 2015. Available at: http://www.ameriburn.org/preven/PediatricScalds_2-27-15.pdf. Accessed July 17, 2016.

27. Nationwide Children's Hospital. Burn Prevention: pre-school and school age. 2015. Available at: http://www.nationwidechldrens.org/burn-prevention-preschool-and-school-age. Accessed July 17, 2016.

28. U.S. Census Bureau. Current population survey, annual social and economic supplement, 2011. 2012. Available at: http://www.census.gov/population/age/data/2011comp.html. Accessed July 17, 2016.

29. American Burn Association. National Burn Repository 2014 report version 10. 2014. Available at: http://ameriburn.org/2014NBRAnnualReport.pdf. Accessed July 17, 2016.

30. Davidge K, Fish J. Older adults and burns. Geriatr Aging 2008;11(5):270–5.

31. Grant, E. J., Burn prevention. In Flynn M.B., editor. Critical care nursing clinics of North America 16(1) 127–138. Philadelphia: Elsevier Saunders: 2004.

32. Appy M. The home safety council and its challenge. Am J Prev Med 2005;28(1):70–1.

33. U. S. Department of Health and Human Services, ADA National Network. What is the American with Disabilities Act? Available at: https://adata.org/learn-about-ada. Accessed July 17, 2016.

34. U. S. Department of Commerce. American with disabilities: 1994-95. Economic and statistic administration, U.S> Bureau of Census, Household Economic Studies. 1997: Washington, DC; Current Population Report #. p. 70–61.

35. United States Fire Administration. Fire risks for the blind and visually impaired. Emmitsburg (MD): Tri-Data Corp; 1999.

Negligent and Inflicted Burns in Children

Zachary J. Collier, BA[a],*, Michelle C. Roughton, MD[b], Lawrence J. Gottlieb, MD[c]

KEYWORDS

- Inflicted burn • Negligent burn • Noninflicted burn • Maltreatment burn • Child abuse

KEY POINTS

- Child abuse is common, affecting 1 in 4 children, and is underreported.
- Burn injury is a common form of lethal child abuse.
- Establishing the cause of burn injury (ie, inflicted, noninflicted, or negligent) is challenging.
- Detailed examination of the burn wound, including source, location, depth, size, margins, and concomitant injury, helps to determine the cause.
- Multidisciplinary care teams involving pediatricians who specialize in child abuse, social and welfare services, and law enforcement are critical for thorough investigations of abuse.

BACKGROUND

The physical stigmata of child abuse were first described in 1946 by pediatric radiologist John Caffey.[1] He described a cluster of physical findings, including multiple metaphyseal fractures, subdural and subarachnoid hemorrhage, and retinal hemorrhage, in what he termed "whiplash shaken-baby syndrome."[1] It was not until 20 years later that Kempe and colleagues'[2] description of battered child syndrome brought national awareness to pediatric abuse, its spectrum of manifestations, and the frequently severe sequelae. Subsequently, all 50 states implemented laws requiring health care providers to report suspicions of abuse and neglect.[3,4]

Numerous studies have determined that 1 in 4 children in the United States experience some form of physical abuse during childhood, with as many as 5 deaths per day as a result of these injuries.[5,6] Despite these high numbers, the problem is underreported. As many as 50% of abuse-related injuries and fatalities are misdiagnosed or not properly reported to local and state agencies.[5,6]

Complex nuances and variations between cases make it difficult to consistently diagnose abuse with an appropriate degree of confidence. Discerning injury mechanism is difficult, and, given the associated risks of an incorrect determination of inflicted versus noninflicted injuries, it is critical that children receive evidence-based evaluations and interventions. Up to 30% of children returned to abusive homes experience ongoing abuse.[7–9] In contrast, and more difficult to measure, children who sustain noninflicted injuries may be wrongly removed from their families.[10]

Compared with other forms of child abuse, negligent and inflicted burns are a particularly difficult diagnostic problem.[11,12] Burns were not recognized in the literature as manifestations of child neglect or abuse until battered child syndrome was described in 1962.[13,14] Burns are a leading cause of abuse-related fatalities in children (6%–20%), thus it is critical to discern negligent and inflicted presentation patterns.[15–17]

[a] Biological Sciences Division, Pritzker School of Medicine, University of Chicago, 924 East 57th Street, Chicago, IL 60637, USA; [b] Division of Plastic and Reconstructive Surgery, Department of Surgery, University of North Carolina at Chapel Hill, 7040 Burnett-Womack, Chapel Hill, NC 27599, USA; [c] Section of Plastic and Reconstructive Surgery, Department of Surgery, University of Chicago, 5841 South Maryland Avenue, Room J-641, Chicago, IL 60637, USA
* Corresponding author.
E-mail address: zcollier@uchicago.edu

Clin Plastic Surg 44 (2017) 467–477
http://dx.doi.org/10.1016/j.cps.2017.02.022
0094-1298/17/© 2017 Elsevier Inc. All rights reserved.

TERMINOLOGY

Pediatric burn injury is grouped into 3 categories: noninflicted, negligent, and inflicted. Often clinicians group negligent and inflicted burns under the umbrella term of abuse. However, the circumstances under which negligent and inflicted burns occur are distinct. Negligent burns occur in the setting of inadequate knowledge, attention, or resources (an act of omission), whereas inflicted burns occur because of the action of a caregiver (an act of commission). Differentiation between these two burn causes is essential from a child welfare perspective because it dictates intervention. **Table 1** provides key characteristics of negligent and inflicted burns.[18]

When grouping the 2 causes for brevity or convenience, it is most appropriate to use the term maltreatment. In addition, care must be taken to avoid the use of identifiers such as intentional when describing burns because this is a legal term and requires proof of motive or intent.

Patient Presentation and Evaluation

Characteristic presentations and patterns often accompany neglect and inflicted causes (**Fig. 1**). Cases with single-parent providers, historical inconsistencies, delayed presentations, genital and perineal injuries, immersion lines or circumferential burns, clearly defined contact wounds, and concomitant or variably aged injuries are strong indicators that the burns resulted from negligent or inflicted causes (**Table 2**).[9,12–14,18]

BURN HISTORY

During the initial history and physical examination, it is critical to evaluate for negligent and inflicted burns. Components of the burn history should include:

- Preceding events
- Setting of injury
- Sequence of events during burn injury
- Status of patient's clothing
- Burn source
- Time and temperature of exposure
- First aid administration
- Initial burn appearance
- Interpretation of severity
- Time from injury to medical care

Historical inconsistencies should raise suspicions for maltreatment burns. History from multiple sources is valuable and documentation is critical. Only 10% of noninflicted cases reveal inconsistency, whereas 78% of patients with inflicted burns and 27% of patients with negligent burns do (see **Table 2**).[18,19] Caregivers likely falsify their stories to avoid punishment but injured children may also report an untrue history because of fear of retaliation or relocation. Following discovery of historical inconsistences, the health care team must collaborate with local law enforcement and child welfare agencies because they often signal a need to evaluate for other signs of abuse (ie, skeletal surveys, urine and hair toxicology, field investigations).[20]

Maltreatment burns are also associated with delayed presentation to care without sufficient reason.[19] Although noninflicted burns may occur days before presentation, usually clear evidence exists of the use of first aid with anticipated recovery and/or receipt of outpatient medical attention.[16,19]

DEVELOPMENTAL AND MEDICAL HISTORY

Close attention to the child's physical and mental development relative to expected milestones is crucial to understand the potential for noninflicted injury (eg, pulling to stand on a stove, climbing into a tub).[21] Incorporating knowledge of the average ages at which children can roll (3 months), sit-up (6 months), crawl (9 months), walk (12 months), and develop certain motor skills (eg, grasp and pinch) allows providers to determine whether or not a child is capable of performing the actions that a caregiver reports during the burn history

Table 1
Distinguishing features between negligent and inflicted burns

Burn Features	Negligent (%)	Inflicted (%)
Historical Details		
Historical inconsistency	27	78[a]
Burn Pattern		
Bilateral	33	67[a]
Burn Location		
Lower legs	3	22[a]
Concomitant Injuries		
Fracture	3	13[a]
Hematoma	3	13[a]
Postadmission Interventions		
Split-thickness skin graft applied	33	66[a]

All of the listed features are significantly more common in inflicted burns than in negligent burns.
[a] P value less than .05.

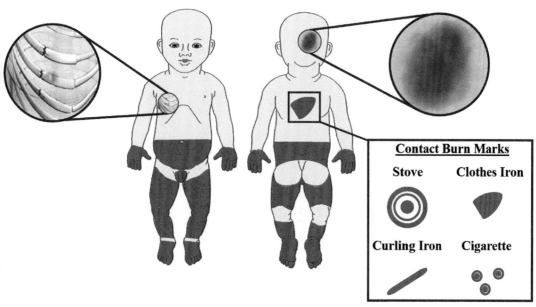

Fig. 1. The numerous burn patterns consistent with abusive causes, including immersion lines, circumferential burns, spared skin creases, a halo or ring sign on the buttocks, and well-defined contact burn marks. Other manifestations of concomitant abuse include bruises and multiple rib fractures of varying ages.

Table 3).[22] The same concept holds true for consideration of intellectual development and the capacity for a child to perform certain functions or tasks (eg, using a stove or microwave). In addition, other medical conditions, including seizure disorders, dermatologic conditions, and a prior history of trauma or surgery, may also complicate interpretation of the burn story.[9,23]

SOCIAL HISTORY

Family dynamics and composition are predictive of abuse or neglect burns.[24] Mothers are most frequently the perpetrators of negligent (37%) and inflicted (31%) burns; however, this is confounded by mothers being much more likely to be the sole caregivers of infants and toddlers.[20] Most noninflicted burns (49%) also occur in

Table 2
Classic features of negligent and inflicted burns

Classic Features	Noninflicted	Negligent	Inflicted
Historical Details			
Historical inconsistency (%)	0	27[a]	78[a]
Delay seeking care (%)	2	17[a]	28[a]
Burn age at presentation (h)	4 ± 1	18 ± 7[a]	28 ± 6[a]
Single parent (%)	48	87[a]	87[a]
Prior child welfare history (%)	8	40[a]	50[a]
Burn Mechanism			
Tap water (%)	20	56[a]	70[a]
Burn Pattern			
Immersion lines/circumferential (%)	4	17[a]	38[a]
Bilateral (%)	23	33[a]	69[a]
Concomitant injuries (%)	0	10[a]	28[a]

All of the listed features are significantly more common in negligent and inflicted burns than in noninflicted burns.
[a] P value less than .05.

Table 3
Developmental milestones

Age	Gross Motor	Fine Motor	Speech/Language	Cognitive	Social/Emotional
Newborn	Primitive reflexes: step, place, Moro, Babinski, flexor posture	Primitive reflexes: grasp	Primitive reflexes: root, suck, alerts/startles to sound, variable cries	Visual focal length ~25 cm (10″) Fix and follow slow horizontal arc Prefers contrast, colors, faces	Bonding (parent→child) Self-regulation
2 mo	Head steady when held, head up 45° at prone	Hands open half of the time Bats at objects	Orients to voice Cooing	Prefers usual caregiver Attends to moderate novelty Follows past midline	Attachment (child → parents) Social smile
4 mo	Sits with support Head up 90° prone, arms out Rolls front→back	Palmar grasp Reaches and obtains items Bring objects to midline	Laugh, squeal	Anticipates routines Purposeful sensory exploration of objects	Turn-taking conversations Explores parents' faces
6 mo	Postural reflexes Sits tripod Rolls both ways	Raking grasp Transfers hand to hand	Babble (nonspecific)	Stranger anxiety Looks for dropped or hidden objects	Expresses emotions Memory lasts 24 h
9 mo	Gets from all fours→sitting Sits with hands free Pulls to stand	Inferior pincer grasp Pokes at objects	Mama, Dada Gestures goodbye Gesture games	Object permanence Uncovers toy	Separation anxiety
12 mo	Walks a few steps Wide-based gait	Fine pincer (fingertips) Voluntary release Throws objects Finger-feed self	Additional words Inhibits with "No" Responds to name 1-step command with gesture	Cause and effect Trial and error Imitates gestures and sounds Uses objects functionally	Explore from secure base Points at wanted items Narrative memory begins

Age	Gross motor	Fine motor	Speech/language	Cognitive	Social/emotional
15 mo	Walks well	Uses spoon, open-top cup Tower of 2 blocks	Points to 1 body part 1-step command no gesture 5 words	Looks for hidden object Experiments with toys	Shared attention: points at interesting items Brings toys to parents
18 mo	Stoops and recovers Runs	Carries toys while walking Removes clothes Tower of 4 blocks Scribbles, fisted pencil grasp	Points to object, 3 body parts 10–25 words Labels familiar objects	Imitates housework Symbolic play with toys	Increased independence Parallel play
2 y	Jumps on 2 feet Up and down stairs	Handedness established Uses fork Tower of 6 blocks Imitates vertical stroke	Follows 2-step commands ≥50 words 2-word phrases	New problem-solving without rehearsal	Testing limits, tantrums Negativism Possessive
3 y	Pedals trike Upstairs alternating feet	Undresses Toilet trained (2.5–3.5 y) Draws circles Turns pages of books	3-step commands 200 words 3–4 word phrases Knows name, age, gender	Simple time concepts Identifies shapes Compares 2 items Counts to 3	Separates easily Sharing, empathy Cooperative play Role play
4 y	Hops on 1 foot Down stairs with alternating feet	Cuts shapes with scissors Uses buttons	Sentences Tells stories Past tense	Counts to 4 Opposites Identifies 4 colors	Has preferred friend Elaborate fantasy play
5 y	Balance on 1 foot for 10 s Skips, may learn to bicycle	Draws person Tripod pencil grasp Independent ADLs	5000 words Future tense Word play, jokes Phonemic awareness	Counts to 10 Recite ABCs Preliteracy	Has group of friends Follows group rules Games with rules

This table provides the key developmental milestones for gross and fine motor, speech/language, cognitive, and social/emotional skills across a 5-year period.
Abbreviation: ADLs, activities of daily living.

children under the care of their mothers and transpire at higher rates than negligent and inflicted injuries.

Children from intact families are less likely to experience burn-related and/or other forms of pediatric abuse.[15] Inflicted burns are more likely to occur in the care of foster parents, minors, and nonparental adults compared with noninflicted burns.[20] Thus, not only is it vital to identify the family structure during initial burn history but it is also equally important to integrate resources for single parents or those with many children in order to reduce future risk of such events.

It is also important to inquire about drug and alcohol use, which may influence the circumstances surrounding the injury. Children can be accidentally or intentionally exposed to these substances and caregiver use of drugs and/or alcohol is a red flag of abuse and neglect. Hair and urine toxicology from the patient can be helpful to identify or confirm concerns.[20]

CHILD AND FAMILY WELFARE SERVICES HISTORY

Patients with negligent and inflicted burns are more likely to have child welfare histories compared with patients with noninflicted burns. Recurrent interactions with child welfare services suggest the phenomenon of repeated abuse or battered child syndrome.[2,6,9,18] Even in scenarios in which no child welfare history exists for that child, prior involvement of the care provider or other family members should increase suspicion for abuse.

BURN WOUND EXAMINATION AND FORMULATING A MECHANISM

Perhaps the most valuable objective evidence for or against an inflicted or negligent cause is derived from examination of the burn wound. Documentation of burn source, location, depth, size, and

margins must be recorded in the greatest detail possible. Photographs are helpful and strongly recommended. Each examination component contributes to the overall burn story or probable mechanism of injury used to corroborate or refute the story provided by the patient and caregivers. **Fig. 1** provides an overview of well-known findings in abusive burns as they relate to the burn wound and additional or concomitant injuries.

Source

Tap water scalds are the most common source of maltreatment burn injury.[19,25] Scalds from stove-heated and microwave-heated liquids, including instant noodles, are more often the source in non-inflicted burns than in inflicted scalds.[20] Accidental scald sources are much more likely to present with splash patterns (**Fig. 2**A) and lack bilateral distributions, immersion line or stocking glove patterns, and the ring sign that are seen in negligent and inflicted groups (see **Fig. 2**B; **Fig. 3**).

Contact burns are also commonly seen in the maltreatment groups (**Fig. 4**).[26,27] They may be more common than scalds because they are underreported. Often, studies strictly include hospitalized patients and many abusive contact burns (eg, from cigarettes, irons, and other small surfaces) do not require admission.[28,29]

Maltreatment burns occur from all sources (ie, scald, contact, flame, chemical, electric, friction),[30] thus it is critical to analyze the burn presentation and how well it fits into the injury narrative provided.

Location

Buttocks, genitalia/perineum, and lower extremity burns are more commonly seen in maltreatment injury.[29] A common theme involves toilet-training accidents and children punished with a hot bath (**Fig. 5**).[18,20] In addition, the inflicted group has more involvement of the lower legs and feet.

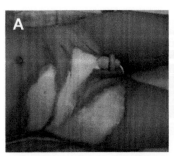
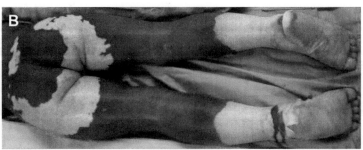

Fig. 2. (*A*) The noninflicted scald more closely resembles a true splash pattern without any clearly defined immersion lines and spared skin creases. (*B*) The inflicted scald shows the spared circular region of buttock skin ring sign and bilateral ankle immersion lines caused by forced submersion into a scalding bathtub.

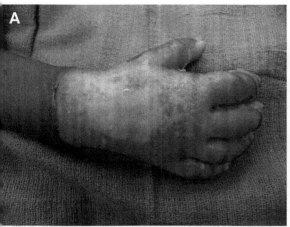
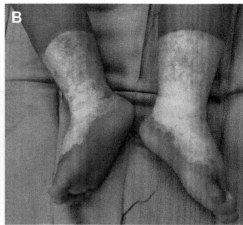

Fig. 3. Common distribution patterns observed in inflicted scald burns with submersion: circumferential stocking glove (*A*) and bilateral immersion lines (*B*).

Mechanistically, noninflicted spills tend to occur from superiorly based locations (eg, child reaches up for hot liquid) and thus resultant burns are on the head, neck, and anterior torso. In contrast, negligent and inflicted burns have a higher proportion of lower torso and extremity involvement caused by immersion-based exposures. An intimate understanding of the distribution patterns associated with specific burn mechanisms is critical to integrate into the corroboration of the caregivers burn narrative.

Depth

Differential depths within a burn wound and its distribution across the body can provide meaningful information regarding exposure vectors for the burn source as well as exposure time. For scalds, the point of initial contact is deeper compared with distal or peripheral sites, which are exposed to liquid after heat has dissipated. Skin across the body varies in epidermal thickness and degree of cutaneous circulation. Both factors influence burn depth.[31,32] Accordingly, scald injuries with uniform depth, symmetry, well-defined margins, and/or immersion lines should prompt further investigation for a potentially inflicted cause.[19]

In contrast with scalds, contact burns have reduced depth gradients throughout the injury because they have less potential for heat loss between contact sites. Noninflicted contact burns are more likely to have poorly defined margins with variable depths because the children attempt to withdraw from the source unless precluded by medical or developmental factors. For example, children may present with uniform, bilateral palmar contact burns after pulling to stand and reflexively grasping rather than releasing on contact with radiators. Accounting for the child's developmental state would thus support such a scenario as noninflicted rather than inflicted despite the concerning bilateral pattern. Burns with consistent depth and clear margins matching the outline of cigarettes, irons, and hairdryers are most often associated with inflicted injuries,[30] although inflicted contact burns from radiators, stoves, and many other sources have also been reported.[33]

Maltreatment burns are more often deeper and result in greater morbidity compared with noninflicted injury (**Table 4**).[20,28]

Size

Inflicted or abusive burns are more likely to involve larger total body surface area (TBSA).[20,29,32]

Margins

Burns with well-defined or linear borders are suspicious for abuse. Most accidental or noninflicted injuries occur in situations in which the child has

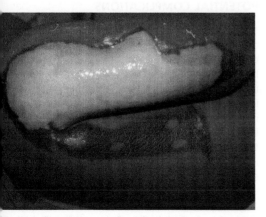

Fig. 4. Inflicted iron contact burn with clear pattern margins.

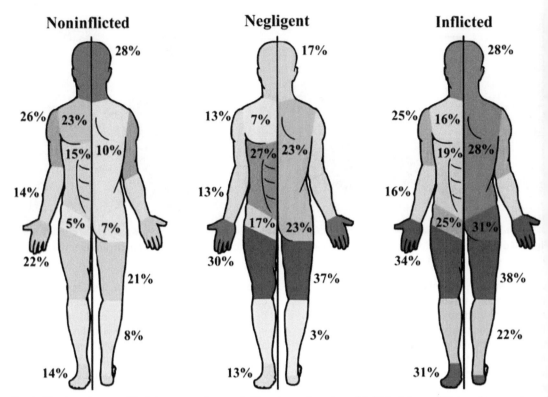

Fig. 5. The location-specific injury rates for noninflicted, negligent, and inflicted burns. Higher frequencies or rates of injury are associated with darker red colors on the heat map.

some degree of mobility or freedom and attempts to withdraw from or avoid the burn source. Because of that reflexive aversion and withdrawal, accidental injuries rarely present with clearly demarcated margins or nonorganic shapes unless explained by the child's clothing (eg, cuff line, diaper, or shoes) or environment (eg, high chair or booster seats). While examining borders and transition zones, it is important to look for any contact burns that may have been intentionally hidden within a larger scald burn.

Concomitant Injuries

Other injuries presenting concurrently with pediatric burns provide meaningful evidence for negligent or abusive causes. Concomitant injuries occur at sufficiently high frequencies to support supplemental studies (ie, skeletal surveys, liver function tests [LFTs: Bilirubin, Total Protein, Albumin, ALP, ALT, AST]) to evaluate for inflicted trauma.[33] Cutaneous manifestations of abuse include genital trauma and lacerations, contusions, bite marks, abrasions, and signs of healed burns.[2,15,22] Other manifestations; occult rib fractures, with or without multiple healing stages; increased LFTs; intracranial or retinal

hemorrhage; and splenic lacerations are all potential signs of abuse.[1,2,15,32] Although an isolated finding may not raise suspicion of abuse, accounting for the entire presentation and pattern of injuries in the setting of burn injury is an important component of the examination. When appropriately assimilated into the overarching medical and social context, suspicious findings warrant further investigation on discovery.

POTENTIAL COMPLICATIONS

Maltreatment burns have significantly higher rates of complications (eg, wound infections, sepsis) compared with noninflicted burns.[20] Inflicted burns also require more systemic antibiotics than noninflicted patients during hospitalization, which is likely a surrogate for increased infection rates in this group (see **Table 4**). In turn, the increased infectious complication rate is likely related to time to presentation. Immediately after thermal injury the burn wound is sterile, but staphylococcal species colonize the wound by 48 hours postburn, whereas polymicrobial (gram-positive, gram-negative, fungal) contamination occurs in up to 87% of burns within 5 to 7 days.[34,35] In addition, maltreatment burns are more likely to have larger

Table 4
Features of severity in negligent and inflicted burns

Features	Noninflicted	Negligent	Inflicted
Burn Size and Depth			
TBSA (%)	5 ± 0.4	7 ± 1.4	10 ± 2.0[a]
Burn Depth			
Superficial partial (%)	73	47[a]	38[a]
Deep partial (%)	15	33[a]	25
Full thickness (%)	9	20[a]	38[a]
Postadmission Interventions			
Surgeries (%)	51	53	75[a]
STSG (%)	36	33	66[a]
FTSG (%)	1	3	6[a]
Allograft (%)	3	10[a]	19[a]
Burn Care Complications			
Complications (%)	4	17[a]	22[a]
Wound infection (%)	1	3	19[a]
Sepsis (%)	1	7[a]	6[a]
Systemic antibiotics (%)	4	7	22[a]
Length of stay (days)	7 ± 0.4	11 ± 1.8[a]	15 ± 2.3[a]

The listed features are either primary or secondary markers of burn severity. Many of these features present more frequently with negligent and/or inflicted burns.

Abbreviations: FTSG, full-thickness skin graft; STSG, split-thickness skin graft; TBSA, total body surface area.

[a] *P* value less than .05.

TBSA, which is correlated with higher rates of bacterial colonization and infection.[36,37]

INVESTIGATIONAL PARADIGM

It is critical for burn team members to appreciate the nontrivial risk of overdiagnosis and underdiagnosis of maltreatment burns and the substantial psychological and physical ramifications for diagnostic error in either direction. Standardized investigation protocols reduce provider bias and ensure that substantial interventions are pursued only when the highest quality evidence has been obtained.

Perhaps most important is effective collaboration between the burn team, child abuse pediatricians, social services, and law enforcement. Law enforcement may assist with field investigations of the household or setting in which the burn occurred. Documentation of the environment (eg, sink or bath size, stove anchors, faucet shapes), child accessibility (eg, counter heights, cabinet knobs, climbable furniture), and water temperatures with attention to time-dependent heating curves (**Fig. 6**) are all extremely valuable and corroborate or refute the reported burn narrative.

Regardless of overt concern for a negligent or abusive cause, investigation by a multidisciplinary team is recommended for all children 3 years of age and younger. This investigation removes bias inherent in the current system, which relies on the health care team to notify child welfare of suspicious behavior. This

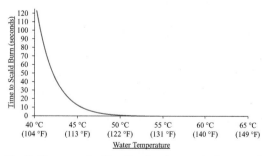

Fig. 6. Time required for the development of a second degree scald burn relative to water temperature. This graph represents data from adults. The respective curve for children is shifted to the left as a result of thinner epidermis. (*Adapted from* Moritz AR, Henriques FC. Studies of thermal injury: II. The relative importance of time and surface temperature in the causation of cutaneous burns. Am J Pathol 1947;23(5):695–720.)

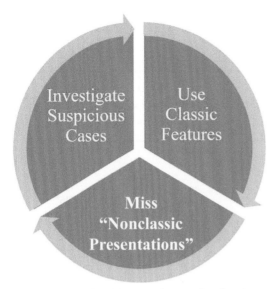

Fig. 7. Age-mandated abuse evaluations for all pediatric burns in patients younger than a specific age (≤3 years) regardless of suspicion circumvents the circular logic used in referral-based investigational paradigms.

process may continually miss nonclassic presentations and reinforce that decision-making process; that is, people only find what they are looking for (**Fig. 7**).[28,29]

SUMMARY

Each year 700,000 injuries and 1600 fatalities occur in the United States as a result of child abuse. Twenty percent of these injuries result from burns. Health care providers must be able to correctly identify children with noninflicted, negligent, and inflicted injuries in order to appropriately allocate medical and child welfare resources. Noninflicted burns may be distinguished from negligent and inflicted injuries following recognition of historical inconsistencies, delayed presentations, genital and perineal involvement, immersion lines, deeper injuries, bilateral patterns, clearly defined contact wounds, and concomitant or variably aged injuries. Inflicted injuries are significantly more likely to present with historical inconsistencies, bilateral distributions, lower extremity involvement, concomitant injuries, and greater depth compared with negligent burns.

Implementation of mandated multidisciplinary investigation for every child regardless of suspicion for abuse is the most effective method for ensuring that all negligent and inflicted injuries are properly diagnosed. Assessment of the aforementioned history and examination findings with a multidisciplinary burn team approach enables burn providers to deliver effective, evidence-based care to pediatric patients.

REFERENCES

1. Caffey J. Multiple fractures in the long bones of infants suffering from chronic subdural hematoma. Am J Roentgenol Radium Ther 1946;56(2): 163–73.
2. Kempe C, Silverman FN, Steele BF, et al. The battered-child syndrome. JAMA 1962;181(1):17–24.
3. Gil DG. Physical abuse of children. Pediatrics 1969; 44(5):857–64.
4. Gregg GS. Physician, child-abuse reporting laws, and injured child. Psychosocial anatomy of childhood trauma. Clin Pediatr (Phila) 1968;7(12): 720–5.
5. Administration for Children and Families, Administration on Children, Youth and Families: Children's Bureau. Child maltreatment 2013 [Internet]. Washington, DC: US Department of Health and Human Services; 2013. Available at: http://www.acf.hhs.gov/programs/cb/resource/child-maltreatment-2013.
6. Stoltenborgh M, Bakermans-Kranenburg MJ, Alink LRA, et al. The prevalence of child maltreatment across the globe: review of a series of meta-analyses. Child Abuse Rev 2015;24(1):37–50.
7. Fluke JD, Yuan Y-YT, Edwards M. Recurrence of maltreatment: an application of the National Child Abuse and Neglect Data System (NCANDS). Child Abuse Negl 1999;23(7):633–50.
8. Paul AR, Adamo MA. Non-accidental trauma in pediatric patients: a review of epidemiology, pathophysiology, diagnosis and treatment. Transl Pediatr 2014;3(3):195–207.
9. Hindley N, Ramchandani PG, Jones DPH. Risk factors for recurrence of maltreatment: a systematic review. Arch Dis Child 2006;91(9):744–52.
10. Biehal N, Sinclair I, Wade J. Reunifying abused or neglected children: decision-making and outcomes. Child Abuse Negl [Internet]. Available at: http://www.sciencedirect.com/science/article/pii/S0145213415001520. Accessed September 25, 2015.
11. Phillips PS, Pickrell E, Morse TS. Intentional burning: a severe form of child abuse. J Am Coll Emerg Physicians 1974;3(6):388–90.
12. Chester DL, Jose RM, Aldlyami E, et al. Non-accidental burns in children—are we neglecting neglect? Burns 2006;32(2):222–8.
13. Fontana VJ, Donovan D, Wong RJ. The maltreatment syndrome in children. N Engl J Med 1963;269(26): 1389–94.
14. Gillespie RWMD. The battered child syndrome: thermal and caustic manifestations. J Trauma Inj Infect 1965;5(4):523–34.

5. Hight DW, Bakalar HR, Lloyd JR. Inflicted burns in children: recognition and treatment. JAMA 1979; 242(6):517–20.

16. Peck M, Priolo-Kapel D. Child abuse by burning: a review of the literature and an algorithm for medical investigations. J Trauma 2002;53(5):1013–22.

17. Korbin JE, Krugman RD, editors. Handbook of child maltreatment [Internet]. Dordrecht (the Netherlands): Springer Netherlands; 2014. Available at: http://link.springer.com/10.1007/978-94-007-7208-3. Accessed January13, 2016.

18. Collier ZJ, Ramaiah V, Glick JC, et al. A 6-year case-control study of the presentation and clinical sequelae for noninflicted, negligent, and inflicted pediatric burns. J Burn Care Res 2016;38(1): e101–24.

19. Maguire S, Moynihan S, Mann M, et al. A systematic review of the features that indicate intentional scalds in children. Burns 2008;34(8):1072–81.

20. Wibbenmeyer L, Liao J, Heard J, et al. Factors related to child maltreatment in children presenting with burn injuries. J Burn Care Res 2014;35(5): 374–81.

21. Urquiza AJ, Wirtz SJ, Peterson MS, et al. Screening and evaluating abused and neglected children entering protective custody. Child Welfare 1994; 73(2):155–71.

22. US Centers for Disease Control and Prevention. Developmental milestones. 2013. Available at: http://www.cdc.gov/ncbddd/actearly/milestones/index.html. Accessed June 5, 2016.

23. Letson MM, Tscholl JJ. Bruises, burns, and other blemishes: diagnostic considerations of physical abuse. Clin Pediatr Emerg Med 2012; 13(3):155–65, 11p.

24. Bakalar HR, Moore JD, Hight DW. Psychosocial dynamics of pediatric burn abuse. Health Soc Work 1981;6(4):27–32.

25. Yeoh C, Nixon JW, Dickson W, et al. Patterns of scald injuries. Arch Dis Child 1994;71(2):156–8.

26. Kumar P. Child abuse by thermal injury—a retrospective survey. Burns 1984;10(5):344–8.

27. Showers JED, Garrison KM. Burn abuse: a four-year study. J Trauma Inj Infect 1988;28(11):1581–3.

28. Pawlik M-C, Kemp A, Maguire S, et al. Children with burns referred for child abuse evaluation: burn characteristics and co-existent injuries. Child Abuse Negl 2016;55:52–61.

29. Thombs BD. Patient and injury characteristics, mortality risk, and length of stay related to child abuse by burning: evidence from a national sample of 15,802 pediatric admissions. Ann Surg 2008; 247(3):519–23.

30. Hobbs CJ, Wynne JM. The sexually abused battered child. Arch Dis Child 1990;65(4):423–7.

31. Manchot C. The cutaneous arteries of the human body. New York: Springer; 1983.

32. Crisan M, Lupsor M, Crisan D, et al. Ultrasonographic assessment of skin structure according to age. Indian J Dermatol Venereol Leprol 2012; 78(4):519.

33. Petersen HD, Wandall JH. Evidence of physical torture in a series of children. Forensic Sci Int 1995;75(1):45–55.

34. Wysocki AB. Evaluating and managing open skin wounds: colonization versus infection. AACN Clin Issues 2002;13(3):382–97.

35. Erol S, Altoparlak U, Akcay MN, et al. Changes of microbial flora and wound colonization in burned patients. Burns 2004;30(4):357–61.

36. Fleming RYD, Zeigler ST, Walton MA, et al. Influence of burn size on the incidence of contamination of burn wounds by fecal organisms. J Burn Care 1991;12(6):510–5.

37. Jeschke MG, Pinto R, Kraft R, et al. Morbidity and survival probability in burn patients in modern burn care. Crit Care Med 2015;43(4):808–15.

Burn Care in Low- and Middle-Income Countries

Anthony G. Charles, MD, MPH[a],*, Jared Gallaher, MD, MPH[b], Bruce A. Cairns, MD[b]

KEYWORDS

- Burn care • Low- and middle-income countries • Societal impact • Global burden of disease

KEY POINTS

- Burn injury is a disease of poverty.
- Increased burn incidence and mortality in low- and middle-income countries.
- Deficient health care system and early resuscitation leads to increased mortality.
- Local wound care and improved nutrition is critical to survival.
- Early excision and grafting be used if health system permits.

BURDEN OF DISEASE

Burn injuries are one of the most devastating injuries and a major global public health issue particularly in low- and middle-income countries (LMIC), where 95% of fire-related burn deaths occur.[1] Annually, more than 300,000 people die from fire-related burn injuries worldwide, and millions more suffer from burn-related disabilities and disfigurements. Fire-related burns account for a loss of 10 million disability-adjusted life-years (DALY) annually.[2]

The burden of burn injury falls predominantly on the world's poor. The high incidence of burn among the global poor is driven by several factors, including migration to urban areas, disorganized urban development, inadequate electrification of homes, the use of paraffin as a primary energy source, and failure of preventative programs. The incidence of burn injury in LMICs is 1.3 per 100,000 population compared with an incidence of 0.14 per 100,000 population in high-income countries (HIC).[3] The rate of burn injury is even more severe in some developing countries such as Bangladesh, where the incidence of nonfatal burn injury is 166.3 per 100,000 per year.[4] The epidemiology of burn injuries in LMICs is different than in HIC, predominantly affecting children and women, with children aged less than 5 years suffering the highest risk of any group among burn victims.[5,6]

In LMICs, the vast majority of childhood burns are reported to occur in the home in comparison to adult burns, which occur equally at home, outdoors, and at workplaces.[7] Women aged 16 to 35 years sustain most domestic burns, due to the traditional practice of floor-level cooking or the use of an open fire.[8,9]

HEALTH CARE SYSTEMS AND PERSONNEL

Countries with a high gross national product per capita often have a relatively healthier population due to higher health care expenditures.[10] Poor health care infrastructure is a common denominator in most LMICs. Most existing burn centers are situated in large cities and have insufficient capacity for the high-burn injury incidence. Although management in these centers is based primarily on standard principles, hospitals are ill equipped with staff and support facilities. In addition to inadequate physical structures, these centers are

a Department of Surgery, North Carolina Jaycee Burn Center, School of Medicine, University of North Carolina at Chapel Hill, 4008 Burnett Womack Building, CB 7228, Chapel Hill, NC, USA; b Department of Surgery, North Carolina Jaycee Burn Center, University of North Carolina at Chapel Hill, 4004 Burnett Womack Building, 101 Manning Drive, Chapel Hill, NC 27599, USA
* Corresponding author.
E-mail address: anthchar@med.unc.edu

Clin Plastic Surg 44 (2017) 479–483
http://dx.doi.org/10.1016/j.cps.2017.02.007

plasticsurgery.theclinics.com

invariably plagued with a lack of resources, inadequate operating room availability, and a shortage of blood products for transfusion. Resuscitation is often delayed, because patients have to travel long distances, and ambulances and prehospital services are nonexistent.[6,11] There is also limited coordination between district hospitals and tertiary burn centers. Furthermore, in many developing countries, a lack of human resources remains the greatest challenge to providing surgical care. Often there are no dedicated burn surgeons, leaving the management of burn patients primarily to general surgeons without formal burn training. Burn nursing is also not a recognized field.

EFFECTIVE BURN CARE RESUSCITATION

Prehospital care of burn victims with simple measures such as irrigation with clean, cool water and clean dressings is of particular importance where access to hospital care is commonly delayed. Initial appropriate burn treatment aimed at conserving scarce resources includes emphasis on early fluid resuscitation and ensuring proper compliance to established resuscitation protocols such as the Parkland formula.[12] Patients with burns less than 10% total body surface area (TBSA) can be hydrated orally, unless there is trauma or burns to the mouth or airway. Burns greater than 10% TBSA requires 1 to 2 large-bore intravenous lines (or intraosseous lines) for fluid resuscitation. The Parkland formula (4 mL isotonic crystalloid solution × kilogram of body weight × [% TBSA] = total milliliter in the first 24 hours) may be used to initiate fluids for ongoing resuscitation and fluid losses.[13] Half of this total is given during the first 8 hours after injury, and the remaining given during the next 16 hours. Patients have highly variable systemic responses to burn injury so formulaic calculations of fluid deficits are merely guides to resuscitation.

MEDICATIONS

Provision of pain relief in the face of limited resources is very challenging. In those without substantial risk of renal injury, mild pain can be treated with nonsteroidal anti-inflammatory agents or acetaminophen. Moderate to severe pain will likely require opioids.[14] In a study of the patterns of pediatric analgesic use in Africa, acetaminophen and ibuprofen were widely used, constituting approximately 60% of all analgesics, whereas opioids were only used in 0.2%, falling well short of the World Health Organization standards.[15]

Because of a paucity of published studies, the role of prophylactic systemic antibiotics in preventing infectious complications is unclear. However, available evidence does not support their use.[16] The appropriate administration of a tetanus immunization is mandatory.

EARLY BURN EXCISION AND GRAFTING

Surgical debridement may be required for deep partial-thickness and full-thickness wounds. In the acute phase, these wounds need simple coverage. Saline bandages or cling wrap is often sufficient to cover wounds and keep patients warm and dry. In HICs, increasingly aggressive surgical approaches with early tangential excision and wound closure are standard practice in burn units. This approach represents the most significant change in recent years, leading to improvement in mortalities of burn victims at a substantially lower cost. However, in the absence of proper health care infrastructure, insufficient blood banking and supplies such as dressings, and inadequately trained health care personnel, such aggressive therapy in burn victims, can induce further trauma and result in a poor outcome.[17] In fact, evidence from sub-Saharan Africa suggests that early excision may have a much higher mortality compared with late excision in a resource-poor environment.[18] Consequently, smaller burns over critical areas such as joints are better suited for this technique.[19] For many burn patients in most LMICs, early excisional surgery, although feasible, is rarely wise.

Given the realities of inadequate operating room access, closed burn wound dressing, eschar separation, and delayed skin grafting will help separate patients with small- and medium-sized burn wounds (<40% TBSA) with the potential for survival from those with extensive wounds (>50%) that should be triaged to palliative care in a resource-poor environment.[12] A delayed operative strategy is especially important considering that the mortality for burns of greater than 40% TBSA in most LMICs approaches 100%.[2] The inability to practice early tangential excision and skin grafting may explain the high incidence of burn-related sequelae, such as disfiguring hypertrophic or keloid scarring, and disabling contractures.[20,21]

LOCAL WOUND CARE

Local wound care in the developing countries is one of the greatest barriers to effective burn wound management because wound care products and dressing supplies are not easily obtainable or far too expensive. Cool running water at a temperature between 10°C and 15°C for 20 to

0 minutes is considered adequate first-aid treatment for burn injury.[22]

Superficial burns do not require antibiotics or wound dressings. All deeper burns require topical antimicrobials or an absorptive occlusive dressing. Silver-based dressing and ointment should be used if available. However, the use of locally available and effective wound care alternatives such as amniotic membranes is cost-effective and ideal as a burn biological dressing.[23,24] They remarkably reduce the cost of dressing changes and hospital length of stay while also significantly reducing nursing time and cost.[25,26]

The medicinal properties of honey have been well described for treatment of burn wounds. The beneficial effects of honey include the cleansing of wounds, absorption of edema fluids, antimicrobial activity, promotion of granulation tissue, epithelialization, and the improvement of nutrition.[27] Another cost-effective, locally available burn dressing is the banana leaf dressing (BLD). Its preparation is very simple and can be easily taught to previously treated patients, relatives of patients, and literate as well as illiterate individuals. More importantly, BLD is a nonadherent dressing.[28] More recently, moist exposed burn ointment (MEBO), a traditional Chinese burn ointment, was reported to provide an adequate moist environment for optimal healing without the need of a cumbersome and expensive overlying protective dressing. Its primary active component is -sitosterol in a base of beeswax and sesame oil. MEBO is a useful alternative in the treatment of partial-thickness burns because of its convenient method of application and should be considered a valuable treatment modality in LMICs.[29,30]

Exposure therapy is often the method of choice because gauze dressings are considered to be expensive. The exposure method is particularly suitable for the treatment of pediatric burn injuries, especially in a tropical climate where patients are nursed under mosquito nets to keep flies and other insects away from open burn wounds. In a recent observational study by Gosselin and Kuppers[31] comparing open versus closed dressings in burn wounds, the open method had as good or better early outcomes than the closed method and at significantly lower costs. This treatment is the recommended therapy for burns in this particular environment.

NUTRITION

The development of a strategy for assessing and screening burn patients for malnutrition is imperative and should be implemented in all burn units. Burn injury healing requires a great deal of energy. Appropriate nourishment, including adequate protein, calories, vitamins, and micronutrients, is essential in supporting wound healing. Some burn units have started to use "Plumpy'nut," a high-protein and high-energy peanut-based food that is readily available as an existing nutritional supplement for malnourished children. A 2-month Plumpy'nut regimen for a child costs $60.[32]

REHABILITATION AND RECONSTRUCTION

In addition to burn-related mortality, burn-related disability causes a marked functional and economic impact. Functional disability is defined in the global burden of disease reported as DALY or the number of years lost due to poor health, disability, or early death. Burns greater than 20% TBSA rank first among injury types as a cause of short- or long-term disability globally. There are an estimated 116 million cases of such burns, roughly 4 times the global prevalence of HIV/AIDS (31 million).[33]

Rehabilitation is a critical issue when addressing cost-effective burn care. It must begin immediately after the injury, and the delay between inpatient and outpatient therapy should be minimized to ensure a quick return of a functional patient to society.[34] Moreover, part of the rehabilitation process is the prevention and treatment of after-burn scarring, the most common and frustrating complication due to aesthetic and functional consequences.[35] The ability to train family members in basic physical and occupational therapy skills such range-of-motion exercises is likely a cost-effective method to reduce disability. With effective rehabilitation, the need for reconstruction should be minimized. However, when reconstruction is needed, available local surgeons will need to be trained in basic plastic surgical techniques such as contracture release.

BURN SURVEILLANCE AND PREVENTION

Mandatory reporting of burn admissions to a central registry can generate data invaluable for evaluating existing strategies and building targeted prevention programs by identifying regional populations most affected by burn injury and characterizing injury patterns.[36] Surveillance systems can be established by optimizing current information systems through customization of coding developments already in use. Although challenging, combining data from various health care and development agencies to form a national burn injury database provides the best national overview of burn injury.

A recent systematic review of burn preventions strategies in LMICs identified 3 broadly researched approaches: education-based, safety device distribution, and media or population-based initiatives.[37] Current evidence largely supports education-based methods, which target small groups of people or individual homes. In regions like sub-Saharan Africa, these strategies target safer meal preparation and basic fire safety and can include individualized home assessments. They can also be combined with safety device distribution programs that are also often specific to safer cooking. Large-scale population-based programs aimed at policymakers, health care professionals, and the public are useful for communicating the burden, impact, and societal losses due to burns, but the effectiveness of these strategies has been less studied. Regardless, the recognition of burns as a national public health problem at a policy level is critical for ensuring that sufficient funds are available for evidence-based prevention programs that are culturally sensitive and tailored to the regional population most burdened by burn injury.

Last, an important subset of burn patients is the victims of abuse or assault who often suffer in silence for fear of further abuse at the hands of perpetrators. In cases of domestic abuse, the social stigma associated with disfigurement and disability from burns can create an even greater financial dependency for victims on their husbands by limiting employment opportunities. Tougher laws that ensure the prosecution of perpetrators and limit the sale of hazardous materials used in burn assaults can deter potential assailants and provide better protection for victims. Many resource-poor environments also lack the necessary social support infrastructure to ensure the safety of victims of violence and provide appropriate medical care.[38] Consequently, any burn injury prevention strategy must also acknowledge and address these deficiencies.

FUTURE DIRECTION

Acute evaluation of burn patients can be performed accurately by telemedicine. The advantages of telemedicine include reduction of inappropriate triage for transport, improve resource utilization, and both enhance and extend burn center expertise to many rural communities at a low cost.[39] Data specific to burn assessment and diagnosis using telemedicine would suggest that this is a safe, reliable, and affordable method to attain consultation from specialists for patients in underserved areas.[40]

SUMMARY

Each low- or middle-income country has different needs that depend on varying geographic,

demographic, and political factors. In addition, each burn patient is a distinctive entity that requires individualized care. Therefore, in resource-poor environments, it is of paramount importance for clinicians and policymakers to carefully and meticulously balance the relationship between quality and affordable burn care.

REFERENCES

1. Forjuoh SN. Burns in low-and middle-income countries: a review of available literature on descriptive epidemiology, risk factors, treatment, and prevention. Burns 2006;32(5):529–37.
2. WHO. The injury chartbook: a graphical overview of the global burden of injuries. Geneva (Switzerland): World Health Organization; 2002. Available at: http://whqlibdoc.who.int/publications/924156220X.pdf. Accessed May 12, 2016.
3. WHO. Global burden of disease 2004 summary tables. Geneva (Switzerland): World Health Organization; 2008. Available at: www.who.int/healthinfo/global_burden_disease/estimates_regional/en/index.html. Accessed March 20, 2016.
4. Mashreky SR, Rahman A, Chowdhury SM, et al. Non-fatal burn is a major cause of illness: findings from the largest community-based national survey in Bangladesh. Inj Prev 2009;15(6):397–402.
5. Ahuja RB, Bhattacharya S. An analysis of 11,196 burn admissions and evaluation of conservative management techniques. Burns 2002;28(6):555–61.
6. Atiyeh B, Masellis A, Conte C. Optimizing burn treatment in developing low- and middle-income countries with limited health care resources (part 1). Ann Burns Fire Disasters 2009;22(3):121–5.
7. Ferrara MM, Masellis M, Conte F. The philosophy of a burns prevention campaign. In: Masellis M, Gunn SWA, editors. The management of mass burn casualties and fire disasters. Netherlands: Kluwer Academic Publishers; 1992. p. 314–6.
8. Sawhney CP. Flame burns involving kerosene pressure stoves in India. Burns 1989;15:362–4.
9. Gupta RK, Srivastava AK. Study of fatal burns cases in Kanpur (India). Forensic Sci Int 1988;37:81–9.
10. Olaitan PB, Olaitan JO. Burns and scalds - epidemiology and prevention in a developing country. Niger J Med 2005;14:9–16.
11. Opaluwa AS, Orkar SK. Emphasize burns prevention in developing countries. BMJ 2004;329:801.
12. Ahuja RB, Bhattacharya S. Burns in the developing world and burn disasters. BMJ 2004;329(7463):447–9.
13. Singer AJ, Dagum AB. Current management of acute cutaneous wounds. N Engl J Med 2008;359(10):1037–46.

14. Stoddard FJ, Sheridan RL, Saxe GN, et al. Treatment of pain in acutely burned children. J Burn Care Rehabil 2002;23(2):135–56.

15. Madadi P, Enato EF, Fulga S, et al. Patterns of paediatric analgesic use in Africa: a systematic review. Arch Dis Child 2012;97(12):1086–91.

16. Burgner FL. What is the role of prophylactic antibiotics in the management of burns. International Child Health Review Collaboration. 2006. Available at: http://www.ichrc.org/sites/default/files/antibioticburns.pdf. Accessed May 12, 2016.

17. Munster AM, Smith-Meek M, Sharkey P. The effect of early surgical intervention on mortality and cost-effectiveness in burn care (1978-1991). Burns 1994;20:61–4.

18. Gallaher JR, Mjuweni S, Shah M, et al. Timing of early excision and grafting following burn in sub-Saharan Africa. Burns 2015;41(6):1353–9.

19. Mock C, Peck M, Juillard C, et al, editors. Burn prevention: success stories, lessons learned. World Health Organization; 2011. Available at: http://apps.who.int/iris/bitstream/10665/97938/1/9789241501187_eng.pdf. Accessed March 20, 2017.

20. Forjuoh SN, Guyer B, Ireys HT. Burn-related physical impairments and disabilities in Ghanaian children: prevalence and risk factors. Am J Public Health 1996;86(1):81–3.

21. Hamanova H, Broz L. Influence of inadequate prehospital and primary hospital treatment on the maturation of scars after thermal injuries. Acta Chir Plast 2002;45(1):18–21.

22. Skinner A, Peat B. Burns treatment for children and adults: a study of initial burns first aid and hospital care. N Z Med J 2002;115:199.

23. Sinha R. Amniotic membrane in the treatment of burn injury. Indian J Surg 1990;52:11–7.

24. Shahin A, Shadata G, Franka MR, et al. Complications of burns in children–a study of 266 severely burned children admitted to a burns centre. Ann Burns Fire Disasters 1998;11(1):8–15.

25. Ravishanker R, Bath AS, Roy R. "Amnion Bank"—the use of long term glycerol preserved amniotic membranes in the management of superficial and superficial partial thickness burns. Burns 2003; 29(4):369–74.

26. Atiyeh BS, Gunn SWA, Hayek SN. New technologies for burn wound closure and healing - review of the literature. Burns 2005;31:944–56.

27. Subrahmanyam M. Topical application of honey in treatment of burns. Br J Surg 1991;78(4):497–8.

28. Jurjus A, Atiyeh BS, Inaya A, et al. Pharmacological modulation of wound healing in experimental burns. Burns 2007;33:892–907.

29. Ang ES, Lee ST, Gan CS, et al. The role of alternative therapy in the management of partial-thickness burns of the face - experience with the use of moist exposed burn ointment (MEBO) compared with silver sulphadiazine. Ann Acad Med Singapore 2000;29:7.

30. Atiyeh BS, Ioannovich J, Magliacani G, et al. A new approach to local burn wound care: moist exposed therapy. A multiphase, multicenter study. J Burns Surg Wound Care 2003;2:18.

31. Gosselin RA, Kuppers B. Open versus closed management of burn wounds in a low-income developing country. Burns 2008;34(5):644–7.

32. Médecins Sans Frontières. MSF: Nutriset patent impeding access to treatment of Severe Acute Malnutrition. 2009. Available at: http://www.msfaccess.org/content/msf-nutriset-patent-impeding-access-treatment-severe-acute-malnutrition. Accessed March 4, 2016.

33. GBD 2004 summary tables prevalence for selected causes, in WHO Regions (a), estimates for 2004. Geneva (Switzerland): Health Statistics and Informatics Department, World Health Organization; 2008. Available at: http://www.who.int/healthinfo/global_burden_disease/GBD_report_2004update_full.pdf. Accessed March 20, 2017.

34. Takayanagi K, Kawai S, Aoki R. The cost of burn care and implications for efficient care. Clin Perform Qual Health Care 1999;7(2):70–3.

35. Van den Kerckhove E, Stappaerts K, Boeckx W, et al. Silicones in the rehabilitation of burns: a review and overview. Burns 2001;27(3):205–14.

36. Bane M, Kaima R, Mapala S, et al. Qualitative evaluation of paediatric burn injury in Malawi: assessing opportunities for injury prevention. Trop Doct 2016; 46(3):165–7.

37. Rybarczyk MM, Schafer JM, Elm CM, et al. Prevention of burn injuries in low- and middle-income countries: a systematic review. Burns 2016;42(6):1183–92.

38. Seedat M, Van Niekerk A, Jewkes R, et al. Violence and injuries in South Africa: prioritising an agenda for prevention. Lancet 2009;374(9694):1011–22.

39. Saffle JR, Edelman L, Theurer L, et al. Telemedicine evaluation of acute burns is accurate and cost-effective. J Trauma 2009;67(2):358–65.

40. Kiser M, Beijer G, Mjuweni S, et al. Photographic assessment of burn wounds: a simple strategy in a resource-poor setting. Burns 2013;39(1):155–61.

Global Burn Care
Education and Research

Anna Schoenbrunner, MAS[a], Wone Banda, MD, FCS(plast)-ECSA, MSc[b],
Amanda A. Gosman, MD[a],*

KEYWORDS

- Global health • Telemedicine • Volunteerism

KEY POINTS

- Burns account for a significant proportion of global health morbidity and mortality, most significantly in low and middle income countries (LMICs).
- Global health initiatives should focus on education and research initiatives that facilitate sustainable collaborations between high income countries (HICs) and LMICs.
- Short term medical service trips should be carried out for a specific purpose at the request of a local provider within an educational framework that promotes bidirectional exchange and includes appropriate postoperative follow-up.
- Telemedicine is an underused technology that can improve medical care and educational collaborations.

BACKGROUND

Burns are an often-overlooked health indicator in global health literature, but account for a significant global health burden in lower middle income countries (LMICs).[1] The World Health Organization (WHO) estimates that approximately 11 million individuals required medical attention for burns in 2004, with an estimated 265,000 deaths annually.[2] Most burns and deaths caused by burns occur in LMICs. There are 7 times as many burn-related deaths in children in LMICs compared with high-income countries (HICs). Burns are among the leading causes of disability-adjusted life years in LMICs; morbidity associated with nonfatal burns results in physical disability and societal stigma.

Burn care can be divided into acute and secondary treatment. Acute treatment involves intensive medical management and resuscitation of patients with burns as well as acute surgical treatment, including escharotomy, fasciotomy, and early excision and grafting. Team care is especially important in acute management and requires an interdisciplinary approach with physicians, intensivists, anesthesiologists, nurses, nutritionists, physical and occupational therapists, respiratory therapists, and pharmacists, among others. Secondary burn reconstruction involves contracture release and includes skin grafting, adjacent tissue transfer, tissue expansion, and flaps. Secondary burn care also requires a team approach, especially with regard to wound care, physical and occupational therapy, splinting, and psychological support.

There is a great imbalance in the distribution of plastic surgery services between HICs and LMICs. For example, there is an estimated 1 plastic surgeon per 57,000 people in the United States and Canada versus 3 plastic surgeons in the entire country of Malawi, with a population of 16.4 million.[3] This imbalance leaves a large unmet surgical need for acute and secondary burn care. This article presents exchange models that facilitate collaboration between plastic surgeons from

[a] School of Medicine, University of California San Diego, 200 West Arbor Drive, San Diego, CA 92103-8890, USA; [b] Queen Elizabeth Central Hospital, Meyfag Flats, Kanjedza, Blantyre, Malawi
* Corresponding author.
E-mail address: agosman@ucsd.edu

Clin Plastic Surg 44 (2017) 485–493
http://dx.doi.org/10.1016/j.cps.2017.02.010

HICs and LMICs to improve access and quality of burn care in LMICs.

EDUCATION AND RESEARCH

Research and education go hand in hand to fulfill the United Nations Development Program capacity development objectives and play a central role in realizing the goals of the Paris Declaration and Accra Agenda for Action.[4–6] These development roadmaps underscore that neither education nor research alone is sufficient to effect lasting change in a health care system. The United Nations Development Program states that capacity development must go beyond education and training to also understand the institutions and systems within which local providers operate.[4] By recognizing the primary role that LMIC providers play in identifying areas of clinical improvement, HIC institutions can act as valuable partners to support research and educational efforts to improve access and quality of care.

Education Initiatives

The Lancet Commission has identified continuing medical education as a central facet for the development of a sustainable workforce in LMICs.[1] The report outlines the important role that national health ministries and professional societies in LMICs play in providing this training. It also highlights the need for basic infrastructure to foster a productive educational environment, including Internet access, clinical practice resources, and access to textbooks and scientific literature. The report also points out that regional and international educational exchanges can provide valuable learning opportunities for LMIC surgeons.[7,8] These bidirectional educational exchanges between HICs and LMICs seek to identify areas of need and use expertise and resources from both partners to create learning opportunities.

There are several established global health partnerships that have facilitated collaborations between plastic surgeons from HICs and LMICs. The American Council of Academic Plastic Surgeons (ACAPS) and the Plastic Surgery Educational Network (PSEN) have partnered to create the ACAPS/PSEN Global Health Scholarship for trainees in resource-limited settings.[9] These scholarships provide access to the PSEN online resident education resources. In addition, regional collaborations allow medical students and residents to pursue postgraduate training that is not available in their home countries.[10] International educational partnerships include the National Institutes of Health–backed Medical Education Partnership Initiative and the Research Training

for Career Development of Junior Faculty programs.[8,11,12] These programs seek to support medical education and research for African trainees with the goal of building clinical and research infrastructure. Other, smaller scale, educational exchanges are sponsored by HIC training institutions or organizations and help to provide tuition stipends for LMIC surgeons to complete advanced degrees and training in HICs that are not available in their home countries.[13,14]

Nonprofit plastic surgery organizations can also support international educational collaborations. ReSurge International, formerly Interplast, in partnership with International Medical Corps, has established an international burn program that focuses on prevention, training, and advocacy.[15] The organization has acute and chronic burn care treatment centers in LMICs. In addition, ReSurge International focuses on capacity development in LMICs by providing educational resources to local burn providers. This approach allows ReSurge International to form educational partnerships between LMIC and HIC plastic surgeons to provide comprehensive burn care to patients in resource-limited settings.

Individual HIC academic institutions can also partner with LMIC institutions to offer exchanges for trainees from both institutions and facilitate bidirectional learning. The Accreditation Council for Graduate Medical Education (ACGME) has established guidelines for international rotations.[16] ACAPS has followed suit by promoting formal global health rotations within residency training programs.[17] Current surveys of United States plastic surgery residency programs estimate that 64% of programs sponsor overseas short-term medical service trips (MSTs) and 41% of programs have a global health curriculum.[18,19] The University of Wisconsin Division of Plastic Surgery has a 24-year partnership with the Universidad Nacional Autonoma de Nicaragua that provides educational exchanges with plastic surgery trainees in Nicaragua and the University of Wisconsin and assists with plastic surgery treatment in Nicaragua.[20] The program has created a global health curriculum that encourages development of culturally sensitive and resource-conscious trainees.[21] The University of Southern California partnered with Operation Smile to create the Tsao Fellowship, a 2-year fellowship program for plastic surgery residents.[22] The program has 3 focuses: clinical research, international surgical experience, and a Master of Science in Clinical and Biomedical Investigations. Tsao fellows benefit from long-term international partnerships and an immersive educational and research experience at home and abroad.

There are well-established educational and professional benefits for HIC trainees who volunteer their time in resource-limited settings. Studies have shown a positive correlation between volunteering during training and later volunteering or practice in underserved settings.[21,23,24] The authors found that surgeons who volunteered were 6 times more likely to have volunteered in medical school and 22 times more likely to have volunteered in residency (**Table 1**).[25] In addition, studies have also found that trainees gain technical skills while volunteering abroad.[24] Campbell and colleagues[26] reported that international volunteer trips not only promote professionalism and cultural sensitivity but also fulfill all 6 core competencies as set forth by the ACGME.

The authors' research on international volunteerism among ASPS members shows that quality markers on international educational exchanges with residents are, overall, higher.[25] Trips with residents and without residents had high use of follow-up care, medical records, and host affiliation (**Fig. 1**). Trips with residents had higher use of international safety surgery guidelines and improved scope of practice compared with trips without residents. In addition, surgeons who traveled with residents on international trips were 3 times more likely to report the use of any anesthesiologist. Children were 3 times more likely to be cared for by a pediatric anesthesiologist on international trips with residents compared with trips without residents. However, surgeons who reported bringing residents on trips were 2 times more likely to report a death or major complication on any trip. This finding must be interpreted with caution, because it is not known whether this finding is caused by more accurate reporting, riskier cases, or resident involvement.

Plastic surgeons from both LMICs and HICs have raised concerns about the safety and ethics of short-term MSTs. Many ethical violations can be traced back to competing priorities and cultural biases. The Volunteers in Plastic Surgery (VIPS) Guidelines and Ethical Considerations directly address many of these issues.[27,28] Surgeons should not perform a procedure on a MST that they do not perform at home and for which they do not have the appropriate training or experience. This calls to mind the ethical principle of "first, do no harm" and the concept elucidated in the VIPS Ethical Considerations that "'doing something is better than nothing' is neither acceptable nor ethical."[28] In our ASPS survey, 68% of visiting surgeons practiced outside their scope of practice on short-term MSTs.[25] In addition, residents and fellows must be supervised by attendings as they would be at their home institutions. Follow-up care must be provided by qualified visiting and/or local surgeons and multidisciplinary teams when appropriate.

Surgical treatment of burn injuries without appropriate follow-up care can often leave patients worse off than they were before surgical treatment. The patient shown in **Fig. 2** was initially treated for a severe burn of his upper extremities with excision and skin grafting. He was sent back to his remote village without any follow-up care, wound care, splinting, or rehabilitation and this resulted in severe burn scar contractures. This patient was unable to use his arms or hands and experienced recurrent infections within his hypertrophic scar contractures. Additional treatment of his burn scars was only undertaken when a

Table 1
Predictors of volunteering

	Never Participated in MST as Attending (%)	Participated in MST as Attending (%)	OR (95% CI)	P Value
Medical School				
Never volunteered in medical school	40.0	60.0	Reference	
Volunteered in medical school	9.8	90.2	6.12 (3.36, 12.31)	<.001
Residency				
Never volunteered in residency	53.5	46.5	Reference	
Volunteered in residency	4.9	95.1	22.30 (12.87, 42.08)	<.001

Abbreviations: CI, confidence interval; OR, odds ratio.

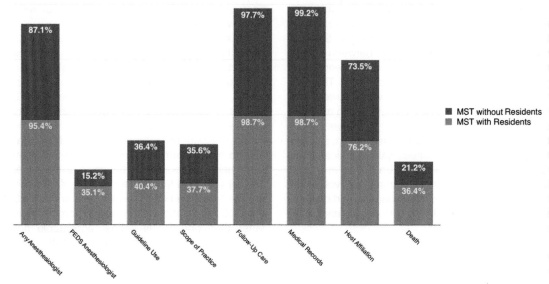

Fig. 1. Quality markers on international volunteer trips. PEDS, pediatric.

viable system of follow-up care was established through telemedicine and after local providers were trained in wound care, splinting, and rehabilitation.

Educational exchanges can provide valuable experiences to HIC and LMIC trainees. There are numerous such programs in existence through academic institutions and national organizations. Short-term MSTs have a role in global surgery education and are most effective when they have clear objectives that were developed through equal and respectful partnership with local providers. Ideally, MSTs should be for a specific purpose at the request of a local provider within an educational framework that promotes bidirectional exchange and includes appropriate postoperative follow-up.

There are several important considerations if surgeons are to plan a short-term MST for burn surgery in an LMIC. Readers are referred to the VIPS Guidelines and the ACGME Criteria for Approved International Rotations for specific and comprehensive guidance.[16,27] Special considerations include:

- Scope of practice: visiting surgeons from HICs must be trained to provide burn care and have experience performing these procedures in their home practices.
- Adherence to safe surgery guidelines: adherence to VIPS Guidelines, WHO Guidelines for Safe Surgery, or Safety Standards in International Anesthesia.[27,29,30]
- Anesthesia: pediatric anesthesiologists must be present when operating on children.

- Equipment: availability of electric (not nitrogen-powered) dermatomes. Wound care and splinting supplies must also be available.
- Supportive care: availability of intensive care unit (ICU) level care, including ventilators and high-protein nutritional supplementation.
- Multidisciplinary follow-up: regular follow-up to provide wound care, rehabilitation, and splinting after burn contracture release. If this is not available, use of telemedicine to provide physical therapy.
- Impact on local health care infrastructure: visiting surgeons must evaluate their impact on local operating room, hospital/ICU beds, and nursing/support staff use such that the routine and emergency provision of local health care is not impeded.

Research Initiatives

The Lancet Commission on Global Surgery has identified health research as one of the key opportunities for improving surgical care.[1] The Commission states that, "research collaborations between well resourced academic institutions with research skills and clinicians in low-resource settings with high clinical loads and important research questions can be a powerful aspect of global health partnerships."[1] Collaborations between HIC and LMIC institutions play a vital role in supporting research efforts directed at improving access and quality of care in resource-limited settings. These efforts should focus on developing and supporting research infrastructure in LMICs. Nayar and colleagues[21]

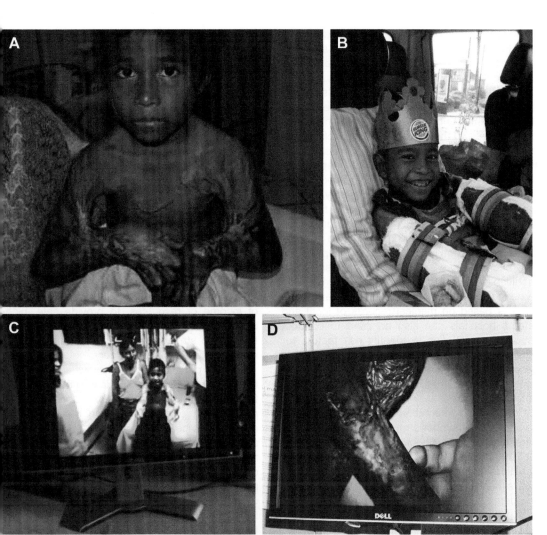

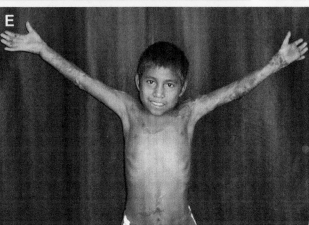

Fig. 2. (*A*) Guatemalan patient with burns after receiving appropriate acute treatment with excision and grafting but with no follow-up care. (*B*) After appropriate follow-up was established through a telemedicine system, the patient underwent burn scar contracture release, skin grafting, and splint placement. (*C, D*) Local providers were trained to provide wound care, splinting, and therapy. The patient and the providers were monitored weekly by a telemedicine videoconference system connected to the University of California San Diego Plastic Surgery Clinic. (*E*) Multidisciplinary outcome after burn scar contracture release and telemedicine follow-up care.

argue that HIC academic institutions should play a vital role in the sustainable development of global surgery. HICs can assist these efforts by supporting access to Internet, clinical resource

databases, and software with which to build research databases. Research databases can be used to track surgical diseases and outcomes by local providers. Specific research projects should then focus on questions identified by providers in LMICs because local surgeons are more apt to understand each community's needs and resource limitations.

With regard to burn research in LMICs, efforts should not only focus on the acute and secondary management of burns but also the epidemiology of burn injuries and the effectiveness of public health interventions. Effective research partnerships between HICs and LMICs necessarily depend on the partnership with local providers to understand the unique challenges of the community. Strategies for effective burn research should focus on supporting local and national research initiatives through establishment and maintenance of injury databases that can identify vulnerable populations and modifiable risk factors for burn injuries. These modifiable risk factors can then be targeted through public health interventions. Research databases based on medical records of local and referral hospitals can also be used to conduct retrospective studies to identify risk factors for acute burn mortality. Research initiatives targeting secondary burn reconstruction should focus on access to reconstructive surgery and the quality of follow-up care.

ConnectMed International, a humanitarian organization that supports multidisciplinary medical care and educational outreach, partnered with Dr Wone Banda, the first plastic surgery resident in Malawi, to support her burn research in Malawi. The aim of Banda's research was to determine the demographic characteristics of children less than 14 years of age with admissions to a burn unit in Malawi for treatment of acute burns and to identify factors predicting mortality.[31] Banda and Kumiponjera[31] conducted a retrospective chart review and found that mortality was 27%. Total body surface area burn (TBSA), patient age, and patient epileptic status were significantly predictive of mortality. Burns greater than 40% TBSA were fatal. This study allowed the local hospital to identify burn prevention strategies. Children less than 5 years of age were most vulnerable because of open-fire cooking on the ground. Prevention strategies focused on education campaigns to cook above ground level and to invest in solar energy to reduce the need for open-fire cooking. Infrastructure limitations that prevented adequate treatment of burns were also identified, including lack of access to blood transfusions, operating room space, ICU beds, skin graft blades, dermatomes, physiotherapists, and high-protein nutrition. Access to nutrition was identified as the single most important modifiable risk factor for acute burn mortality. This issue was addressed by providing tube feeds of nutritional supplements. By partnering with a local plastic surgeon in Malawi, the local hospital was able to identify burn care needs that served as the basis for future partnerships and interventions.

INFRASTRUCTURE

Infrastructure with regard to global surgical care refers to the equipment, resources, and personnel required to perform safe surgery, including basic necessities such as electricity, water, oxygen, blood, anesthetic and surgical equipment, medications, and staff. Multiple organizations, including the WHO, the Lancet Commission, and VIPS, have published guidelines and checklists to ensure provision of the basic infrastructure required for safe surgery.[1,27,29,30,32] These guidelines serve to guide all health systems, regardless of income or resources, to provide safe, high-quality surgical care. Resource-limited health systems often struggle to provide the infrastructure needed to perform safe surgery.[1]

Medical donations from HICs, when judiciously donated, can improve surgical infrastructure in LMICs. The WHO medical device donation guide provides an exhaustive outline on responsible medical device donation (**Fig. 3**).[33] The WHO and Lancet Commission have identified common pitfalls of ineffective device donation. These causes include, but are not limited to, lack of partnership between donor and recipient, lack of awareness of infrastructure limitations, lack of long-term technical support, and insufficient training.[1,34,35] Successful device donations result when local providers in LMICs identify a need and communicate that need to donors who then work with local staff to recondition, transport, integrate, and train local providers to use and service the equipment.[35] The successful implementation of donated devices therefore depends on a strong partnership between donor and recipient that takes into account needs and resource limitations.

Important limitations to be aware of when partnering with LMICs on burn projects include patient transportation to burn centers, power sources for dermatomes (electrical vs nitrogen), availability of maintenance for equipment such as dermatomes, backup power supply or generator, access to ventilators and oxygen, availability of blood for transfusion, laboratory facilities and capacity, nutritional support, access to dressing supplies and other consumables, and availability of medications and antibiotics. These challenges underscore the importance of communication between HIC and LMIC organizations to understand the

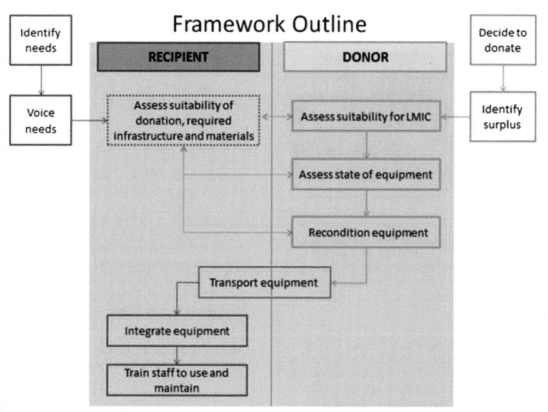

Fig. 3. WHO conceptual framework for donation of medical supplies. (*Data from* WHO. Donation of medical equipment. Available at: http://www.who.int/medical_devices/management_use/manage_donations/en/. Accessed November 16, 2016.)

resource limitations before undertaking research or educational partnerships.

TELEMEDICINE

Telemedicine is the use of technology to provide clinical care from a distance to remote or immobile populations and to overcome logistical and geographic barriers. This system can take the form of sharing digital images or health information, videoconference consultations, or telesurgery. The technology is also especially suited to providing burn care in LMICs because the technology can overcome geographic barriers to remotely provide access to specialists or follow-up care.[36] Telemedicine is also a valuable educational resource that can be used for educational collaborations as well as virtual surgical training.[37] The Lancet Commission on Global Surgery has identified telemedicine as a key intervention for improving access to safe surgery.[1]

Telemedicine has been used in educational collaborations by providing interactive teaching sessions, mentoring, and surgical training. Audiovisual technology can allow educational conferences

for international trainees without the expense and time required for traveling. The technology can also be used to broadcast live surgeries to a remote conference room with a surgeon moderator. This ability allows a unique learning opportunity in a low-stress environment. Studies have found that trainees ask more questions in these environments and rate these experiences as valuable learning experiences.[38] Telemedicine is able to provide valuable learning experiences and foster educational collaborations.

Telemedicine is also uniquely applicable to burn care, particularly in secondary burn reconstruction. The technology can be used as a resource for local surgeons in perioperative planning, follow-up care, and multispecialty team care. Telemedicine can be particularly useful in burn care follow-up by providing regular physical therapy and wound monitoring to patients who are unable to travel to hospitals. The authors have used this technology by collaborating with local providers in Guatemala to provide remote postoperative evaluations of patients who underwent secondary burn contracture release (see **Fig. 2**; **Fig. 4**). We were able to monitor wound healing remotely

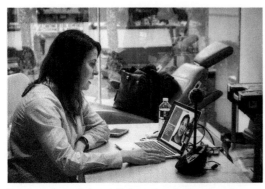

Fig. 4. Telemedicine collaboration in Guatemala.

and provided wound care recommendations to local providers. The technology also allowed us to provide remote physical therapy sessions and allowed us to closely monitor patients' progress.

SUMMARY

Burns represent a significant disease burden in LMICs. Global burn care in LMICs faces challenges because of resource and infrastructure limitations. Education and research initiatives from LMIC providers will guide sustainable improvements in burn care. Awareness of resource limitations and health system needs can guide investments in medical infrastructure. Short-term MSTs should be for a specific purpose at the request of a local provider within an educational framework that promotes bidirectional exchange. Telemedicine is an underused technology that can improve medical care and educational collaborations.

REFERENCES

1. Meara JG, Leather AJM, Hagander L, et al. Global Surgery 2030: evidence and solutions for achieving health, welfare, and economic development. Lancet 2015;386:569–624.
2. World Health Organization. Burns fact sheet. Available at: http://www.who.int/mediacentre/factsheets/fs365/en/. Accessed November 10, 2016.
3. Semer NB, Sullivan SR, Meara JG. Plastic surgery and global health: how plastic surgery impacts the global burden of surgical disease. J Plast Reconstr Aesthet Surg 2010;63:1244–8.
4. Programme, U. N. D. Understanding capacity development. Available at: http://www.undp-globalfund-capacitydevelopment.org/en/functional-capacities/understanding-capacity-development/. Accessed November 16, 2016.
5. OECD. Accra Agenda for Action Organization for Economic Cooperation and Development, 2008.
6. GBD 2013 DALYs and HALE Collaborators, Murray CJ, Barber RM, Foreman KJ, et al. Global, regional, and national disability-adjusted life years (DALYs) for 306 diseases and injuries and healthy life expectancy (HALE) for 188 countries, 1990-2013: quantifying the epidemiological transition. Lancet 2015;386:2145–91.
7. Binagwaho A, Kyamanywa P, Farmer PE, et al. The Human Resources for Health Program in Rwanda — a new partnership. N Engl J Med 2013;369: 2054–9.
8. Olapade-Olaopa EO, Baird S, Kiguli-Malwadde E, et al. Growing partnerships: leveraging the power of collaboration through the medical education partnership initiative. Acad Med 2014;89:S19–23.
9. ACAPS/ASPS 2017 PSEN global scholarship. Available at: http://www.psenetwork.org/psen-global-scholarship. Accessed November 16, 2016.
10. Sawatsky AP, Parekh N, Muula AS, et al. Specialization training in Malawi: a qualitative study on the perspectives of medical students graduating from the University of Malawi College of Medicine. BMC Med Educ 2014;14:1–10.
11. Medical Education Partnership Initiative (MEPI). 2016. Available at: https://www.fic.nih.gov/Programs/Pages/medical-educationafrica.aspx. Accessed November 20, 2016.
12. MEPI Junior Faculty Research Training. Available at: https://www.fic.nih.gov/Programs/Pages/mepi-junior-faculty.aspx. Accessed November 20, 2016.
13. Bajunirwe F, Twesigye L, Zhang M, et al. Influence of the US President's Emergency Plan for AIDS Relief (PEPfAR) on career choices and emigration of health-profession graduates from a Ugandan medical school: a cross-sectional study. BMJ Open 2013;3:1–7.
14. Baird R, Poenaru D, Ganey M, et al. Partnership in fellowship: comparative analysis of pediatric surgical training and evaluation of a fellow exchange between Canada and Kenya. J Pediatr Surg 2016;51: 1704–10.
15. International, R. Expanding burn care with a comprehensive approach. Available at: http://www.resurge.org/transforming_lives/story_expanding_burn_care.cfm. Accessed December 25, 2016.
16. Criteria for approved international rotations Review Committee for Plastic Surgery. Accreditation Council for Graduate Medical Education, 2015.
17. Nayar H, Mount D, Bentz M. The state of global health training in plastic surgery residency: pragmatic considerations and future directions. In 93rd annual meeting of the American Association of Plastic Surgeons, Miami, FL. April 5 – 8th, 2014.
18. Nayar HS, Salyapongse AN, Mount DL, et al. The current state of global surgery training in plastic surgery residency. Plast Reconstr Surg 2015;136: 830–7.

9. Ho T, Bentz M, Brzezienski M, et al. The present status of global mission trips in plastic surgery residency programs. J Craniofac Surg 2015;26:1088–90.

0. Plastic Surgery Residency International Training Program: The University of Wisconsin and Nicaplast. Available at: http://www.surgery.wisc.edu/education-training/residencies/plastic-surgery-residency/international-training-program/. Accessed December 21, 2016.

1. Nayar HS, Bentz ML, Baus GH, et al. The imperative of academia in the globalization of plastic surgery. J Craniofac Surg 2015;26:1102–5.

2. Yao CA, Taro TB, Wipfli HL, et al. The Tsao Fellowship in Global Health: a model for international fellowships in a surgery residency. J Craniofac Surg 2016;27:282–5.

3. Aziz S, Ziccardi V, Chuang S. Survey of residents who have participated in humanitarian medical missions. J Oral Maxillofac Surg 2012;70:e147–57.

4. Thompson M, Huntington M, Hunt D, et al. Educational effects of International Health Electives on U.S. and Canadian Medical Students and Residents: a literature review. Acad Med 2003;78:342.

5. Schoenbrunner A, Kelley K, McIntyre J, et al. Quality markers in residents' international surgical experiences and impact on future volunteering: results from a Comprehensive Survey of American Society of Plastic Surgery (ASPS) Members In ACAPS Winter Retreat, Chicago, IL, February 7, 2016.

6. Campbell A, Sherman R, Magee W. The role of humanitarian missions in modern surgical training. Plast Reconstr Surg 2010;126:295–302.

7. Schneider WJ, Politis GD, Gosain AK, et al. Volunteers in plastic surgery guidelines for providing surgical care for children in the less developed world. Plast Reconstr Surg 2011;127:2477–86.

8. Schneider WJ, Migliori MR, Gosain AK, et al. Volunteers in plastic surgery guidelines for providing surgical care for children in the less developed world: part II. Ethical considerations. Plast Reconstr Surg 2011;128:216e–22e.

29. Haynes AB, Weiser TG, Berry WR, et al. A surgical safety checklist to reduce morbidity and mortality in a global population. N Engl J Med 2009;360:491–9.

30. Merry AF, Cooper JB, Soyannwo O, et al. International standards for a safe practice of anesthesia 2010. Can J Anaesth 2010;57:1027–34.

31. Banda W, Kumiponjera D. Demographic characteristics and outcomes of paediatric burns at a large referral centre in Blantyre, Malawi. Paper presented at: ANZBA 2015 Annual scientific meeting. Melbourne, Australia, October 23.

32. WHO. WHO guidelines for safe surgery 2009: safe surgery saves lives. 2009.

33. WHO. Medical device donations: considerations for solicitation and provision. WHO Medical device technical series. Geneva, Switzerland: WHO; 2011.

34. LeBrun DG, Chackungal S, Chao TE, et al. Prioritizing essential surgery and safe anesthesia for the Post-2015 Development Agenda: operative capacities of 78 district hospitals in 7 low- and middle-income countries. Surgery 2014;155:365–73.

35. WHO. Donation of medical equipment. Available at: http://www.who.int/medical_devices/management_use/manage_donations/en/. Accessed November 16, 2016.

36. Gosman, A. Telemedicine technology in plastic surgery practice. Available at: http://www.plasticsurgerypulsenews.com/7/article_dtl.php?QnCategoryID=71&QnArticleID=152&QnCurPage=12016. Accessed November 16, 2016.

37. Gosman AA, Fischer CA, Agha Z, et al. Telemedicine and surgical education across borders: a case report. J Surg Educ 2009;66:102–5.

38. McIntyre T, Monahan T, Villegas L, et al. Teleconferencing surgery enhances effective communication and enriches medical education. Surg Laparosc Endosc Percutan Tech 2008;18:45–8.

Resuscitation

Acute Fluid Management of Large Burns

Pathophysiology, Monitoring, and Resuscitation

Justin Gillenwater, MD, MS, Warren Garner, MD*

KEYWORDS

- Fluid resuscitation • Burn shock and burn edema • Colloid • Crystalloid

KEY POINTS

- The systemic inflammatory response caused by large burns requires resuscitation to maintain tissue perfusion.
- While the endpoints of resuscitation are still debated, the mean arterial pressure and hourly urine output remain standard markers for adequate perfusion in most patients.
- Newer technologies may lead to improvements in guided resuscitation, but their use is not yet widespread. More research is required to validate their use in patients with burns.

INTRODUCTION

This article discusses the underlying mechanistic reasons for fluid resuscitation after a burn injury and a suggested algorithm for achieving restoration of normal fluid stasis. Like many important medical treatments, there is much information, consensus on general points, and some remaining controversies. The single most important suggestion is that each patient and injury is unique. The best result is achieved by individualizing treatment to each specific patient.

PATHOPHYSIOLOGY

Overview

The response to burn injury occurs on a local and systemic level. Large burns (>20%) result in release of inflammatory mediators from damaged tissue that can exert their effects on the body as a whole. Predictable alterations of major organ systems are the result, leading to hypovolemic

shock in the short term and multiple organ system dysfunction in the subacute setting.

In the first 24 hours after a massive burn, increased vascular permeability leads to migration of water into the interstitium. This decreases the intravascular fluid volume and necessitates replacement to maintain perfusion. If intravascular losses are not replaced, there is generalized and organ-specific hypoperfusion. Cardiac output (CO) is suppressed because of fluid shifts and changes in systemic vascular resistance as catecholamine release occurs on a large scale. Gastrointestinal and renal systems are the first to evidence dysfunction but eventually all organ systems are affected. Electrolyte imbalances are common and intercellular ion shifts occur from cellular death in thermally damaged tissues. Endocrine function is depressed, insulin and cortisol requirements increase, and hyperglycemia is common. The initial massive inflammatory response is followed by a period of immunosuppression. An effective therapeutic response requires knowing

Division of Plastic Surgery, Department of Surgery, Keck School of Medicine, University of Southern California, 1510 San Pablo Street, Suite 415, Los Angeles, CA 90033, USA
* Corresponding author.
E-mail address: wgarner@med.usc.edu

Clin Plastic Surg 44 (2017) 495–503
http://dx.doi.org/10.1016/j.cps.2017.02.008
0094-1298/17/© 2017 Elsevier Inc. All rights reserved.

the physiologic changes that occur locally and systemically.

Local Response: Burn Wound Edema and Tissue Loss

Thermal injury to the skin results in cell death through coagulation, protein denaturation, and cell rupture. Cellular injury and death cause the release of many inflammatory mediators. Histamine, bradykinin, and prostaglandins act locally to promote tissue edema by altering connections in the basement membrane and increasing endothelial cell permeability. This results in transudation of large, osmotically active intravascular proteins out of the capillaries and into the burned tissues. Plasma oncotic pressure is reduced and water is leaked from the microvascular capillary circulation into burned tissue.[1,2] Additionally, interstitial hydrostatic pressure is increased as integrins are broken and cell-to-cell adhesion is disrupted. This leads to exposure of hydrophilic proteoglycans, which further drive water into the interstitial space. The sum total of these interactions leads to profound and immediate edema in burn-injured tissue.

In addition, within thermally damaged tissue, the release of cytokines, such as interleukin-1, interleukin-8, and tumor necrosis factor-α, attracts leukocytes to the wound. Neutrophil degranulation results in release of proteases and reactive oxygen species. Although in small burns this serves as a useful microbicide, in large burns these are cytotoxic to normal tissue. Complement activation occurs, which furthers disruption of dermal microvasculature and perpetuates local tissue ischemia and necrosis.[3,4]

Systemic Response: Burn Shock and Burn Edema

Burns greater than 20% of total body surface area cause a system-wide inflammatory response. The large volume release of inflammatory mediators and cytokines into the circulation leads to leaky microvasculature, vasodilation, and decreased CO. Simplistically, the local response overwhelms the microenvironment and becomes systemic.

As in burned tissue, capillary integrity becomes compromised systemically. Low-flow state coupled with osmotic pressure generated by transudate of proteins and electrolytes results in a profound efflux of intravascular volume into the interstitial space. Hematocrit increases as intravascular volume rapidly decreases. Changes in cell membrane integrity cause additional sequestration of fluid within the cellular space. The result

is rapid onset total body edema, with maximal fluid shifts occurring at around 12 hours postburn.[5,6]

In contrast to burned tissue, capillary integrity in nonburned tissue returns to near normal within 24 hours, and transudation of colloids out of the vascular space decreases. However, water continues to collect in the interstitial space in nonburned tissue even after capillary integrity has been restored because of loss of normal oncotic gradient. The loss of plasma proteins into burned tissue is significant enough to decrease vascular oncotic pressure, resulting in ongoing third spacing of water.

Burn shock is multifactorial because of the interplay between loss of intravascular volume, cardiac dysfunction, and vascular changes. Although hypovolemia is common early, vasodilatation also develops, caused by large volume release of inflammatory mediators. Cardiac dysfunction is common in large burns.[7] This can be a primary cardiac dysfunction as a result of massive cytokine release or decreased circulating blood volume from serum loss.[8] These changes in preload, contractility, and after-load can alone or in combination result in low CO and hypoperfusion. The kidney is most vulnerable to damage from burn shock.[9,10] Increased blood viscosity from the elevated hematocrit and myoglobinemia from deeper tissue damage coupled with intravascular volume loss lead to poor perfusion and acute renal failure. Furthermore, injured tissue within the "zone of stasis" dies.[11]

RESUSCITATION

The mainstay of treatment of acute burn shock is providing supportive care with fluid resuscitation until vascular permeability is restored and interstitial fluid losses are minimized. The goal is to maintain end organ perfusion while limiting fluid overload. Overresuscitation has undesirable sequelae, such as conversion of partial-thickness burns to full thickness, pulmonary edema, and abdominal compartment syndrome. There is ongoing debate as to the optimal fluid used for resuscitation, the timing of fluid administration, and the volume of fluid to administer. Similarly, precise end points of resuscitation are controversial. However, two guiding principles are clear. First, resuscitation should involve the least amount of fluid necessary to provide organ perfusion. Second, the resuscitation should be continuously adjusted to prevent overresuscitation and underresuscitation.[3]

Two determinants that guide initial efforts at resuscitation are the size of the burn and the size of the person burned. The larger the burn, the larger the person, the more fluid needed to resuscitate.[12] Multiple formulas have been advocated using these two variables, of which the Parkland formula is the most popular. Using this formula, fluid needs are estimated at 4 mL/kg/% burn for the first 24 hours, with half of the total volume given within the first 8 hours. Lactated Ringer (LR) solution is the crystalloid of choice using this formula. The less popular modified Brooke formula and consensus formulas are other popular crystalloid-based resuscitations that advocate 2 and 3 mL/kg/total body surface area, respectively. As resuscitation efforts proceed, the rate of fluid given is titrated based on predetermined end points. In our center, we begin with the Parkland formula, and adjust fluid rates using vital signs, such as mean arterial pressures (MAP) and hourly urine output (UOP), with goal UOP between 0.5 and 1 mL/kg in adults. Strictly adhering to the Parkland formula may result in underresuscitation or overresuscitation.

Alternate forms of monitoring in addition to simply measuring UOP may lend to improved resuscitative efforts and are discussed later.[12–14] Larger burn size, depth of burn, and presence of inhalational injury have also all been correlated with fluid requirements greater than predicted by the Parkland formula.[15]

Other formulas that guide resuscitation are described, some incorporating the use of colloids. The debate on crystalloids versus colloids is as old as the history of burn care. Although arguments are made to support either position, the supporting evidence is contradictory and no consensus recommendation exists.

Crystalloids Alone

Proponents of crystalloid resuscitation argue that the solutions are inexpensive, readily available, and have a proven track record. Physiologically, capillaries in burned tissue remain leaky for more than 48 hours. Theoretically, colloids continue to leak into the burned tissue, which only perpetuates the osmotic drive of water into the interstitial space and worsens edema. Although logical, this thesis is not been proven to occur in human burn tissue.

There is no consensus statement regarding appropriate choice of crystalloid. LR solution is a balanced crystalloid and is the most popular, providing 130 mEq/L of sodium and 4 mEq of potassium. Although hypo-osmolar when compared with serum plasma it is effective at restoring extracellular sodium deficits.[16] The lactate in the solution is metabolized by the liver to bicarbonate and thus the solution is alkalinizing. On the contrary, normal saline with 154 mEq of sodium and 154 mEq of chloride induces academia because of the dissociation of these ions in solution. In the setting of the lactic acidosis that accompanies

burn injuries, this is undesirable and can potentiate the acidosis, rather than correct it. Our burn unit uses LR for crystalloid resuscitation. In the setting of hyperkalemia, sodium bicarbonate solution may be used. We never resuscitate with normal saline.

Hypertonic Saline

Hypertonic saline is a largely historic alternative to traditional crystalloid. In theory hypertonic saline acts osmotically to draw water from the interstitium into the intravascular space, thereby lessening fluid requirements. First popularized in the 1970s for use in the burn population, its use has been shown to reduce the amount of volume needed to maintain a target UOP.[17] More recent reports suggest that increasing the intravascular osmolality by using hypertonic saline limits edema formation and reduces the incidence of abdominal compartment syndrome.[18] Other authors, however, have reported that hypertonic saline does not reduce total fluid loads.[19,20] Alarmingly, studies have also associated increased incidence of hypernatremia, renal failure, and mortality when hypertonic saline was used in burn resuscitation.[21] Given these potentially devastating consequences, it is our opinion that hypertonic saline solutions have no role in the resuscitation of the burned patient and their use should be avoided. In 1996 Monafo[22] recommended not using hypertonic as a burn resuscitation fluid.

Colloids and Starches

The use of colloids, starches, and plasma in burn resuscitation remains controversial. Proponents of colloids assert that these fluids are osmotically active intravascularly, require less volume to achieve a given end point, and may lead to less edema. In theory, the capillary beds in nonburned tissue return to baseline levels of permeability at 5 to 8 hours after initial thermal injury.[23] Resuscitation after this time with colloids, such as albumin, fresh frozen plasma (FFP), or long chain polysaccharides, could provide circulating intravascular volume and lessen fluid needs.[24,25] Decreased fluid volumes during initial resuscitation would lead to less global tissue edema and therefore decreased risks of compartment syndromes or other sequelae of overresuscitation.

The evidence for use of albumin or other colloids in burn resuscitation is plentiful and many burn institutions use them regularly in their resuscitation protocols. In a retrospective study, albumin use has been linked with decreased mortality when controlling for age, burn size, and inhalational injury.[26] In another retrospective study specific to patients with large burns, albumin use has been demonstrated to decrease the incidence of extremity compartment syndrome and renal failure.[20] A recent meta-analysis of albumin use in acute burn resuscitation found that its use was associated with decreased mortality and decreased incidence of compartment syndrome.[27]

A prospective, randomized trial, comparing the use of LR alone against LR and FFP demonstrated that use of FFP was correlated with less total volume used and that patients had lower intra-abdominal pressures.[28]

However, the evidence against use of colloids is equally plentiful. Cochrane systematic reviews have concluded that in resuscitation of critically ill patients, there is no improvement in mortality when using colloids over crystalloids alone.[29] Similarly there is no difference in outcomes among the various colloid solutions.[30] Moreover, in burned patients, colloid use has been associated with increased lung water after finishing resuscitation.[31] A double blind, randomized clinical trial has demonstrated that hydroxyethyl starch is not superior to LR alone.[32] FFP can cause transfusion-associated lung injury and allergic and anaphylactic reactions.

Given that colloids are more expensive and may have drawbacks when compared with iso-osmotic crystalloid solutions alone, the clinician should be judicious in their use. They may have a role in the patient with fluid-sensitive comorbidities, such as in chronic renal or heart failure.

In our burn unit albumin is used during resuscitation in two situations: symptomatic low oncotic pressure after massive crystalloid resuscitation, and when resuscitation is failing. With massive burn injuries, the volume of crystalloid needed to maintain tissue perfusion predictably dilutes the albumin remaining in the intravascular space. The result is an imbalance between intravascular and extracellular oncotic and hydrostatic pressures. This leads to ongoing loss of intravascular volume and excessive resuscitation. Depending on the patient, this occurs when albumin levels drop lower than 1.2 to 1.5 g/dL. In some patients with serious burns, standard Parkland formula resuscitation is not successful. In many patients the use of a 5% albumin solution results in restoration of effective perfusion. Although the mechanistic rationale for this treatment is not known, senior members of the burn community supported this algorithm at the National Institutes of Health state of the art consensus conference.

Adjuncts to Resuscitation

The massive inflammatory reaction to burn injury is acknowledged by all. A component of this is neutrophil degranulation, which releases large qualities of oxygen free radicals. Some have proposed this as a mechanism for burn wound progression in well-resuscitated patients. Antioxidants could therefore play a role in decreasing the effect of reactive oxygen species in burned tissue. The data for use of ascorbic acid (vitamin C) are clear in experimental models and are suggestive enough to support its use in the acutely burned patient.[33] High-dose ascorbic acid delivered during the first 24 hours after a large burn has been shown to reduce fluid volume needed for adequate resuscitation.[34,35] Although administration of vitamin C has been complicated by oxalate nephropathy, we believed the evidence is sufficient to recommend the use of ascorbic acid as an adjunct to resuscitation.[36]

MONITORING AND END POINTS TO RESUSCITATION

Monitoring of the patient with large burns is critical to determine end points of resuscitation. Assessing end organ perfusion is accomplished using clinical, hemodynamic, renal, and biochemical parameters. These, in turn, guide resuscitative efforts. Outcomes are improved when resuscitation is guided by end point monitoring rather that strict adherence to a single formula (eg, Parkland).[37,38] The precise nature of those end points, however, is still controversial.

New technologies in hemodynamic monitoring and tissue perfusion may add critical data to help finely tune resuscitative efforts and limit consequences of imperfect resuscitation. However, the effectiveness of these technologies has not been validated in patients with large burns. The next sections review traditional methods of monitoring and include new methods that could be used to guide resuscitative efforts in the future.

Traditional Methods

Noninvasive

In the patient with a large burn, hourly UOP monitored via a Foley catheter has been the consensus parameter that guides resuscitation. UOP indicates adequate perfusion of the kidney, a surrogate marker for overall volume status and CO. Optimal UOP has been suggested to be between 0.5 and 1 mL/kg but this has never been verified experimentally.[16] A systematic review suggested UOP alone has similar outcomes on mortality when compared with more invasive hemodynamic monitoring.[39]

The use of only UOP and vital signs alone to evaluate successful resuscitation has been called into question. A retrospective study comparing ital signs and UOP with oxygen consumption, oxygen delivery, and CO suggests that these traditional parameters alone do not sufficiently represent adequate resuscitation has occurred.[40]

Lactate is released from damaged or poorly perfused cells and causes a metabolic acidosis. Elevated serum lactates or base deficits have been shown to correlate with mortality in critically ill patients and in burned patients. However, their use as guides for resuscitation is yet to be determined.[41] Following these markers over time can serve to confirm that resuscitation is occurring and that tissue perfusion is adequate. Normalization of base deficit after 24 hours has been associated with improved survival.[42] Elevated serum lactate after 48 hours is associated with increased mortality.[43]

Invasive

Vital signs obtained through noninvasive methods may be sufficient to supplement UOP. Often, especially in the case of burned extremities or with significant soft tissue edema, these data may be imprecise and unreliable. Central line and arterial lines are more invasive methods that provide basic data about hemodynamic and volume status, including MAP, central venous pressure (CVP), and heart rate. However, CVP is more influenced by external or abdominal pressures and may not be a true monitor of intravascular volume.[44]

In the patient with pre-existing cardiac or renal disease, the pulmonary artery catheter (PAC) can be used to determine heart function and volume status. Hemodynamic data are obtained, such as pulmonary capillary wedge pressure (PCWP), pulmonary artery pressures, CO, cardiac index, systemic vascular resistance, and oxygen consumption (Vo_2). The CO and cardiac index are useful in determining cardiac sufficiency. PCWP and systemic vascular resistance are markers of volume status and shock. Vo_2 determines whether sufficient oxygen is delivered to tissues and whether these tissues are extracting the oxygen from the circulation. Taken together these parameters are a reflection of the cardiovascular system and end organ perfusion.

In the burned patient, PCWP has been shown to be more reliable as a resuscitative marker than CVP.[45] Resuscitating to target CO has been linked to improved survival in burned patients.[46] Routine placement of the PAC and use of the previously mentioned variables correlates with improved survival.[47] However, there are potential complications to PAC placement, such as arrhythmias, blood clots, and damage or tearing of the pulmonary artery. Clearly, risks of placement of the PAC must be weighed against the benefits when guiding resuscitation.

New Adjuncts or Alternatives

Newer technologies provide the opportunity to assess volume status in patients without the need for traditional invasive methods, such as the PAC. Such technologies can provide new data with less risk to the patient. Transpulmonary thermodilution (TPTD), pulse contour analysis (PCA), and transesophageal echocardiography (TEE) are methods of obtaining hemodynamic parameters without the need for invasive maneuvers. Markers of tissue perfusion, such as subcutaneous gas tension or gastric tonometry, are also newly developing technologies that can add data to understanding burn resuscitation.

Requiring only a central line and an arterial line, TPTD can provide similar information as a PAC without the need for floating a balloon through the heart. Its use in burned patients has been studied and is reproducible and correlates well to data from the PAC.[48,49] These technologies have been studied in burned patients, but the evidence for their use as end points for resuscitation is contradictory. Their accuracy requires that a patient have no pre-existing cardiac disease and be paralyzed and on a mechanical ventilator.

Intrathoracic blood volume (ITBV) is a measurement obtained from TPTD that can be used to assess volume status and is a reflection of cardiac preload.[50] Other investigators have guided resuscitation based on ITBV end points. They found that ITBV targets were reached, whereas MAPS and UOP were below common end points. Thus, early resuscitation guided by ITBV targets seems safe and avoids unnecessary fluid input.[51]

However, there are competing data that show that resuscitating using ITBV results in using more fluid, more tissue edema, and shows no benefit to survival. Holm and colleagues[52,53] have investigated ITBV as an end point of resuscitation in observational and prospective randomized studies. Their research indicates that volumetric resuscitation to ITBV goals resulted in use of more fluid than predicted by the Baxter formula. With similar results, other researchers found that, in a comparative trial between resuscitation using the Parkland formula and traditional end points or resuscitation using ITBV, the group that received guided resuscitation by ITBV required more fluids and had subjectively more edema with no benefit to survival.[54]

PCA is another semi-invasive method of measuring CO and vital signs using thermodilution from a peripheral arterial catheter. Their use in burned patients is contradictory. Reid and Jayamaha[55] first described the use in a case study in 2007 where they found it useful to adjust rates of fluid resuscitation based on measurements. In 2013, other authors measured the variation of stroke volume by PCA as it correlates with fluid administration.[56] These authors found that improvements in the pulse contour of patients with low CO were noted after rapid infusion of fluid, indicating a positive correlation to the volume given. Thus, they concluded that measuring stroke volume variation (SVV) by PCA might be a way to predict volume responsiveness in the early postburn period. Moreover, a small 21-patient randomized controlled trial was conducted comparing goal-directed resuscitation in patients with PCA and SVV versus traditional end points, such as UOP and MAP. Outcomes were similar but patients randomized to resuscitation based on the SVV received statistically significantly less crystalloid during the first 24 hours while having similar overall outcomes in terms of intensive care unit stay, duration of ventilation, and mortality.[57] In summary, PCA may be a useful adjunct to aid in resuscitation but, standing alone, may not be superior to traditional end points. More data are needed.

Transthoracic echocardiography and TEE allow direct visualization of the heart and intrathoracic vascular structures. As with a PAC and PCA, echo allows assessment of cardiac parameters, such as CO and SVV, but gives additional information, such as cardiac valvular function, ejection fraction, and size and compressibility of the vena cava. These data are also available in real time and can be monitored to evaluate real-time responsiveness to resuscitation efforts. However, the quality of data is limited in that the study is operator and assessor dependent. Furthermore, placing a TEE probe is not without serious risk, such as esophageal perforation.

Studies for the use of TEE as a guide for resuscitation in burned patients are nonexistent. In 2003 researchers showed that patients are persistently hypovolemic according to TEE data, whereas other indicators of perfusion seem normal.[58] In 2008 researchers retrospectively studied a cohort of patients that had routinely received TEE during the acute phase of resuscitation. They concluded that TEE was valuable to assess real-time changes in hemodynamics but that the quality of data from TEE is not sufficient to replace traditional end points of resuscitation.[59] They suggested that TEE was useful as an adjunct in patients with pre-existing cardiac or renal function. Similarly, Bak and colleagues[60] recorded hemodynamic variables on 10 consecutive patients including with a TEE and a PAC but did not use those as end points to resuscitation, instead relying on UOP and MAP. They found that there was hypovolemia according to the TEE and PAC measurements during the first 12 hours of resuscitation. These measurements did not correlate with traditional measures of end organ perfusion, such as UOP, and corrected by 24 hours with no additional fluid resuscitation outside of what is recommended by the Parkland formula. They concluded that traditional methods are sufficient to guide resuscitation and that correcting for hypovolemia based on TEE measurements may lead to increased fluid administration without clinical benefit. Lastly, Maybauer and colleagues[61] conducted a systematic review of the research on TEE in burned patients. These authors corroborated the conclusions of others, namely that TEE was good at evaluating the cardiac function and anatomy but did not improve outcomes when used as an end point guiding resuscitation.

Maintaining adequate end organ perfusion is the goal of burn resuscitation. Underperfusion leads to conversion of partial thickness burns to full thickness. Devices that directly monitor the perfusion of the skin could therefore help guide resuscitation and improve salvage of deep partial-thickness burns. Subcutaneous tissue gas tension is measured with a fiberoptic device in the skin. Tissue pH, O_2, and CO_2 reflect perfusion of these tissues.

Venkatesh and coworkers[62] studied subcutaneous gas tensions in a prospective series of 10 patients. This research found that perfusion in burned and unburned skin was similar during the resuscitation. Also, the research demonstrated deteriorating oxygenation, and therefore perfusion, of burned and unburned tissue despite adequate resuscitation as assessed by traditional markers. A second small cohort study evaluated tissue gas tension and perfusion of a burned wound in response to resuscitation. In this series, the measured subcutaneous pH, a marker of poor wound perfusion, occurred before and predicted decreases in global markers of hypoperfusion, such as UOP, MAP, and lactates.[63]

Although using markers of tissue perfusion may lead to salvage of partial-thickness burns, resuscitating to these end points may lead to unnecessary administration of more fluid. A balance must be struck between maintaining perfusion of the skin against the multiple consequences of overresuscitation, namely pulmonary edema and abdominal compartment syndrome.

SUMMARY

Understanding the need and causes for fluid resuscitation after burn injury helps the clinician develop an effective plan to balance the competing goals of normalized tissue perfusion and limited tissue edema. Thoughtful, individualized treatment is the best answer and the most effective compromise.

REFERENCES

1. Cartotto R, Callum J. A review of the use of human albumin in burn patients. J Burn Care Res 2012; 33(6):702–17.

2. Demling RH, Kramer G, Harms B. Role of thermal injury-induced hypoproteinemia on fluid flux and protein permeability in burned and nonburned tissue. Surgery 1984;95(2):136–44.

3. Warden GD. Fluid resuscitation and early management. In: Herndon DN, editor. Total burn care. 4th edition. London: W.B. Saunders; 2012. p. 115–24.e3.

4. Kao CC, Garner WL. Acute burns. Plast Reconstr Surg 2000;105(7):2482–92 [quiz: 2493; discussion: 2494].

5. Tricklebank S. Modern trends in fluid therapy for burns. Burns 2009;35(6):757–67.

6. Kramer GC. Pathophysiology of burn shock and burn edema. In: Herndon DN, editor. Total burn care. 4th edition. London: W.B. Saunders; 2012. p. 103–13.e104.

7. Hilton JG, Marullo DS. Effects of thermal trauma on cardiac force of contraction. Burns Incl Therm Inj 1986;12(3):167–71.

8. Horton JW, Maass DL, White DJ, et al. Effects of burn serum on myocardial inflammation and function. Shock 2004;22(5):438–45.

9. Holm C, Hörbrand F, Donnersmarck von GH, et al. Acute renal failure in severely burned patients. Burns 1999;25(2):171–8.

10. Chrysopoulo MT, Jeschke MG, Dziewulski P, et al. Acute renal dysfunction in severely burned adults. J Trauma 1999;46(1):141–4.

11. Garner WL, Magee W. Acute burn injury. Clin Plast Surg 2005;32(2):187–93.

12. Cancio LC, Chávez S, Alvarado-Ortega M, et al. Predicting increased fluid requirements during the resuscitation of thermally injured patients. J Trauma 2004;56(2):404–13 [discussion: 413–4].

13. Ivy ME, Atweh NA, Palmer J, et al. Intra-abdominal hypertension and abdominal compartment syndrome in burn patients. J Trauma 2000;49(3):387–91.

14. Blumetti J, Hunt JL, Arnoldo BD, et al. The Parkland formula under fire: is the criticism justified? J Burn Care Res 2008;29(1):180–6.

15. Grunwald TB, Garner WL. Acute burns. Plast Reconstr Surg 2008;121(5):311e–9e.

16. Pham TN, Cancio LC, Gibran NS, American Burn Association. American Burn Association practice guidelines burn shock resuscitation. J Burn Care Res 2008;29(1):257–66.

17. Monafo WW. The treatment of burn shock by the intravenous and oral administration of hypertonic lactated saline solution. J Trauma 1970;10(7): 575–86.

18. Oda J, Ueyama M, Yamashita K, et al. Hypertonic lactated saline resuscitation reduces the risk of abdominal compartment syndrome in severely burned patients. J Trauma 2006;60(1):64–71.

19. Gunn ML, Hansbrough JF, Davis JW, et al. Prospective, randomized trial of hypertonic sodium lactate versus lactated Ringer's solution for burn shock resuscitation. J Trauma 1989;29(9):1261–7.

20. Dulhunty JM, Boots RJ, Rudd MJ, et al. Increased fluid resuscitation can lead to adverse outcomes in major-burn injured patients, but low mortality is achievable. Burns 2008;34(8):1090–7.

21. Huang PP, Stucky FS, Dimick AR, et al. Hypertonic sodium resuscitation is associated with renal failure and death. Ann Surg 1995;221(5):543–54 [discussion: 554–7].

22. Monafo WW. Initial management of burns. N Engl J Med 1996;335(21):1581–6.

23. Vlachou E, Gosling P, Moiemen NS. Microalbuminuria: a marker of endothelial dysfunction in thermal injury. Burns 2006;32(8):1009–16.

24. Wisner DH, Street D, Demling R. Effect of colloid versus crystalloid resuscitation on soft tissue edema formation. Curr Surg 1983;40(1):32–5.

25. Du GB, Slater H, Goldfarb IW. Influences of different resuscitation regimens on acute early weight gain in extensively burned patients. Burns 1991;17(2):147–50.

26. Cochran A, Morris SE, Edelman LS, et al. Burn patient characteristics and outcomes following resuscitation with albumin. Burns 2007;33(1):25–30.

27. Navickis RJ, Greenhalgh DG, Wilkes MM. Albumin in burn shock resuscitation: a meta-analysis of controlled clinical studies. J Burn Care Res 2016; 37(3):e268–78.

28. O'Mara MS, Slater H, Goldfarb IW, et al. A prospective, randomized evaluation of intra-abdominal pressures with crystalloid and colloid resuscitation in burn patients. J Trauma 2005; 58(5):1011–8.

29. Perel P, Roberts I, Ker K. Colloids versus crystalloids for fluid resuscitation in critically ill patients. Cochrane Database Syst Rev 2013;(2):CD000567.

30. Bunn F, Trivedi D. Colloid solutions for fluid resuscitation. Cochrane Database Syst Rev 2012;(7): CD001319.

31. Goodwin CW, Dorethy J, Lam V, et al. Randomized trial of efficacy of crystalloid and colloid resuscitation on hemodynamic response and lung water following thermal injury. Ann Surg 1983;197(5): 520–31.

32. Béchir M, Puhan MA, Fasshauer M, et al. Early fluid resuscitation with hydroxyethyl starch 130/0.4 (6%) in severe burn injury: a randomized, controlled,

double-blind clinical trial. Crit Care 2013;17(6): R299.

33. Matsuda T, Tanaka H, Shimazaki S, et al. High-dose vitamin C therapy for extensive deep dermal burns. Burns 1992;18(2):127–31.

34. Tanaka H, Matsuda T, Miyagantani Y, et al. Reduction of resuscitation fluid volumes in severely burned patients using ascorbic acid administration: a randomized, prospective study. Arch Surg 2000; 135(3):326–31.

35. Kahn SA, Beers RJ, Lentz CW. Resuscitation after severe burn injury using high-dose ascorbic acid: a retrospective review. J Burn Care Res 2011; 32(1):110–7.

36. Buehner M, Pamplin J, Studer L, et al. Oxalate nephropathy after continuous infusion of high-dose vitamin C as an adjunct to burn resuscitation. J Burn Care Res 2016;37(4):e374–9.

37. Greenhalgh DG. Burn resuscitation. J Burn Care Res 2007;28(4):555–65.

38. Arlati S, Storti E, Pradella V, et al. Decreased fluid volume to reduce organ damage: a new approach to burn shock resuscitation? A preliminary study. Resuscitation 2007;72(3):371–8.

39. Paratz JD, Stockton K, Paratz ED, et al. Burn resuscitation–hourly urine output versus alternative endpoints: a systematic review. Shock 2014;42(4):295–306.

40. Dries DJ, Waxman K. Adequate resuscitation of burn patients may not be measured by urine output and vital signs. Crit Care Med 1991;19(3):327–9.

41. Cartotto R. Fluid resuscitation of the thermally injured patient. Clin Plast Surg 2009;36(4): 569–81.

42. Andel D, Kamolz L-P, Roka J, et al. Base deficit and lactate: early predictors of morbidity and mortality in patients with burns. Burns 2007;33(8):973–8.

43. Cochran A, Edelman LS, Saffle JR, et al. The relationship of serum lactate and base deficit in burn patients to mortality. J Burn Care Res 2007;28(2): 231–40.

44. Küntscher MV, Germann G, Hartmann B. Correlations between cardiac output, stroke volume, central venous pressure, intra-abdominal pressure and total circulating blood volume in resuscitation of major burns. Resuscitation 2006;70(1):37–43.

45. Aikawa N, Martyn JA, Burke JF. Pulmonary artery catheterization and thermodilution cardiac output determination in the management of critically burned patients. Am J Surg 1978;135(6):811–7.

46. Agarwal N, Petro J, Salisbury RE. Physiologic profile monitoring in burned patients. J Trauma 1983;23(7): 577–83.

47. Schiller WR, Bay RC. Hemodynamic and oxygen transport monitoring in management of burns. New Horiz 1996;4(4):475–82.

48. Küntscher MV, Blome-Eberwein S, Pelzer M, et al. Transcardiopulmonary vs pulmonary arterial thermodilution methods for hemodynamic monitoring of burned patients. J Burn Care Rehabil 2002;23(1):21–6.

49. Holm C, Mayr M, Hörbrand F, et al. Reproducibility of transpulmonary thermodilution measurements in patients with burn shock and hypothermia. J Burn Care Rehabil 2005;26(3):260–5.

50. Wiesenack C, Prasser C, Keyl C, et al. Assessment of intrathoracic blood volume as an indicator of cardiac preload: single transpulmonary thermodilution technique versus assessment of pressure preload parameters derived from a pulmonary artery catheter. J Cardiothorac Vasc Anesth 2001; 15(5):584–8.

51. Sánchez M, García-de-Lorenzo A, Herrero E, et al. A protocol for resuscitation of severe burn patients guided by transpulmonary thermodilution and lactate levels: a 3-year prospective cohort study. Crit Care 2013;17(4):R176.

52. Holm C, Melcer B, Hörbrand F, et al. Intrathoracic blood volume as an end point in resuscitation of the severely burned: an observational study of 24 patients. J Trauma 2000;48(4):728–34.

53. Holm C, Mayr M, Tegeler J, et al. A clinical randomized study on the effects of invasive monitoring on burn shock resuscitation. Burns 2004;30(8): 798–807.

54. Aboelatta Y, Abdelsalam A. Volume overload of fluid resuscitation in acutely burned patients using transpulmonary thermodilution technique. J Burn Care Res 2013;34(3):349–54.

55. Reid RD, Jayamaha J. The use of a cardiac output monitor to guide the initial fluid resuscitation in a patient with burns. Emerg Med J 2007; 24(5):e32.

56. Lavrentieva A, Kontakiotis T, Kaimakamis E, et al. Evaluation of arterial waveform derived variables for an assessment of volume resuscitation in mechanically ventilated burn patients. Burns 2013; 39(2):249–54.

57. Tokarik M, Sjöberg F, Balik M, et al. Fluid therapy LiDCO controlled trial-optimization of volume resuscitation of extensively burned patients through noninvasive continuous real-time hemodynamic monitoring LiDCO. J Burn Care Res 2013;34(5): 537–42.

58. Papp A, Uusaro A, Parviainen I, et al. Myocardial function and haemodynamics in extensive burn trauma: evaluation by clinical signs, invasive monitoring, echocardiography and cytokine concentrations. A prospective clinical study. Acta Anaesthesiol Scand 2003;47(10):1257–63.

59. Wang G-Y, Ma B, Tang H-T, et al. Esophageal echo-Doppler monitoring in burn shock resuscitation: are hemodynamic variables the critical standard guiding fluid therapy? J Trauma 2008;65(6): 1396–401.

60. Bak Z, Sjöberg F, Eriksson O, et al. Hemodynamic changes during resuscitation after burns using the Parkland formula. J Trauma 2009; 66(2):329–36.

61. Maybauer MO, Asmussen S, Platts DG, et al. Transesophageal echocardiography in the management of burn patients. Burns 2014;40(4):630–5.

62. Venkatesh B, Meacher R, Muller MJ, et al. Monitoring tissue oxygenation during resuscitation of major burns. J Trauma 2001;50(3):485–94.

63. Jeng JC, Jaskille AD, Lunsford PM, et al. Improved markers for burn wound perfusion in the severely burned patient: the role for tissue and gastric Pco2. J Burn Care Res 2008;29(1):49–55.

Inhalation Injury
Pathophysiology, Diagnosis, and Treatment

Samuel W. Jones, MD[a],*, Felicia N. Williams, MD[a],
Bruce A. Cairns, MD[a], Robert Cartotto, MD, FRCS(C)[b]

KEYWORDS

- Inhalation injury • Pneumonia • Respiratory failure • Bronchodilators • Heparin

KEY POINTS

- Determinants of mortality in burns are size of burn, age, and the presence of inhalation injury.
- Inhalation injury with or without cutaneous burn increases morbidity and mortality for burn survivors.
- Resuscitation efforts are significantly altered by the presence of inhalation injury.
- There is no consensus among leading burn centers on the optimal mechanical ventilation modes for these patients. Supportive care remains the mainstay of treatment.
- Despite research gains in nutrition, and the hypermetabolic response to burn injury, there remains a lack of understanding of the pathophysiology of inhalation injury and the long-term physiologic consequences.

INTRODUCTION

There is no greater trauma than a large burn. No single injury affects more organ systems than a severe burn injury. The subsequent supraphysiologic responses to that injury lead to full-body catabolism and increased morbidity and mortality. Advances in critical care management, nutrition, wound coverage, and antimicrobial therapies have substantially improved outcomes for burn survivors regardless of burn size. However, when burns are accompanied by inhalation injury, health care providers and clinical scientists have yet to make major impacts on survival.

Inhalation injury is present in up to one-third of all burn injuries; however, it accounts for up to 90% of all burn-related mortality.[1–3] Inhalation injury causes localized damage via direct cellular damage, changes in regional blood flow and perfusion, airway obstruction, as well as toxin and proinflammatory cytokine release.[2,4] Inhalation injuries significantly incapacitate mucociliary clearance and impair alveolar macrophages.[5] They predispose patients to bacterial infection, specifically and primarily pneumonia, a leading cause of death for patients with burns.[6,7] Burn critical care units have the highest rates of ventilator-associated pneumonia in the country, and those patients with concomitant cutaneous injuries with inhalation injury have double the rates of ventilator-associated pneumonia.[5] Moreover, the probability of death increases from 40% to 60% when a burned patient with inhalation injury has pneumonia compared with patients with just cutaneous injuries.[8]

[a] Department of Surgery, North Carolina Jaycee Burn Center, University of North Carolina at Chapel Hill, 3007D Burnett Womack Building, CB 7206, Chapel Hill, NC 27599-7206, USA; [b] Department of Surgery, Ross Tilley Burn Centre, Sunnybrook Health Sciences Centre, University of Toronto, Room D712, 1075 Bayview Avenue, Toronto, Ontario M4N 3M5, Canada
* Corresponding author.
E-mail address: Samuel_Jones@med.unc.edu

Clin Plastic Surg 44 (2017) 505–511
http://dx.doi.org/10.1016/j.cps.2017.02.009
0094-1298/17/© 2017 Elsevier Inc. All rights reserved.

PATHOPHYSIOLOGY

The mechanism of destruction can be classified in 4 ways: (1) upper airway injury, (2) lower airway injury, (3) pulmonary parenchymal injury, and (4) systemic toxicity. The extent of damage from an inhalation injury depends on the environment and the host: the source of injury, temperature, concentration, and solubility of the toxic gases generated, and the response to that injury by the individual.[9] Inhalation injuries cause formation of casts, reduction of available surfactant, increased airway resistance, and decreased pulmonary compliance,[10] leading to acute lung injury and acute respiratory distress syndrome (ARDS).[11]

The major pathophysiology seen in upper airway inhalation injuries is induced by microvascular changes from direct thermal injury and chemical irritation.[6] The heat denatures protein, which subsequently activates the complement cascade causing the release of histamine.[9,12] Subsequently, there is the formation of xanthine oxidase and release of reactive oxygen species (ROS), which combine with nitric oxide in the endothelium to induce upper airway edema by increasing the microvascular pressure and local permeability.[9,13,14] Proinflammatory cytokines, ROS, and eicosanoids attract polymorphonuclear cells to the area, further amplifying ROS and signaling proteases.[15–17] There is a substantial increase in microvascular hydrostatic pressure, a decrease in interstitial hydrostatic pressure, and an increase in interstitial oncotic pressure.[9] The hallmark of burn resuscitation is the administration of large amounts of crystalloid, which reduces plasma oncotic pressure affecting the oncotic pressure gradient in the microcirculation causing significantly more airway edema.[9] Barring steam inhalation injuries and blast injuries, the upper airway efficiently protects the lower airway via heat exchange to limit distal damage to the lower airway.

Injury to the lower airway is caused by the chemicals in smoke. The heat capacity of air is low and the bronchial circulation very efficient in warming or cooling the airway gases, so that most gases are at body temperature as they pass the glottis.[18] In order to induce thermal injury to the airway, flames must be in direct contact.[19] Accelerants, or burned biological materials, are caustic to the airways and induce an initial response to trigger a proinflammatory response. There is a 10-fold increase in bronchial blood flow within minutes of an inhalation injury,[20] which is sustained and causes increased permeability and destruction of the bronchial epithelium.[9] There is a subsequent increase in pulmonary transvascular fluid and a decrease in Pao_2/fraction of inspired oxygen

(Fio_2) ratio less than or equal to 200 nearly 24 hours after injury.[21] There is a subsequent hyperemia of the tracheobronchial tree and lower airways, and that very prevalent clinical finding is used to diagnose the injury.[22–25] Early in the injury, the secretions from goblet cells are copious and foamy. In hours to days these secretions solidify, forming casts and airway obstruction.[9]

Changes to lung parenchyma are delayed, and depend on the severity of injury and the patient's response to the injury. Parenchymal injuries are associated with an increase in pulmonary transvascular fluid, which is directly proportional to the duration of exposure of smoke and toxins. As stated previously, injury to the lower airways and lung parenchyma is rarely caused by direct thermal contact. Only steam can overcome the very efficient upper airway heat dissipating capabilities.[6] There is a reduction to the permeability of protein, an increase in the permeability to small particles, an increase in pressure in the pulmonary microvasculature pressure, and a loss of hypoxic pulmonary vasoconstriction.[9] The key pathologic derangements in inhalation injury are edema, decreased pulmonary compliance from extravascular lung water and pulmonary lymph, and immediate inactivation of surfactant. There is a subsequent ventilation-perfusion mismatch that can lead to profound hypoxemia and ARDS.[6]

Systemic toxic changes are caused by the inhalation of chemicals and cytotoxic liquids, mists, fumes, and gases. Smoke combines with these toxins and increases mortality by increasing tissue hypoxia, metabolic acidosis, and decreasing cerebral oxygen consumption and metabolism.[26,27]

DIAGNOSIS

In the past, the diagnosis of inhalation injury has rested on both subjective and objective measures. History and physical are important factors because they may help prognosticate the host response and comorbidities. For example, the elderly population that is unable to escape from danger may have prolonged exposure to smoke and toxins. Key factors in diagnosis from history are the mechanism (flame and smoke or steam), exposure (duration), location (enclosed space), and disability. For the physical examination, facial burns, singed nasal or facial hair, carbonaceous sputum, soot, stridor, or edema.[6,23] There are no changes in chest radiograph on admission. Oxygen saturation by pulse oximetry (Spo_2) is usually not initially affected and may be misleading, even in the presence of carbon monoxide poisoning, in which the Spo_2 is typically normal. Similarly, arterial blood gases are nondiagnostic. Even in the presence of carbon monoxide poisoning, the Pao_2 is normal or increased and only the arterial oxygen saturation is decreased.[9]

Other adjuncts used for confirming inhalation injury include carboxyhemoglobin measurements, chest computed tomography, fiberoptic bronchoscopy (FOB), radionuclide scan with 133 xenon, and pulmonary function testing.[23] To date, these tools have substantial variability within and between institutions and lack sensitivity. Of the aforementioned studies, FOB prognosticates risk of acute lung injury, resuscitative needs, and mortality most accurately and is the focus of this article.[28]

FOB is the standard technique for diagnosis of inhalation injury. It is readily available and allows a longitudinal evaluation. The presence of hyperemia, edema, and soot on FOB are diagnostic of inhalation injury but there remains a discordance of determining severity of injury. Severity of injury depends on the material inhaled, length of exposure, and the host response to this trauma. To further underscore the problem with grading inhalation injury, FOB, which is the most widely accepted diagnostic tool, cannot access distal airways. Hence, damage in the most distal airways is assumed and hypothesized to be the explanation of inconsistent severity of bronchoscopic findings and mortality.

The most widely used approach for grading the severity of an inhalation injury is the abbreviated injury score (AIS), popularized by Endorf and Gamelli.[29] The AIS assigns a severity score from 0 (no injury) to 4 (massive injury) based on the findings at the initial FOB examination. The AIS grading scale for inhalation injury on bronchoscopy has shown variable results with respect to predicting outcome. Higher-grade injuries have been associated with poorer oxygenation in some studies[30,31] but not others.[32–34] Similarly, a higher (worse) grade of inhalation injury was associated with a longer duration of mechanical ventilation in 1 study,[32] whereas other investigators have not been able to show this relationship.[29,31] Surprisingly, the AIS grade of inhalation injury severity has not been found to be associated with fluid resuscitation requirements.[29,31,32] In addition, the grade of inhalation injury severity does not consistently correlate with an increase in mortality.[29,31,32] A recent study has found that clinically relevant trends toward worse oxygenation, more prolonged mechanical ventilation, and higher fluid resuscitation volumes were associated with patients with high-grade inhalation injuries (former grades 3 and 4) compared with those with low-grade inhalation injury (former grades 1 and 2).[35] Further refinement of this approach is

required and it is worth noting that serial bronchoscopic evaluations over the first 24 to 48 hours after the burn may yield more accurate information than a single examination at burn center admission.[28,31,32]

Laboratory values used to determine severity include Pao_2/Fio_2 and alveolar-arterial gradients but these can be arbitrarily high or low depending on ventilation modes and other clinical parameters.[23]

TREATMENT

Although mortalities for inhalation injury have not changed significantly over the last 50 years, the improvements in standards of care for severe burn injuries have. Thus, survival is standard. There is no consensus among leading burn centers about the optimal treatment protocol for inhalation injury. The fundamental tenet of treatment of inhalation injury is supportive care through the acute hospitalization and rehabilitation. This article outlines key evidence in the literature for common treatment modalities for patients with inhalation injury.

SUPPORTIVE CARE

Inhalation injuries cause formation of casts, reduction of available surfactant, increased airway resistance, and decreased pulmonary compliance.[10] Patients require aggressive pulmonary toilet, chest physiotherapy, airway suctioning, therapeutic serial bronchoscopies, and early aggressive ambulation, and these define our current treatment options.

Bronchodilators

Bronchodilators decrease airflow resistance and improve airway compliance. β2-Adrenergic agonists such as albuterol and salbutamol decrease airway pressure by relaxing smooth muscle and inhibiting bronchospasm, thereby increasing the Pao_2/Fio_2 ratio.[36]

Muscarinic Receptor Antagonists

Muscarinic receptor antagonists such as tiotropium decrease airway pressures and mucus secretion and limit cytokine release by causing smooth muscle constriction within the airways, and stimulation of submucosal glands.[37,38]

Both beta agonists and muscarinic receptor antagonists decrease the host inflammatory response after inhalation injury. Anatomically, there are muscarinic and adrenergic receptors lining the respiratory tract. How that affects the inflammatory response and host response is largely unknown. They have been shown to decrease proinflammatory cytokine levels after stress.[39]

Inhaled (Nebulized) Mucolytic Agents and Anticoagulants

The airway obstruction secondary to mucus, fibrin cast formation, and cellular debris after inhalation injury are addressed by mucolytic agents, specifically, N-acetylcysteine (NAC).[40] NAC is an antioxidant and free radical scavenger with antiinflammatory properties.[41] It is a powerful mucolytic agent that attenuates ROS damage.[23]

Inhaled anticoagulants are also used to mitigate airway obstruction from fibrin casts. Heparin has antiinflammatory properties, it prevents the formation of fibrin, and inhibits cast formation. The available evidence, from a limited number of human studies,[42–45] is controversial. Some studies suggest that, among mechanically ventilated patients with burns with inhalation injury, 1 week of therapy with nebulized heparin (5000–10,000 units) alternating with 3 mL of 20% NAC every 4 hours is beneficial, leading to improved oxygenation and lung compliance, lower reintubation rates, and higher survival.[42,44,45] Other studies have found no improvements in outcome with this therapeutic intervention.[43]

RESPIRATORY SUPPORT

Without consistent reproducible data to support the use of the pharmacologic adjuncts discussed earlier, other centers have focused on the risks and benefits of different modes of ventilation. Ideally, aggressive pulmonary toilet without the use of mechanical ventilation improves outcomes. However, there is often such significant upper airway edema from the inhalation injury, or the resuscitation of the cutaneous injury, that it leads to worsening airway edema. This physiologic consequence can be deadly and may progress expeditiously.[6] It is thus paramount to obtain and sustain a definitive airway early in treatment.

The only mechanical ventilation strategies shown to improve morbidity and mortality from ARDS and acute lung injury come from the ARDSNET trial, which showed in a large randomized controlled trial that lung-protective strategies of limited tidal volumes of 6 to 8 mL/kg body weight and plateau pressures of less than 30 cm H_2O improved outcomes.[46] However, this study excluded patients with burns with greater than 30% total body surface area. Conventional mechanical ventilation modes, to include control mode ventilation, assist-control mode, synchronized intermittent mandatory ventilation, pressure control mode, and pressure support mode are limited in patients with inhalation injury. In patients with airway obstruction from fibrin casts, decreased airway compliance, extensive chest wall thermal injuries, or high volumes of resuscitative needs, maintaining the recommended tidal volumes of 6 to 8 mL/kg body weight and plateau pressures of less than 30 cm H_2O can prove impossible with conventional techniques.[10,47] These conventional settings may be inadequate to appropriately oxygenate and ventilate patients with inhalation injury and overcome the obstructive and restrictive physiology. Thus, in order to support these patients and apply lung-protective ventilation strategies in patients with inhalation injury, nonconventional ventilator modes are often used.[48] A recent survey of mechanical ventilation practices in North American burn centers identified wide disparity in ventilation approaches and a lack of consensus with respect to the optimal method of mechanical ventilation, be it conventional or unconventional.

High Tidal Volume Versus Low Tidal Volume

The efficacy of high tidal volumes compared with low tidal volumes (LTVs) in inhalation injury remains a work in progress. Contrary to the lung-protective and mortality findings in the ARDSNET trial,[46] 1 center retrospectively found that pediatric patients treated with high-tidal-volume ventilation had significantly fewer ventilator days, and a lower incidence of atelectasis and ARDS compared with those treated with lower tidal volumes.[10] Of note, strict adherence to an LTV strategy in patients with burns with inhalation injury may not be feasible because of the associated problems of impaired chest wall compliance from restrictive chest wall eschar and edema, along with the problem of bronchospasm and bronchial obstruction related to inhalation injury. In the only randomized controlled trial in which LTV was assessed, a third of patients failed to meet oxygenation and ventilation goals and two-thirds failed when a smoke inhalation injury had occurred.[49] Larger randomized controlled trials will need to be completed in order for a consensus to be made.

High-frequency Percussive Ventilation

High-frequency percussive ventilation (HFPV) was first described by Cioffi and colleagues[50,51] and Pruitt's group in patients with inhalation injury as a means of assisting with clearance of sloughed respiratory mucosa fibrin casts and mucous plugs, as well as decreasing the incidence of pneumonia. It had been classically used as a salvage mode but subsequent studies from this group showed significant benefits from using HFPV preemptively.[50–54]

One of the major findings comparing HFPV with conventional and LTV ventilation is a statistically significant increase in PaO2/FiO2 ratio, a decreased incidence of pneumonia (the leading cause of death), and survival benefit.[50] A randomized controlled trial comparing HFPV with LTV in human patients with burns and inhalation injuries found that although there were no significant differences in ventilator-free days, ventilator-associated pneumonia, or survival between the two ventilation strategies, subjects receiving LTV required significantly more frequent rescue (by crossover to HFPV) to maintain adequate oxygenation and ventilation.[49] Physiologically, HFPV also improves secretion clearance, and allows more gentle (lower) airway pressures and increased functional reserve capacity.[50,51,55,56]

High-frequency Oscillatory Ventilation

High-frequency oscillatory ventilation (HFOV) is not a suitable ventilatory modality following inhalation injury, because bronchial obstructive changes likely impair any ability of HFOV to adequately open and recruit the lung.[57,58] Furthermore, enthusiasm for HFOV has waned following recent large randomized controlled trials, such as the OSCILLATE[59] and OSCAR[60] studies in patients without burns but with ARDS, which found no benefit and potential harm related to HFOV. However, the findings from those studies possibly should not be directly extrapolated to patients with burns, in whom differing causes for ARDS (eg, nonpulmonary) and chest wall mechanics (poor chest wall compliance) may affect the relative benefits and risks related to HFOV.

Airway Pressure Release Ventilation

Airway pressure release ventilation (APRV) is an inverse ratio, pressure-controlled mode of ventilation that allows for spontaneous breaths. It has been shown to recruit alveoli, improve oxygenation and hemodynamics, and is potentially lung protective.[61] In inhalation injury, PaO2/FiO2 ratios were initially lower with APRV compared with conventional mechanical ventilation, but equilibrated in 48 hours. APRV required higher mean airway pressures to maintain oxygenation and there was no survival benefit.[62]

Extracorporeal Membrane Oxygenation

A systematic review and meta-analysis on the use of extracorporeal membrane oxygenation (ECMO) in inhalation injury is currently limited by the number of available studies. Although there is no survival benefit, there is a trend toward increased survival in patients with burns with acute hypoxemic respiratory failure treated with ECMO for less than 200 hours compared with patients receiving greater than 200 hours. There was no mortality benefit if ECMO was delayed and initiated once the PaO2/FiO2 ratio was less than 60.[63]

SUMMARY

Despite gains in burn critical care, nutrition, understanding of the hypermetabolic response to burns, burn wound coverage, and rehabilitative strategies, clinicians have failed to make significant gains in improving outcomes from inhalation injury. Supportive strategies are promising, but large, multicenter trials are needed to show consistent results for many of the pharmacologic adjuncts. Unconventional modes of ventilation, primarily HFPV, show the most promising results and address the physiologic derangements from inhalation injury. Further studies are needed to better understand the pathophysiology and may help guide future therapeutic options.

REFERENCES

1. Haponik EF. Clinical smoke inhalation injury: pulmonary effects. Occup Med 1993;8:430–68.
2. Kadri SS, Miller AC, Hohmann S, et al. Risk factors for in-hospital mortality in smoke inhalation-associated acute lung injury: data from 68 United States hospitals. Chest 2016;150:1260–8.
3. Tan A, Smailes S, Friebel T, et al. Smoke inhalation increases intensive care requirements and morbidity in paediatric burns. Burns 2016;42:1111–5.
4. Reper P, Heijmans W. High-frequency percussive ventilation and initial biomarker levels of lung injury in patients with minor burns after smoke inhalation injury. Burns 2015;41:65–70.
5. Al Ashry HS, Mansour G, Kalil AC, et al. Incidence of ventilator associated pneumonia in burn patients with inhalation injury treated with high frequency percussive ventilation versus volume control ventilation: a systematic review. Burns 2016;42:1193–200.
6. Mlcak RP, Suman OE, Herndon DN. Respiratory management of inhalation injury. Burns 2007; 33:2–13.
7. Pruitt BA Jr, McManus AT. The changing epidemiology of infection in burn patients. World J Surg 1992;16:57–67.
8. Shirani KZ, Pruitt BA Jr, Mason AD Jr. The influence of inhalation injury and pneumonia on burn mortality. Ann Surg 1987;205:82–7.
9. Traber D, Herndon D, Enkhbaatar P, et al. The pathophysiology of inhalation injury. In: Herndon D, editor. Total burn care. 4th edition. Edinburgh: Saunders Elsevier; 2012. p. 219–28.

10. Sousse LE, Herndon DN, Andersen CR, et al. High tidal volume decreases adult respiratory distress syndrome, atelectasis, and ventilator days compared with low tidal volume in pediatric burned patients with inhalation injury. J Am Coll Surg 2015;220:570–8.

11. Jones SW, Ortiz-Pujols SM, Cairns B. Smoke inhalation injury: a review of the pathophysiology, management, and challenges of burn-associated inhalation injury. In: Gilchrist IC, Cheng EY, editors. Current concepts in adult critical care Society of Critical Care Medicine. Mount Prospect (IL): Society of Critical Care Medicine; 2011.

12. Friedl HP, Till GO, Trentz O, et al. Roles of histamine, complement and xanthine oxidase in thermal injury of skin. Am J Pathol 1989;135:203–17.

13. Granger DN. Role of xanthine oxidase and granulocytes in ischemia-reperfusion injury. Am J Physiol 1988;255:H1269–75.

14. Granger DN, Kvietys PR. Reperfusion injury and reactive oxygen species: the evolution of a concept. Redox Biol 2015;6:524–51.

15. Demling RH, Lalonde C. Topical ibuprofen decreases early postburn edema. Surgery 1987;102:857–61.

16. Herndon DN, Abston S, Stein MD. Increased thromboxane B2 levels in the plasma of burned and septic burned patients. Surg Gynecol Obstet 1984;159:210–3.

17. Katz A, Ryan P, Lalonde C, et al. Topical ibuprofen decreases thromboxane release from the endotoxin-stimulated burn wound. J Trauma 1986;26:157–62.

18. Baile EM, Dahlby RW, Wiggs BR, et al. Role of tracheal and bronchial circulation in respiratory heat exchange. J Appl Physiol (1985) 1985;58:217–22.

19. Moritz AR, Henriques FC, McLean R. The effects of inhaled heat on the air passages and lungs: an experimental investigation. Am J Pathol 1945;21:311–31.

20. Abdi S, Herndon D, McGuire J, et al. Time course of alterations in lung lymph and bronchial blood flows after inhalation injury. J Burn Care Rehabil 1990;11:510–5.

21. Herndon DN, Barrow RE, Traber DL, et al. Extravascular lung water changes following smoke inhalation and massive burn injury. Surgery 1987;102:341–9.

22. American Burn Association. Inhalation injury: diagnosis. J Am Coll Surg 2003;196:307–12.

23. Walker PF, Buehner MF, Wood LA, et al. Diagnosis and management of inhalation injury: an updated review. Crit Care 2015;19:351.

24. Woodson LC. Diagnosis and grading of inhalation injury. J Burn Care Res 2009;30:143–5.

25. You K, Yang HT, Kym D, et al. Inhalation injury in burn patients: establishing the link between diagnosis and prognosis. Burns 2014;40:1470–5.

26. Moore SJ, Ho IK, Hume AS. Severe hypoxia produced by concomitant intoxication with sublethal doses of carbon monoxide and cyanide. Toxicol Appl Pharmacol 1991;109:412–20.

27. Pitt BR, Radford EP, Gurtner GH, et al. Interaction of carbon monoxide and cyanide on cerebral circulation and metabolism. Arch Environ Health 1979;34:345–9.

28. Hassan Z, Wong JK, Bush J, et al. Assessing the severity of inhalation injuries in adults. Burns 2010;36:212–6.

29. Endorf FW, Gamelli RL. Inhalation injury, pulmonary perturbations, and fluid resuscitation. J Burn Care Res 2007;28:80–3.

30. Davis CS, Janus SE, Mosier MJ, et al. Inhalation injury severity and systemic immune perturbations in burned adults. Ann Surg 2013;257:1137–46.

31. Mosier MJ, Pham TN, Park DR, et al. Predictive value of bronchoscopy in assessing the severity of inhalation injury. J Burn Care Res 2012;33:65–73.

32. Albright JM, Davis CS, Bird MD, et al. The acute pulmonary inflammatory response to the graded severity of smoke inhalation injury. Crit Care Med 2012;40:1113–21.

33. Davis CS, Albright JM, Carter SR, et al. Early pulmonary immune hyporesponsiveness is associated with mortality after burn and smoke inhalation injury. J Burn Care Res 2012;33:26–35.

34. Albright JM, Romero J, Saini V, et al. Proteasomes in human bronchoalveolar lavage fluid after burn and inhalation injury. J Burn Care Res 2009;30:948–56.

35. Spano S, Hanna S, Li Z, et al. Does bronchoscopic evaluation of inhalation injury severity predict outcome? J Burn Care Res 2016;37:1–11.

36. Lange M, Hamahata A, Traber DL, et al. Preclinical evaluation of epinephrine nebulization to reduce airway hyperemia and improve oxygenation after smoke inhalation injury. Crit Care Med 2011;39:718–24.

37. Dries DJ, Endorf FW. Inhalation injury: epidemiology, pathology, treatment strategies. Scand J Trauma Resusc Emerg Med 2013;21:31.

38. Jonkam C, Zhu Y, Jacob S, et al. Muscarinic receptor antagonist therapy improves acute pulmonary dysfunction after smoke inhalation injury in sheep. Crit Care Med 2010;38:2339–44.

39. van der Poll T, Coyle SM, Barbosa K, et al. Epinephrine inhibits tumor necrosis factor-alpha and potentiates interleukin 10 production during human endotoxemia. J Clin Invest 1996;97:713–9.

40. Suter PM, Domenighetti G, Schaller MD, et al. N-acetylcysteine enhances recovery from acute lung injury in man. A randomized, double-blind, placebo-controlled clinical study. Chest 1994;105:190–4.

41. Villegas L, Stidham T, Nozik-Grayck E. Oxidative stress and therapeutic development in lung diseases. J Pulm Respir Med 2014;4.

42. Desai MH, Mlcak R, Richardson J, et al. Reduction in mortality in pediatric patients with inhalation injury

with aerosolized heparin/N-acetylcystine [correction of acetylcystine] therapy. J Burn Care Rehabil 1998; 19:210–2.

53. Holt J, Saffle JR, Morris SE, et al. Use of inhaled heparin/N-acetylcystine in inhalation injury: does it help? J Burn Care Res 2008;29:192–5.

54. Miller AC, Elamin EM, Suffredini AF. Inhaled anticoagulation regimens for the treatment of smoke inhalation-associated acute lung injury: a systematic review. Crit Care Med 2014;42:413–9.

45. Miller AC, Rivero A, Ziad S, et al. Influence of nebulized unfractionated heparin and N-acetylcysteine in acute lung injury after smoke inhalation injury. J Burn Care Res 2009;30:249–56.

46. Ventilation with lower tidal volumes as compared with traditional tidal volumes for acute lung injury and the acute respiratory distress syndrome. The Acute Respiratory Distress Syndrome Network. N Engl J Med 2000;342:1301–8.

47. Petrucci N, Iacovelli W. Lung protective ventilation strategy for the acute respiratory distress syndrome. Cochrane Database Syst Rev 2007;(3):CD003844.

48. Fitzpatrick JC, Cioffi WG Jr. Ventilatory support following burns and smoke-inhalation injury. Respir Care Clin N Am 1997;3:21–49.

49. Chung KK, Wolf SE, Renz EM, et al. High-frequency percussive ventilation and low tidal volume ventilation in burns: a randomized controlled trial. Crit Care Med 2010;38:1970–7.

50. Cioffi WG Jr, Rue LW 3rd, Graves TA, et al. Prophylactic use of high-frequency percussive ventilation in patients with inhalation injury. Ann Surg 1991;213: 575–80 [discussion: 80–2].

51. Cioffi WG, Graves TA, McManus WF, et al. High-frequency percussive ventilation in patients with inhalation injury. J Trauma 1989;29:350–4.

52. Cioffi WG, deLemos RA, Coalson JJ, et al. Decreased pulmonary damage in primates with inhalation injury treated with high-frequency ventilation. Ann Surg 1993;218:328–35 [discussion: 35–7].

53. Cortiella J, Mlcak R, Herndon D. High frequency percussive ventilation in pediatric patients with inhalation injury. J Burn Care Rehabil 1999;20:232–5.

54. Hall JJ, Hunt JL, Arnoldo BD, et al. Use of high-frequency percussive ventilation in inhalation injuries. J Burn Care Res 2007;28:396–400.

55. Jones SW, Short KA, Hanson WJ, et al. Evaluation of a new circuit configuration for the VDR-4 high-frequency percussive ventilator. J Burn Care Res 2010;31:640–5.

56. Tiffin NH, Short KA, Jones SW, et al. Comparison of three humidifiers during high-frequency percussive ventilation using the VDR-4(R) Fail-safe Breathing Circuit Hub. J Burn Care Res 2011;32:e45–50.

57. Cartotto R, Walia G, Ellis S, et al. Oscillation after inhalation: high frequency oscillatory ventilation in burn patients with the acute respiratory distress syndrome and co-existing smoke inhalation injury. J Burn Care Res 2009;30:119–27.

58. Cartotto R. Use of high frequency oscillatory ventilation in inhalation injury. J Burn Care Res 2009;30: 178–81.

59. Ferguson ND, Cook DJ, Guyatt GH, et al. High-frequency oscillation in early acute respiratory distress syndrome. N Engl J Med 2013;368:795–805.

60. Young D, Lamb SE, Shah S, et al. High-frequency oscillation for acute respiratory distress syndrome. N Engl J Med 2013;368:806–13.

61. Daoud EG, Farag HL, Chatburn RL. Airway pressure release ventilation: what do we know? Respir Care 2012;57:282–92.

62. Batchinsky AI, Burkett SE, Zanders TB, et al. Comparison of airway pressure release ventilation to conventional mechanical ventilation in the early management of smoke inhalation injury in swine. Crit Care Med 2011;39:2314–21.

63. Asmussen S, Maybauer DM, Fraser JF, et al. Extracorporeal membrane oxygenation in burn and smoke inhalation injury. Burns 2013;39:429–35.

Management of Pulmonary Failure after Burn Injury: From VDR to ECMO

 CrossMark

Apoorve Nayyar, MBBS, Anthony G. Charles, MD, MPH, Charles Scott Hultman, MD, MBA*

KEYWORDS

- Inhalation injury • High frequency ventilation • Extracorporeal membrane oxygenation

KEY POINTS

- Inhalation injury at the time of burn injury increases both morbidity and mortality.
- Pulmonary failure after burn injury can be managed by airway pressure release ventilation (APRV), pressure regulated volume control (PRVC), volumetric diffuse respiratory (VDR) ventilation, or even extracorporeal membraneous oxygenation (ECMO).
- Weaning respiratory support remains a critical component of providing oxygenation and ventilation for burn patients.

INTRODUCTION

In recent years, survival from burn injury has increased with effective fluid resuscitation, respiratory management, and early surgical excision of the burned tissue. The mortality from burn trauma, however, continues to be high, with progressive pulmonary failure being one of the major determinants of morbidity and mortality in burn patients, both from inhalation injury and from secondary complications after burn injury. In 1 study, pulmonary failure was demonstrated to be the cause of death in 29% of pediatric burn patients.[1]

This article reviews the diagnostic and therapeutic interventions along with the recent advances in management of pulmonary failure in burn patients.

Inhalation Injury

Inhalation injury is generally defined as injury to the respiratory tract from inhalation of smoke and chemical products of combustion. It is, along with age and total body surface area (TBSA), one of the three most significant predictors of mortality after thermal injury. The incidence of inhalation injury varies from about 2.2% in patients with less than 20% TBSA burn to 14% in those with 80% to 99% TBSA burn injury.[2] In addition, disasters such as the Station Nightclub Fire in Rhode Island in 2005,[3] or the devastating terrorism attacks on the World Trade Center in New York[4,5] and Pentagon have significantly higher incidence of inhalation injury. For example, out of the 790 injured survivors from the World Trade Center attack, 49% suffered from inhalation injury.

Combined with cutaneous burns, inhalation injury increases fluid resuscitation requirements,[6] incidence of pulmonary complications like prolonged ventilator days, pneumonia and acute respiratory distress syndrome (ARDS),[7] and mortality.[8]

Inhalation injury can be classified into 3 types: thermal injury, chemical injury of the respiratory tract and systemic toxicity due to metabolic asphyxiants, or a combination of these insults. Thermal injury is primarily restricted to the upper airways, causing damage to the mouth, oropharynx, and supraglottic larynx. In the setting of steam, however, the injury is pervasive, causing damage

Department of Surgery, University of North Carolina School of Medicine, Suite 7038, Burnett Womack, CB#7195, Chapel Hill, NC 27599, USA
* Corresponding author.
E-mail address: cshult@med.unc.edu

Clin Plastic Surg 44 (2017) 513–520
http://dx.doi.org/10.1016/j.cps.2017.02.011
0094-1298/17/© 2017 Elsevier Inc. All rights reserved.

plasticsurgery.theclinics.com

to both upper airways and direct thermal injury to lung parenchyma. Chemical injury caused by particulate matter and chemical constituents of smoke like sulfur dioxide, nitrogen dioxide, ammonia, or toxic aldehydes damages the epithelial and capillary endothelial cells of lower airways and lung parenchyma leading to inflammatory changes, bronchiolar edema, and eventually airway obstruction. Increased capillary permeability amplifies the pulmonary edema.[9] Systemic toxicity is most often caused by incomplete products of combustion, most commonly carbon monoxide and hydrogen cyanide. Carbon monoxide poisoning compromises the delivery of oxygen to tissues by reducing the oxygen carrying capacity of blood and less efficient dissociation at the tissue level. Hydrogen cyanide, produced most often by combustion of household materials, inhibits the cytochrome oxidase pathway, causing hypoxia, acidosis, and decreased cerebral oxygen consumption.[10]

DIAGNOSIS OF INHALATION INJURY

Before transferring the patient to a burn center, it is important to assess the patient's risk for airway and respiratory problems and secure the airway, if required. Classically, the diagnosis of inhalation injury was subjective and made mainly on the basis of reported history and clinical findings. The physician should thoroughly review the history and the reported mechanism of burn injury. Pertinent information that provide clues to likelihood of an inhalation injury include exposure to smoke, flame, noxious fumes, and chemicals (household and industrial) at the scene of fire; duration of exposure; exposure in an enclosed space; loss of consciousness; and disability.[11]

In addition, it should be determined if the patient has been exposed to an explosion, as this can cause lung barotrauma. Pertinent symptoms indicating inhalation injury include facial burns, singed nasal vibrissae, carbonaceous sputum, and changes in voice. Clark and colleagues[12] retrospectively reviewed the presenting symptoms in patients with inhalation injury (**Table 1**).

Fiberoptic bronchoscopy (FOB) remains the gold standard to assess the presence and severity of smoke inhalation injury. The relative ease and availability allows FOB to be used for initial diagnosis (**Fig. 1**) and to serially follow-up the changes.[11] FOB is used to visualize the pathognomic mucosal hyperemia, edema, and the presence or absence of carbonaceous material (soot) in the airways. In addition, patients may have copious or no secretions and may progress from necrosis to sloughing of the airway. Repeat bronchoscopy within 24 to 48 hours may be more revealing.[13]

Table 1 Frequency of physical examination findings in patients who had inhalation injury	
Findings	Frequency (%)
Burns, face	65
Carbonaceous sputum	48
Soot, nose and mouth	44
Wheeze	31
Rales, rhonchi	23
Voice change	19
Corneal burn	19
Singed nasal vibrissae	11
Cough	9
Stridor	5
Dyspnea	3
Intraoral burn	2

Adapted from Clark WR, Bonaventura M, Myers W. Smoke inhalation and airway management at a regional burn unit: 1974-1983. Part I: diagnosis and consequences of smoke inhalation. J Burn Care Rehabil 1989;10:52–62.

Several studies have demonstrated that inhalation injury is a graded phenomenon, with increasing severity correlating with worse outcomes. Many authors have described criteria to grade the severity of inhalation injury based on the findings of initial FOB.[14–17] The Abbreviated Injury Score (AIS) (**Table 2**) has been shown to correlate with increased mortality and impaired oxygenation and ventilation. Endorf and colleagues[14] found that patients with higher grades of inhalation injury on initial presentation had worse survival rates than those with lower grades.

Several other modalities that have been described in the literature for diagnosis of inhalation injury include computed tomography (CT), carboxyhemoglobin measurement, and radionuclide imaging with [133]Xenon. Many of these modalities lack sensitivity, are invasive, vary significantly between institutions and hence are not routinely employed for initial diagnosis. Chest radiographs usually appear normal at admission, therefore are a poor indicator of inhalation injury; still, they are important for baseline evaluations.[18] Late findings include alveolar or interstitial edema, diffuse or focal infiltrates, bronchial thickening, consolidation, and atelectasis.

AIRWAY MANAGEMENT

It is imperative for the physician to identify burn patients requiring early intubation. Patients with direct thermal injury to the upper airways (including mouth and oropharynx), higher grades of inhalation injury,

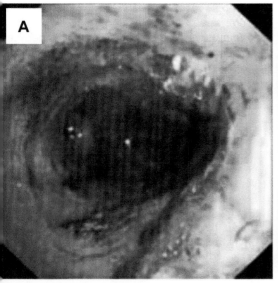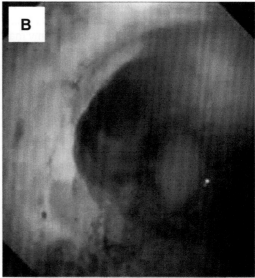

Fig. 1. Bronchoscopic findings in a patient 18 hours after inhalation injury depicting severe edema and congestion of the bronchus along with carbonaceous soot deposition (*A*) and formation of pseudomembrane (*B*). *Adapted from* Bai C, Huang H, Yao X, et al. Application of flexible bronchoscopy in inhalation lung injury. Diagn Pathol 2013;8:174.)

and extensive facial and circumferential neck burns are at a high risk of rapid airway edema formation, which may lead to catastrophic obstruction. Prophylactic intubation in these scenarios is appropriate, as a rapidly developing airway edema may hinder intubation later on, thus requiring immediate cricothyroidotomy at that moment. Ideally, the clinician most experienced in airway management should perform the intubation with the largest available and age-appropriate endotracheal tube. Special consideration should be given to patients who require higher fluid resuscitation volumes as they can develop significant postburn airway edema. Patients with altered mental status due to suspected metabolic asphyxiation and patients with subglottic injury leading to pulmonary failure are also good candidates for early intubation to prevent hypoxic injury. It important to note that not all patients with smoke inhalation injury require intubation; patients with inhalation injury but no facial or neck burns can be carefully observed and later intubated, if neccessary.[19]

After the patient is endotracheally intubated, the tube should be carefully secured. Accidental removal of the endotracheal tube can be severely damaging, if not fatal. A dislodged endotracheal tube may damage the vocal cords, necessitating tracheostomy to prevent further damage. It is important to note that adhesive tape will not stick to extensive burn areas. In that case, cotton ties or even umbilical ties can be used to safely secure the endotracheal tube.

Table 2
Abbreviated injury score grading scale for inhalation injury on bronchoscopy

Grade	Class	Description
0	No injury	Absence of carbonaceous deposits, erythema, edema, bronchorrhea, or obstruction
1	Mild injury	Minor or patchy areas of erythema, carbonaceous deposits, bronchorrhea, or bronchial obstruction.
2	Moderate injury	Moderate degree of erythema, carbonaceous deposits, bronchorrhea, or bronchial obstruction
3	Severe injury	Severe inflammation with friability, copious carbonaceous deposits, bronchorrhea, or obstruction.
4	Massive injury	Evidence of mucosal sloughing, necrosis, endoluminal obstruction

Adapted from Albright JM, Davis CS, Bird MD, et al. The acute pulmonary inflammatory response to the graded severity of smoke inhalation injury. Crit Care Med 2012;40:1113–21.

Although endotracheal intubation is the preferred route for placement of an artificial airway in the immediate postburn period, early tracheostomy may be required as an adjunct to the care of patients with indications of prolonged respiratory failure or acute loss of airway. In a retrospective analysis, it was demonstrated that tracheostomies were more likely to be performed on patients with TBSA greater than 60%, full-thickness burns to the face requiring reconstruction, and patients with pre-existing pulmonary disease.[20] The patient population requiring late tracheostomy includes those with ventilation weaning problems or failed extubation. The complications associated with tracheostomies include chest infection, tracheal stenosis (TS), tracheoesophageal fistula (TEF), tracheoarterial fistula (TAF),[21] and speech problems.

MECHANICAL VENTILATION

Over the past 2 decades, ventilator techniques have increased exponentially, providing new advances for the management of pulmonary failure in burn victims. The classic trial conducted by ARDS Network demonstrated significant benefits of using low tidal volume (6 mL/kg body weight) instead of the higher tidal volumes (10–15 mL/kg body weight) used earlier. The trial concluded that lower tidal volumes demonstrated lower lung inflammation,[22] reduced ventilator associated stretch-induced lung injury, and reduced mortality.[23] However, the trial excluded patients with greater than 30% TBSA burns, which forms an important subset of the authors' patient population. Therefore it is important to be careful when applying the results of the ARDS Trial to a patient population. The patients with inhalation injury not only have a risk of ARDS due to pulmonary edema, but also have increased ventilation perfusion mismatch due to chemical damage to small airways, thereby causing an increased blood flow to poorly ventilated lung areas.[24]

The best mode of ventilation for management of pulmonary failure of burn patients depends on the extent of injury, clinical condition of the patient, and whether there is an associated inhalation injury. The strategy of mechanical ventilation selected must provide adequate oxygenation and ventilation and prevent ventilator-induced lung injury. The author recommends use of lorazepam, vecuronium, and methadone for adequate sedation, neuromuscular blockade, and analgesia, respectively, to improve the patient's comfort level. Adequate attention should be provided to bronchial hygiene, which includes therapeutic coughing, chest physiotherapy, early ambulation, regular airway suctioning, and therapeutic bronchoscopy with aggressive pulmonary toilet to remove copious secretions.[25]

Ventilation protocols vary not only between different burn centers but also between individual physicians. For patients with associated inhalation injury, it can be difficult to maintain the recommended tidal volume of less than 7 mL/kg and peak plateau pressure of less than 30 cm water with conventional modes of ventilation.[26] Thus nonconventional modes are employed.

High-frequency percussive ventilation (HFPV) is a novel mode of ventilation, delivered by means a Volumetric Diffusive Respiratory ventilator (VDR-4, Percussionnaire Corporation, Sagle, Idaho). VDR-4 (**Fig. 2**) is a pneumatically powered, pressure-limited, time-cycled ventilator that provides a lung-protective strategy by facilitating ventilation at lower peak and mean airway pressures. This is accomplished by delivering subtidal volumes in a progressive step-wise manner until a preset oscillatory equilibrium is reached. Exhalation is passive, and the level of continuous positive airway pressure can be selected. The VDR-4 combines both subtidal, high frequency (eg, 400–1000 breaths per minute) and tidal, low-frequency (0–20 breaths per minute) ventilation.[27] This is effective in clearing the sloughed off respiratory mucosa and secretions, provide positive airway pressure throughout the ventilator cycle, and increase functional reserve capacity,[28] thus facilitating better gas exchange.[29]

The initial settings recommended for adults by the US Army Institute for Surgical Research include a peak inspiratory pressure (PIP) of 28 cm H_2O, pulse frequency (PF) of 550 cycles/minute, I:E ratio of 1:1 (time 2 seconds) with the oscillatory positive

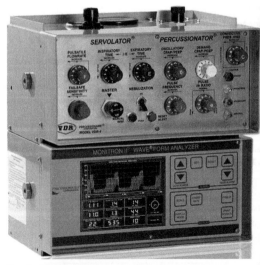

Fig. 2. VDR-4. (*Courtesy of* Percussionnaire, Incorporated, Sagel, ID; with permission.)

end expiratory pressure (PEEP) of 5 cm H_2O. Several retrospective studies have demonstrated reduced mortality and decreased incidence of pulmonary barotrauma[30,31] and pneumonia[28] in patients with inhalation injury using VDR.

Once the clinical condition of the patient begins to improve along with decreased secretions on repeat bronchoscopy and improving chest radiographs, it is a common practice to shift the patient to another mode of ventilation called airway pressure release ventilation (APRV). It is a pressure-regulated mode of ventilation that uses continuous positive airway pressure at high levels and intermittent releases of airway pressure to facilitate CO_2 elimination. This produces lower peak but higher mean airway pressure, resulting in more effective alveolar recruitment. This mode allows for spontaneous breathing while limiting airway pressures and thus may decrease the need for sedative, analgesic, and neuromuscular blocking agents required. However, benefits of APRV over conventional modes have not yet been demonstrated.[29] Possible adverse effects include higher intrinsic PEEP and short expiratory times, resulting in hyperinflation of lungs.[29] Therefore, this is a mode that can be used effectively by clinicians familiar with its rationale and experienced in its use.

For patients with extensive cutaneous burn injury without associated inhalation injury requiring mechanical respiratory support, low tidal volume ventilation with permissive hypercapnia represents the standard of care. One of the modes most frequently employed at the authors' center is the pressure-regulated volume control (PRVC). It is a time- and patient-triggered, volume set/pressure-supported mode of ventilation that adjusts the pressure support over the course of few breaths to achieve a preset tidal volume. This ensures adequate ventilation by augmenting patient efforts to a minimal extent necessary. This reduces the risk of barotrauma; 1 study demonstrated significant decrease in peak inspiratory pressures with PRVC when compared with conventional volume control modes of ventilation.[32] PRVC is basically a pressure control mode with adaptive targeting. Unfortunately, variable pressure alterations on a breath-to-breath basis can cause the ventilator to overestimate or underestimate the optimal pressure support, hence the rationale of employing combined PRVC and synchronized intermittent mandatory ventilation (SIMV) modes together. It combines a preset number of mandatory breaths delivered by the ventilator and intermittent patient-generated spontaneous breaths.[33] This facilitates better patient–ventilator synchrony. With this mode of ventilation, it provides an opportunity for variation in the level of ventilator support, ranging from near-total ventilatory support

to spontaneous breathing. This allows it to be also used as a weaning mode when the patient condition improves. Although the setting of the individual parameters depends on the patient condition and physician preference, a general initial setting includes a tidal volume of 6 to 8 mL/kg, a respiratory rate of 8 to 12 breaths per minute (as per patient condition), PEEP of 8 cm H_2O, Fio_2 of 100% (which can be reduced later on), and I:E ratio of 1:1.

It is important to continuously monitor the patient condition by doing regular arterial blood gas (ABG) analysis, daily chest radiographs, bronchoscopy, and hemodynamic monitoring to guide the course of therapy. It is noteworthy to mention that the authors' center uses the Pulse index Continuous Cardiac Output (PiCCO) catheter (PULSION medical system, Munich, Germany) to monitor important hemodynamic indices like cardiac output, systemic vascular resistance, and extravascular lung water index (ELWI). One should be cognizant of the signs of deteriorating gas exchange like persistently low oxygen saturation levels, increasing peak airway pressures on ventilator, and increasing end tidal carbon dioxide (ETC02), which could indicate progression of the disease process, mandating escalation of respiratory support (after ruling out an acute airway problem [eg, an obstructed, dislodged, or kinked endotracheal tube]).

Despite maximum ventilatory support (Fio_2 of 100% and maximum positive pressure ventilator support), if the patient continues to have signs of pulmonary failure and deteriorating ABGs, the authors administer aerosolized epoprostenol[34] and inhaled nitric oxide as salvage therapy before considering a patient for extracorporeal membrane oxygenation (ECMO). Inhaled nitric oxide has been demonstrated to have an immediate and sustained improvement in Pao_2/Fio_2 ratio (PFR) and pulmonary artery mean pressure in burn patients with severe respiratory failure.[35,36]

Ever since its first successful use in an adult in 1972 for severe respiratory failure in a trauma patient,[37] ECMO has become widely available with significant improvements in the design, cannulae, and oxygenators, resulting in miniaturized systems and improved biocompatibility, allowing for its extended use from days to even months and decreased morbidity and mortality associated with this modality. Until recently, most studies supported the use of ECMO for neonatal and pediatric respiratory failure,[38,39] but the data for adult patients were less convincing. Since the CESAR trial,[40] a multicenter randomized trial, which demonstrated significantly improved outcomes with the use of ECMO in adult patients with severe pulmonary failure, there has been a paradigm shift in use of ECMO in this patient population. As a patient is being considered for ECMO, it is important to take into account comorbidities, neurologic status, duration of mechanical ventilation prior to ECMO,[41,42] patient factors, contraindications, and pre-ECMO support before making a decision. Once a decision is made to cannulate the patient for ECMO, meticulous multiorgan system management is required with the focus on providing time for the lungs to recover, to minimize ventilator-induced lung injury, and prevent oxygen toxicity. The Extracorporeal Life Support Organization (ELSO) guidelines recommend ECMO to be considered for patients with a high predicted mortality (>50%).[41] A Pao_2/Fio_2 less than 150, Murray Score of 2-3[42], and a high APACHE II score (>24) correlate with high predicted mortality. However, the most important consideration is the potential reversibility of the disease process causing persistent hypoxemia.

Veno-venous ECMO is the mode used most commonly in this patient population that drains blood from the patient (usually via internal jugular) and returns blood to the body via the femoral vein, thereby minimizing the risk of embolization. One recent study has demonstrated higher survival with ECMO duration less than 200 hours than with greater than 200 hours.[43] Despite limited data until now, there are a growing number of reports indicating a 70% survival rate in patients with life-threatening respiratory failure. Further investigation is required to establish the criteria regarding the timing of initiation of ECMO. It is important for the physician to use clinical judgment and thorough case-by-case consideration for the use of this potentially life-saving modality.

WEANING RESPIRATORY SUPPORT

As the patient condition stabilizes and begins to resolve, attention must be paid to get the patient off the ventilator as soon as possible. It is essential to assess and move toward weaning and discontinuing mechanical ventilation when the following criteria are met[44]:

- Improving oxygenation (Pao_2/Fio_2 > 200–250)
- Requiring minimal respiratory support (PEEP <5–8 cm H_2O, Fio_2 <40%)
- Ability to initiate inspiratory effort (Negative Inspiratory Force >−30 cm H_2O)
- Hemodynamic stability
- Evidence for reversal of underlying cause of respiratory failure
- Improving ABGs (pH ≥ 7.25)

If patients meet the previously described criteria, they should undergo spontaneous breathing trials (SBTs). The SBT is initiated with pressure support/continuous positive airway pressure (CPAP) for 1 hour per day and gradually increasing the time period of spontaneous breathing over the subsequent days. The tolerance of SBTs lasting 30 to 120 minutes prompts discontinuation of the ventilator support. It is important to assess the patient's capability to protect his or her airway and effectively expel out secretions before removing the endotracheal tube. Doing a swallow study prior to extubation is helpful in this regard.

When the extubation is scheduled, it is necessary to have the reintubation equipment readily available and that the person performing the extubation is experienced in emergency intubations, if need be.

COMPLICATIONS

By far, the most common complication following an inhalation injury and prolonged ventilator support is infection of the respiratory tract. Damage by heat and smoke impairs the mucocilliary clearance mechanisms, combined with decreased functioning of pulmonary macrophages,[34] renders the respiratory tract vulnerable to infection. Persistent hyperthermia and consolidation/infiltrates on chest radiographs should raise the suspicion for pneumonia, and empiric antibiotics should be initiated. The final antibiotic therapy should be tailored based on the results of the sputum culture. Repeat bronchoscopy may be required for bronchoalveolar lavage to remove the secretions and obtain a sample for culture and sensitivity.

Plastic surgeons performing serial reconstructive surgeries may encounter patients with long-term respiratory complications following inhalation injury. The patients are at risk for long-term complications as a combined result of injury, intubation, infection, and chronic inflammation. These include bronchiectasis,[45] tracheobronchial polyposis,[46] main bronchial stenosis, tracheal stenosis, subglottic stenosis,[47] and stricture formation. Pulmonary function testing and stroboscopic laryngeal examination at regular follow-up examination are ideal to monitor for development of any of the complications and intervene accordingly.

METABOLIC ASPHYXIANTS

Smoke inhalation injury may be associated with systemic toxicity with carbon monoxide (CO) and hydrogen cyanide as by products of combustion. CO decreases oxygen delivery at the tissue level and disrupts cellular respiration at the mitochondrial level. Symptoms of CO poisoning include confusion, stupor, coma, seizures, and even myocardial infarction. Administration of 100% oxygen is the mainstay of treatment. The role of hyperbaric oxygen therapy (HBO) is debatable. The administration of HBO, in theory, results in improved outcomes and prevents the neurologic sequelae of CO toxicity. However, logistical factors limit the use of HBO, and data from recent studies do not provide conclusive evidence of prevention of neurologic sequelae.[48]

Hydrogen cyanide is formed from combustion of nitrogen-containing polymers like cotton, wool, and nylon and is common in household fires. Cyanide poisoning can mimic CO poisoning, but a high lactate level should raise the suspicion for cyanide poisoning. Hydroxycobalamin is the most commonly available antidote, which binds to hydrogen cyanide, forming nontoxic cyanocobalamin that is excreted in urine.

BURN CENTER REFERRAL

Many of the modalities mentioned in this article may not be available outside of highly specialized burn centers including respiratory therapists and other personnel trained and experienced in the management of significant burn and/or inhalation injury. It is important for the physician to recognize the extent of injuries and the scope of facilities available. The presence of inhalation injury is one of the criteria for burn center referral as listed by American Burn Association.[49] The presence of inhalation injury warrants, at a minimum, consultation of the regional burn center.

SUMMARY

Pulmonary failure with or without inhalation injury remains a significant cause of morbidity and mortality in burn patients. Advances in critical care have facilitated dramatic improvements in patient outcomes. Appropriate care of burn patients involves a multidisciplinary team involving the physicians, trained nurses, respiratory therapists, physical therapists, and other personnel who contribute to helping patients recover from this difficult injury.

REFERENCES

1. Williams FN, Herndon DN, Hawkins HK, et al. The leading causes of death after burn injury in a single pediatric burn center. Crit Care 2009;13(6):R183.
2. Veeravagu A, Yoon BC, Jiang B, et al. National trends in burn and inhalation injury in burn patients: results of analysis of the nationwide inpatient sample database. J Burn Care Res 2015;36(2):258–65.
3. Harrington DT, Biffl WL, Cioffi WG. The station nightclub fire. J Burn Care Rehabil 2005;26(2):141–3.
4. Yurt RW, Bessey PQ, Bauer GJ, et al. A regional burn center's response to a disaster: September 11, 2001, and the days beyond. J Burn Care Rehabil 2005;26(2):117–24.
5. Centers for Disease Control and Prevention (CDC). Rapid assessment of injuries among survivors of the terrorist attack on the World Trade Center—New York City, September 2001. JAMA 2002;287(7):835–8.
6. Dai NT, Chen TM, Cheng TY, et al. The comparison of early fluid therapy in extensive flame burns between inhalation and noninhalation injuries. Burns 1998;24(7):671–5.
7. Dries DJ, Endorf FW. Inhalation injury: epidemiology, pathology, treatment strategies. Scand J Trauma Resusc Emerg Med 2013;21:31.
8. Smith DL, Cairns BA, Ramadan F, et al. Effect of inhalation injury, burn size, and age on mortality: a study of 1447 consecutive burn patients. J Trauma 1994;37:655–9.
9. Herndon DN, Traber LD, Linares H, et al. Etiology of the pulmonary pathophysiology associated with inhalation injury. Resuscitation 1986;14(1–2):43–59.
10. Moore SJ, Ho IK, Hume AS. Severe hypoxia produced by concomitant intoxication with sublethal doses of carbon monoxide and cyanide. Toxicol Appl Pharmacol 1991;109(3):412–20.
11. Walker PF, Buehner MF, Wood LA, et al. Diagnosis and management of inhalation injury: an updated review. Crit Care 2015;19:351.
12. Clark WR, Bonaventura M, Myers W, et al. Smoke inhalation and airway management at a regional burn unit: 1974 to 1983. II. Airway management. J Burn Care Rehabil 1990;11(2):121–34.
13. Hunt JL, Agee RN, Pruitt BA Jr. Fiberoptic bronchoscopy in acute inhalation injury. Fiberoptic bronchoscopy in acute inhalation injury. J Trauma 1975;15(8):641–9.
14. Endorf FW, Gamelli RL. Inhalation injury, pulmonary perturbations, and fluid resuscitation. J Burn Care Res 2007;28(1):80–3.
15. Albright JM, Davis CS, Bird MD, et al. The acute pulmonary inflammatory response to the graded severity of smoke inhalation injury. Crit Care Med 2012;40:1113–21.
16. Woodson LC. Diagnosis and grading of inhalation injury. J Burn Care Res 2009;30(1):143–5.
17. Hassan Z, Wong JK, Bush J, et al. Assessing the severity of inhalation injuries in adults. Burns 2010;36(2):212–6.
18. Putman CE, Loke J, Matthay RA, et al. Radiographic manifestations of acute smoke inhalation. AJR Am J Roentgenol 1977;129(5):865–70.

19. Demling RH. Smoke inhalation lung injury: an update. Eplasty 2008;8:e27.

20. Aggarwal S, Smailes S, Dziewulski P. Tracheostomy in burns patients revisited. Burns 2009;35(7):962–6.

21. Jones WG, Madden M, Finkelstein J, et al. Tracheostomies in burn patients. Ann Surg 1989;209(4):471–4.

22. Ranieri VM, Suter PM, Tortorella C, et al. Effect of mechanical ventilation on inflammatory mediators in patients with acute respiratory distress syndrome: a randomized controlled trial. JAMA 1999;282:54–61.

23. Ventilation with lower tidal volumes as compared with traditional tidal volumes for acute lung injury and the acute respiratory distress syndrome. The acute respiratory distress syndrome network. N Engl J Med 2000; 342(18):1301–8.

24. Shimazu T, Yukioka T, Ikeuchi H, et al. Ventilation–perfusion alterations after smoke inhalation injury in an ovine model. J Appl Physiol (1985) 1996;81(5): 2250–9.

25. Mlcak RP, Suman OE, Herndon DN. Respiratory management of inhalation injury. Burns 2007;33(1):2–13.

26. Petrucci N, Iacovelli W. Lung protective ventilation strategy for the acute respiratory distress syndrome. Cochrane Database Syst Rev 2013;(2):CD003844.

27. Cancio LC. Airway management and smoke inhalation injury in the burn patient. Clin Plast Surg 2009; 36(4):555–67.

28. Cioffi WG, Rue LW, Graves TA, et al. Prophylactic use of high-frequency percussive ventilation in patients with inhalation injury. Ann Surg 1991;213(6):575–82.

29. Mlcak RP. Airway pressure release ventilation. J Burn Care Res 2009;30(1):176–7.

30. Cortiella J, Mlcak R, Herndon D. High frequency percussive ventilation in pediatric patients with inhalation injury. J Burn Care Rehabil 1999;20(3):232–5.

31. Allan PF, Osborn EC, Chung KK, et al. High-frequency percussive ventilation revisited. J Burn Care Res 2010;31(4):510–20.

32. Guldager H, Nielsen SL, Carl P, et al. A comparison of volume control and pressure-regulated volume control ventilation in acute respiratory failure. Crit Care 1997;1(2):75–7.

33. Weisman IM, Rinaldo JE, Rogers RM, et al. Intermittent mandatory ventilation. Am Rev Respir Dis 1983; 127(5):641–7.

34. Tabrizi MB, Schinco MA, Tepas JJ 3rd, et al. Inhaled epoprostenol improves oxygenation in severe hypoxemia. J Trauma Acute Care Surg 2012;73(2):503–6 [Erratum appears in J Trauma Acute Care Surg 2012;73(5):1354].

35. Musgrave MA, Fingland R, Gomez M, et al. The use of inhaled nitric oxide as adjuvant therapy in patients with burn injuries and respiratory failure. J Burn Care Rehabil 2000;21(6):551–7.

36. Sheridan RL, Hurford WE, Kacmarek RM, et al. Inhaled nitric oxide in burn patients with respiratory failure. J Trauma 1997;42(4):629–34.

37. Hill JD, O'Brien TG, Murray JJ, et al. Prolonged extracorporeal oxygenation for acute post-traumatic respiratory failure (shock-lung syndrome). Use of the Bramson membrane lung. N Engl J Med 1972 286(12):629–34.

38. O'Toole G, Peek G, Jaffe W, et al. Extracorporeal membrane oxygenation in the treatment of inhalation injuries. Burns 1998;24(6):562–5.

39. Bennett CC, Johnson A, Field DJ, et al, UK Collaborative ECMO Trial Group. UK collaborative randomised trial of neonatal extracorporeal membrane oxygenation: follow-up to age 4 years. Lancet 2001;357(9262):1094–6.

40. Peek GJ, Mugford M, Tiruvoipati R, et al, CESAR trial collaboration. Efficacy and economic assessment of conventional ventilatory support versus extracorporeal membrane oxygenation for severe adult respiratory failure (CESAR): a multicentre randomised controlled trial. Lancet 2009;374(9698):1351–63 [Erratum appears in Lancet 2009;374(9698):1330].

41. Extracorporeal Life Support Organization (ELSO). Patient specific guidelines. Available at: http://www.elsonet.org/index.php/resources/guidelines. Html. Accessed April 17, 2017.

42. Pranikoff T, Hirschl RB, Steimle CN, et al. Mortality is directly related to the duration of mechanical ventilation before the initiation of extracorporeal life support for severe respiratory failure. Crit Care Med 1997 25(1):28–32.

43. Asmussen S, Maybauer DM, Fraser JF, et al. Extracorporeal membrane oxygenation in burn and smoke inhalation injury. Burns 2013;39(3):429–35.

44. MacIntyre NR, Cook DJ, Ely EW Jr, et al. Evidence-based guidelines for weaning and discontinuing ventilatory support: a collective task force facilitated by the American College of chest physicians; the American association for respiratory care; and the American College of critical care medicine. Chest 2001;120(6 Suppl):375S–95S.

45. Tasaka S, Kanazawa M, Mori M, et al. Long-term course of bronchiectasis and bronchiolitis obliterans as late complication of smoke inhalation. Respiration 1995;62(1):40–2.

46. Shin B, Kim M, Yoo H, et al. Tracheobronchial polyps following thermal inhalation injury. Tuberc Respir Dis (Seoul) 2014;76(5):237–9.

47. Arakawa A, Fukamizu H, Hashizume I, et al. Macroscopic and histological findings in the healing process of inhalation injury. Burns 2007;33(7): 855–9.

48. Buckley NA, Juurlink DN, Isbister G, et al. Hyperbaric oxygen for carbon monoxide poisoning. Cochrane Database Syst Rev 2011;(4):CD002041.

49. Anonymous. Guidelines for trauma centers caring for burn patients. Available at: www.ameriburn.org BurnCenterReferralCriteria.pdf. Accessed April 17, 2017.

Rational Selection and Use of Antimicrobials in Patients with Burn Injuries

David M. Hill, PharmD, BCPS[a,b,*],
Scott E. Sinclair, MD, FCCP[c,d],
William L. Hickerson, MD, FACS[e,f]

KEYWORDS

- Burn • Antimicrobials • Sepsis • Infections • Biomarkers • Pharmacokinetics • Pharmacodynamics
- Dosing

KEY POINTS

- Caring for patients with burn injuries is challenging secondary to the acute disease process, chronic comorbidities, and underrepresentation in evidence-based literature.
- Much of current practice relies on extrapolation of guidance from different patient populations and wide variations in universal practices.
- Identifying infections or sepsis in this hypermetabolic population is imperfect and often leads to overprescribing of antimicrobials, suboptimal dosing, and multidrug resistance.
- An understanding of pharmacokinetics and pharmacodynamics may aid optimization of dosing regimens to better attain treatment targets.

INTRODUCTION

Over the past century, the armamentarium available to the burn practitioner has dramatically increased.[1] Mortality from a burn injury has been dramatically reduced with the discovery of new technology and medications, development of new surgical philosophies, and the continual expansion of burn-specific literature. Parallel to the expanding repertoire of available antimicrobials is the occurrence of multidrug-resistant (MDR) organisms.[2] The increasing prevalence of MDR organisms is unfortunate, as they are associated with increased morbidity and mortality.[3] Proper selection and use of antimicrobials is imperative for reducing unneeded exposure, cost, resistance, and mortality.[4] Knowledge of existing literature and an understanding of pharmacokinetics and pharmacodynamics will aid appropriate antimicrobial prescribing and optimize patient outcomes.

Disclosure Statement: Drs D.M. Hill and S.E. Sinclair have no disclosures; Dr W.L. Hickerson is on the speaker's bureau for Medline and advisory board for PermeaDerm. He is also on the medical advisory board for Avadim and Alliqua. He holds shares in Avadim.
[a] Department of Pharmacy, Firefighters Regional Burn Center, Regional One Health, 877 Jefferson Avenue, Memphis, TN 38103, USA; [b] Department of Clinical Pharmacy, College of Pharmacy, University of Tennessee Health Science Center, 881 Madison Avenue, Memphis, TN 38163, USA; [c] Department of Medicine, Firefighters Regional Burn Center, Regional One Health, 877 Jefferson Avenue, Memphis, TN 38103, USA; [d] Department of Medicine, College of Medicine, University of Tennessee Health Science Center, Memphis, TN 38163, USA; [e] Department of Plastic Surgery, Firefighters Regional Burn Center, Regional One Health, 877 Jefferson Avenue, Memphis, TN 38103, USA; [f] Department of Plastic Surgery, College of Medicine, University of Tennessee Health Science Center, Memphis, TN 38103, USA
* Corresponding author.
E-mail address: dhill19@uthsc.edu

Clin Plastic Surg 44 (2017) 521–534
http://dx.doi.org/10.1016/j.cps.2017.02.012
0094-1298/17/© 2017 Elsevier Inc. All rights reserved.

DEFINING INFECTION AND SEPSIS

Defining infection in a patient with burn injuries can be challenging in light of the hyperdynamic, hypermetabolic, and proinflammatory presentation. As a result, burn injury is often an exclusion criteria for studies of sepsis identification, treatment, and outcomes. Unfortunately, infection is a frequent accompaniment to acute illness and even more so in patients with burn injuries with a compromised primary immunologic barrier. However, the identification of early signs that distinguish infection from acute burn injury physiology is key for prompt and appropriately targeted intervention.[5]

The diagnosis of pneumonia in a patient in the intensive care unit is controversial.[6,7] Patients with acute burn injury are uniquely challenging in that they are prone to pulmonary dysfunction due to multiple noninfectious mechanisms, such as inhalational injury, pulmonary edema, dysregulated systemic inflammation, and the acute respiratory distress syndrome. Because of these and other noninfectious sources of pulmonary dysfunction, patients with burn injuries often exhibit the clinical signs and symptoms associated with infectious pneumonia. Even in the absence of bacterial pneumonia, many patients with burn injuries will have fever, purulent sputum, leukocytosis (or leukopenia), abnormal gas exchange, and infiltrates on chest imaging. There have been numerous clinical scoring systems created to aid in the diagnosis of pneumonia, such as the clinical pulmonary infection score. Such tools have not been adopted or validated in patients with burn injuries because they use many of the same clinical signs seen in patients with burn injuries without pneumonia.[8] Most burn centers depend on bronchoscopic sampling (protected specimen brush or bronchoalveolar lavage [BAL]) or nonbronchoscopic BAL and quantitative cultures of the samples obtained to make a diagnosis of pneumonia.[6,9–11] Pneumonia should be diagnosed if clinically suspected and BAL results in quantitative culture of $\geq 10^4$ colony-forming units/mL.[12]

Burn wound infections do not occur with the frequency that they did several years ago because of a more aggressive surgical approach, topical antimicrobials, and the appropriate use of systemic antibiotics. The appearance of the burn wound often holds the key to early diagnosis of the infection and thus optimal care. Therefore, it is imperative that constant wound surveillance be performed. It is stated that early eschar separation is indicative of burn wound infections, but this is rarely seen today due to early wound excision.[12] Color changes within the wound are often the first subtle signs of infection. Conversion of partial-thickness wounds to full thickness and the loss of grafts are indicative of localized wound infections. *Pseudomonas* colonization may be a yellow/green exudate in the wound bed, whereas black violent areas suggest invasive infection. Typically, fungal infections are insidious. *Candida* infections may be more purulent in appearance, whereas *Aspergillus* may be gray-brown and *Mucor* appear as black-staining growths on the wound bed itself.[12] Herpetic infections will appear more like punched-out lesions and often occur in healed second-degree burns. With changes occurring subtly, vigilant visual surveillance is vital for survival of tissue and sometimes the person. As Krizek and Robson[13] have noted: "Having preceded man on earth, bacteria continue to exert a 'territorial imperative' and the interaction between man, his environment and his defense system is either a symbiotic relationship or one that is leading to the path of infection."

Systemic Inflammatory Response Syndrome (SIRS) criteria have been repeatedly documented as having poor correlation with infection in patients with burn injuries, with up to 98% of patients fulfilling criteria regardless of clinical stability or infection status.[14–17] Burn injury is traditionally classified in 2 phases: "ebb" and "flow." The first 24 to 48 hours after burn injury is termed the ebb phase and is characterized by the initiation of the inflammatory process. Inflammatory mediators surge to produce local vasodilation and augment vascular permeability. The resulting albumin and fluid shifts into the interstitial space transiently produce a low cardiac output, increase systemic vascular resistance, and potential for reduced organ perfusion.[18] After adequate resuscitation, the flow phase is characterized by the hyperdynamic response to the insult with increased cardiac contractility and output plus a reduced systemic vascular resistance.

SIRS has traditionally been considered a trigger for the initial suspicion of an infectious process in patients without burn injuries. Danger exists when extrapolating definitions and treatment protocols for sepsis validated only in patients without burn injuries, as they can lead to overtreatment with resuscitation volumes and antimicrobials. Early goal-directed therapy has improved outcomes in nonburn septic patients; however, use of recommended resuscitation volumes to reach end hemodynamic targets may lead to new unwanted issues in a fragile and often overresuscitated population.[19–22] To be discussed later, overexposure to antimicrobials also must be avoided in a population with an expected prolonged hospital stay and heightened risk for MDR and fungal pathogens.

Recognizing the irrelevance in application of sepsis criteria to patients with burn injuries, recommendations, largely based on expert opinion, were published in 2007 by the American Burn Association (ABA) to serve as a catalyst.[12] Since the consensus conference, several studies have attempted to either validate or improve the criteria for identifying sepsis in the patient with burn injuries. Mann-Salinas and colleagues[16] suggested the model most predictive of sepsis from bacteremia included 6 variables: heart rate >130 beats per minute, mean arterial pressure <60 mm Hg, base deficit less than −6, temperature <36°C, vasoactive medications, and serum glucose >150 mg/dL. Other investigators disagree on which parameters are most predictive.[15,23] Hypothermia (<36°C) is generally recognized as a predictor of poor prognosis, but disagreement exists for what febrile threshold should trigger suspicion for infection.[14–16,23,24] Despite evident baseline heart rate elevations in patients with burn injuries, tachycardia appears to be an important distinguishing factor for an infectious process, provided appropriate volume repletion. It also seems clear the SIRS threshold of 90 beats per minute should not be used as a trigger in patients with burn injuries. Some studies have validated the ABA threshold, whereas greater than 130 beats per minute also has been reported as most predictive.[15,16,23] Threshold definitions for respiratory rate greater than 25 breaths per minute, thrombocytopenia, and enteral nutrition intolerance also seem unreliable.[14–16,23] Hyperglycemia and particularly glucose variability also appear to have strong correlation with infection.[16,25]

Biomarkers

With white blood cell count and C-reactive protein as unreliable predictors, several clinicians have searched for other biomarkers that would serve as a reliable early indicator of sepsis. Procalcitonin (PCT) is a propeptide for calcitonin with cleavage occurring in the thyroid and storage found in several tissues.[26] Additionally, monocytes and, inherently, macrophages have been shown to produce PCT.[27] PCT's proposed roles for immunologic modulation are to increase monocyte motility, inhibit nitric oxide synthase in vascular smooth muscle, and inactivate certain cytokines.[28] Minimally detected in plasma under normal circumstances, PCT has been shown to release within 3 hours of endotoxin exposure and peak at approximately 14 hours with a half-life of 2.5 hours.[29] In patients with severe renal dysfunction (creatinine clearance <30 mL/min), PCT half-life could extend to 1.5 times longer than nonrenal impairment. Plasma clearance of PCT shows weak, but significant, correlation with creatinine clearance (CrCl), as renal elimination accounts for a little more than one-third of PCT plasma elimination.[30] Some nonseptic conditions may present with marked elevations in PCT, including trauma, burns, prolonged cardiogenic shock, heat stroke, rhabdomyolysis, liver transplantation, and severe pancreatitis.[28]

Elevated baseline values may raise red flags for the utility of PCT in patients with burn injuries. Some investigators have shown PCT as a quality marker for early sepsis identification, whereas others disagree.[14,31–34] Additionally, there is disagreement whether larger total body surface area (TBSA) correlates with augmented admission PCT concentrations.[14,32] Due to elevated baseline values of PCT in patients with burn injuries, it may be best to raise septic thresholds to greater than 1.5 ng/mL to maximize sensitivity and specificity.[14] Furthermore, most PCT studies have been conducted with bacteremic sources and thresholds may be variably dependent on sources with some less systemically invasive infections having lower cutoffs.[35] If most PCT release into the plasma is a result of systemic symptoms from infection, it stands to reason, severe infections would have higher values and may be best to differentiate sepsis from local infection. PCT also has shown utility as a prognostic indicator for mortality and response to antimicrobial therapy.[14,32,36] PCT may best serve as a daily monitored laboratory marker and incorporated as an algorithm component to indicate appropriate response to treatment and reduce duration of antimicrobial therapy.[37,38] It is worth remembering that reduced elimination is expected in renal dysfunction and may reflect as a false-negative response to therapy.[30]

One important factor may be to consider the high interpatient variability that is exhibited in the burn population. Perhaps the best avenue may be to not use a set threshold for any particular clinical or laboratory parameter, but consider each patient individually as his or her own control and monitor for acute changes. Additionally, it must be stressed to not rely on 1 single variable to reliably raise alarm for suspected infection. For the best balance of predictive values, consideration should be given to multiple factors of the complex clinical picture that is the patient with burn injury.

PROPHYLACTIC ANTIMICROBIAL SELECTION
Topicals

Beyond prevention techniques like separate bed enclosures, the shift from immersion to showering hydrotherapy, universal barrier precautions, removal of colonized invasive devices, and tight glycemic control lies the use of prophylactic antimicrobial therapy.[39–43] Topical antimicrobials, like honey, have been used for wound care dating back several millennia. Today's topical arsenal contains a wide range of agents targeted at reducing the incidence of wound infection by controlling microbial contamination at the wound surface. A potential advantage to local antimicrobial therapy is the ability to get high concentrations of the active agent at the site. Deeper thermal injuries may result in damaged blood vessels and impede delivery of systemic agents. Additionally, local therapy offers the theoretic advantage of less systemic toxicities.[44] Most of the data relating to the efficacy of topical antimicrobials are quite dated. Recent literature has focused on disadvantages, like skin reactions, metabolic acidosis, delayed wound healing, toxicities, systemic absorption, and reduced sensitivities.[44–47] Specifics regarding pharmacodynamics is a focus later in this article, but must be a consideration when selecting the most appropriate agent. Eschar penetration, safety profile, desired spectrum of activity, patient tolerance, and projected length of therapy must be balanced.

Honey offers many unique properties that have proven ideal for wound healing. Honey's broad spectrum of activity against many bacteria and fungi is believed to be mainly due to hydrogen peroxide activity.[48] Additional proposed properties are stimulation of tissue growth, reduced inflammatory changes, and debriding action.[49] Unfortunately, honey may not be suitable for deep burns because of poor eschar penetration.

Sodium hypochlorite is a very potent traditional agent with a comprehensive antimicrobial profile. Unfortunately, its potency is not selective and its deleterious effect on human cells can impair wound healing. A concentration of 0.25% is frequently used; however, a dilution down to 0.00025% may provide the best efficacy/toxicity profile.[45,50] Due to a favorable cytotoxic profile, some burn centers have switched product selection to more pH-balanced hypochlorous acid agents. Reduced efficacy against MDR organisms also has been reported.[44]

Silver is another long-standing staple for the treatment of wounds. Several products exist with silver as the active moiety. Silver nitrate, silver sulfadiazine, and silver-based dressings are the most commonly used agents. Silver works quickly and may have one of the broadest spectra of activity that includes gram-positive, gram-negative, and fungal organisms. Interactions with thiol groups, release of intracellular potassium, direct cellular membrane disruption, and microbial DNA interaction are mechanisms attributed to silver's successful antimicrobial properties.[46,51,52] Recent data suggest the emergence of resistance and reduced efficacy to some MDR pathogens.[44,47] Conflicting studies suggest that silver sulfadiazine may delay wound healing, react in sulfa-allergic patients, complicate wound evaluation secondary to the formation of a pseudoeschar, systemically absorb in larger TBSA burns, cause leukopenia and have poor eschar penetration.[46,52–54] Silver-based dressings offer the antimicrobial benefits of topicals with less frequent dressing changes and better patient tolerability.[55–57]

First introduced as a 10% ointment, mafenide is a topical sulfonamide with broad gram-positive and gram-negative activity, particularly *Pseudomonas* spp.[58] Mafenide offers the added benefit of eschar penetration for deep burns. Although rare, adverse reactions in sulfa-allergic patients, painful application, and metabolic acidosis from carbonic anhydrase inhibition have been reported.[59] Side effects and hospital costs are minimized and efficacy retained with dilutions down to 5.0% and 2.5%.[60] Mixed reports exist of mafenide selecting out yeast, yet retaining in vitro activity against some mold.[45,57]

Systemic

Patients with burn injuries often have protracted hospital stays with multiple episodes of infection and, subsequently, spend more than half of their admission on several courses of antibiotics.[38] The use of prophylactic antibiotics on admission for contaminated skin is sometimes used to reduce future infection, but efficacy data are inconclusive and the practice discouraged.[61–63] Patients with a delay in time to presentation after burn injury may offer the best scenario for initiating antibiotics on admission secondary to higher wound-infection rates, but careful assessment of the wounds may prove the term prophylactic misplaced.[64] As previously discussed, antimicrobial exposure can lead to resistance, need for "last resort" or combination antimicrobials, or death.[65] Efficacy also is in question, secondary to poor perfusion in deeper wounds with extensive vessel damage. Easily overlooked, antimicrobial use and resultant changes in flora extend selection effects to the burn unit ecosystem and other patients. Prophylactic antimicrobials on admission may seem like an attractive short-term option, but may lead to a difficult abiding battle.

Burn wound manipulation extending from routine daily cleansing to more invasive burn wound excision carries a risk of bacteremia with rates increasing with invasiveness, TBSA, and time to excision.[66,67] It is debated whether such bacteremia results in clinically significant sepsis or is just transient.[68–71] Additionally, frequency of bacteremia has been scrutinized owing to advances in techniques and the evolution of burn care.[67] As is often the case, current guidance for antimicrobial prophylaxis in surgery require extrapolation for application to patients with burn injuries. Current guidelines recommend using preoperative antibiotics for plastics procedures in patients with risk factors, despite lack of supporting evidence from randomized controlled trials.[72] Considering existing evidence, it is difficult to recommend perioperative prophylaxis, especially for early excision and TBSA less than 40%. If systemic antimicrobials are used, care must be taken for appropriate agent selection, based on the local antibiogram, and frequency of dosing. Improper selection of agents and prolonged exposure may lead to emergence of selected bacteria or resistance.[68,73] Consideration must be given to the differences presented by the patient with burn injuries with regard to pharmacokinetics and pharmacodynamics, as some agents may require redosing depending on length of procedure and antibiotic half-life.[73,74]

EMPIRIC

When choosing empirical antimicrobials, it is critical to consider local flora over national pathogen incidence.[3,75] It is recommended that each unit keep an annual antibiogram that is unit specific and separate from that of the broader institution.[75–77] Technology hurdles and low pathogen yield are frequent preclusions to annual analysis. However, a multiyear format can be used for units with low incidence of certain pathogens of concern.[78] Knowing incidence and sensitivities to unit-specific pathogens will allow more accurate targeting of empirically prescribed antimicrobials (**Table 1**). Exposure to broad-spectrum antibiotics can hasten development of antimicrobial resistance and increases the risk for undesirable adverse drug effects.[78] Empiric antimicrobials should be narrowed and tailored to culture and sensitivity results as soon as they are available.

Patients with burn injuries are also at an increased risk for fungal infections secondary to integument damage, central venous access, and frequent exposure to antimicrobials.[79] Fungal infections also carry a high mortality burden in patients with burn injuries, with an overall decrease in median survivability (LD50) from 65% to 47% TBSA.[80] Mortality is correlated with increased age, TBSA, invasive infection, and presence of mold.[80–82] Special attention to fungus should be afforded in geographic areas of high incidence

and where the burn is extinguished with a garden hose, standing water, or by rolling in dirt.[80,83] Environmental risk factors that should increase suspicion for fungal infection on admission include geographic areas with favorable climates for spore proliferation, seasonal selection differences, and areas with recent natural disaster.[80,83–85] Increased age, diabetes, obesity, immunocompromised states, and significant history of antimicrobial use increase the risk of fungal infection.[86] Fungal infection can emerge early or be delayed for weeks. Diligent attention and frequent visualization of the wounds should occur to better assess occurrence of progression. Progression can be rapid with an ideal environment to flourish, so wound care is critical. Even when prompt empiric treatment is initiated, early aggressive wound excision, and sometimes amputation, is required to preserve life.[80,87] As with antibacterials, empiric antifungal therapy should be tailored to local flora to prevent unwarranted adverse effects, costs, and overexposure.[80]

DOSING
Pharmacokinetics

It is understandable that patients with burn injuries are most often excluded from dosing and outcomes studies because of their large interpatient and intrapatient variability. Some burn-specific dosing studies exist, and the noted extreme differences confirm the need for individualized therapeutic drug monitoring and studies with other medications frequently used in this population.[88–91] In the meantime, an understanding of pharmacokinetic principles allows better extrapolation of dosing studies to ensure adequate dosing by the burn practitioner.

Absorption can be defined by the bioavailability, or percentage of drug that reaches the systemic circulation. Intravenous administration is considered to have 100% bioavailability and provide a control for comparisons with orally administered medications. For example, most β-lactam antibiotics, like penicillin, dicloxacillin, or cefdinir, have poor bioavailability (25%–60%) and require chemical structure or dosage form manipulation to increase systemic absorption.[92–94] Some of the cephalosporins, like cephalexin and cefaclor, approach 90%.[95] Lipophilic drugs generally have higher absorption profiles from better passive diffusion across intestinal membranes, which leads to development of esterified formulations of some β-lactam antibiotics.[96] Considerations also must be given to the impact of food or tube feeds on absorption. Fatty foods delay gastric emptying, and may decrease peak concentrations

Table 1
Example antibiogram

2015 Burn Antibiogram Gram-Positive Percent Strains Susceptible	No. Tested	Oxacillin (%)	Vancomycin (%)	Linezolid (%)	Ampicillin (%)	Gentamicin (Synergy) (%)	Tetracycline (%)	Trimethoprim/ Sulfameth-oxazole (%)	Clindamycin (%)	Synercid (%)
Data Collected 1/15–12/15 (Hospital name)										
Departments of Pharmacy, Laboratory, & Infection Control										
Duplicate organisms excluded										
Blanks indicate susceptibility was not tested, not clinically applicable, or ≤45% susceptible										
Page _____ with questions										
Enterococcus faecalis	8	—	88	100	100	88	—	—	—	—
Enterococcus faecium	6	—	14	75	0	86	—	—	—	100
Staphylococcus aureus	109	41	100	100	—	98	94	99	81	100
Oxacillin-Susceptible *S aureus (MSSA)* 41%	45	100	100	100	—	100	93	96	93	100
Oxacillin-Resistant *S aureus (MRSA)* 59%	64	—	100	100	—	97	95	100	73	—

Gram-Negative Percent Strains Susceptible	No. Tested	Ampicillin/ Sulbactam (%)	Piperacillin/ Tazobactam (%)	Cefazolin (%)	Ceftriax-one (%)	Ceftazidime (%)	Cefepime (%)	Colistin (%)	Imipenem (%)	Aztreonam (%)	Trimethoprim/ Sulfameth-oxazole (%)	Ciproflox-acin (%)	Gentamicin (%)	Tobramycin (%)	Amikacin (%)
Pseudomonas aeruginosa	59	—	96	—	—	87	89	100	83	93	—	93	80	83	100
Enterobacter sp[a]	42	—	100	—	97	97	100	—	100	97	97	100	100	100	100
Acinetobacter sp	33	61	—	—	—	—	—	100	54	—	—	—	—	—	84
Escherichia coli[a,b]	32	45	93	80	97	97	97	—	100	100	73	67	90	90	100
Klebsiella sp[a,b]	30	79	93	86	93	90	93	—	97	89	93	93	97	93	96
Proteus sp	20	95	100	68	90	94	95	—	100	100	100	95	100	90	94

Haemophilus influenzae (7 isolates) 60% susceptible to ampicillin (29% beta lactamase positive).

Stenotrophomonas maltophilia (9 isolates) 100% susceptible to sulfamethoxazole/trimethoprim, 87% to levofloxacin.

Aeromonas sp (2 isolates) 100% susceptible to piperacillin/tazobactam, ceftriaxone, ceftazidime, cefepime, imipenem, ciprofloxacin, gentamicin, tobramycin, amikacin.

[a] Carbapenemase producers: 0% *E coli*, 3% *Klebsiella sp*, 0% *Enterobacter sp*.

[b] Extended-spectrum beta lactamase positive: 3% *E coli*, 7% *Klebsiella sp*.

ut not always the extent of bioavailability.[97] For
ther less soluble medications, bioavailability
may increase with high-fat meals due to enhanced
olubility.[98] Acid lability and pH also can impact
bsorption and guide dosage form selection. For
xample, itraconazole tablets should be taken
with food to increase gastric acidity; however,
the solution should be taken on an empty stom-
ch.[99] Coadministration with cation constituents
may decrease absorption from chelation, as is
een with some tetracyclines.[100] Conversely,
ome medications are ideal because they lack
reat systemic absorption, like vancomycin or
faximin.[101]

Beyond bioavailability issues, some antibiotics
re developed only as intravenous formulations,
s they are generally prescribed for severe infec-
ons. Patients with severe infections may have
ompromised absorption due to changes in perfu-
ion or gut flora, resulting in possible reduced
ioavailability with oral administration.[102] Addi-
onally, severe infections require antibiotics to be
t optimum concentrations immediately. Intrave-
ous loading doses have proven effective for
ttainment of immediate therapeutic concentra-
ons for many antimicrobials; such as vancomy-
in, colistin, and voriconazole.[103,104] Ideally, the
enefit of using a loading dose before initiating
he normal maintenance regimen is for the patient
o quickly achieve and maintain therapeutic con-
entrations. The loading dose is eliminated while
he maintenance dose reaches steady state over
pproximately 5 half-lives.

Distribution is a drug's movement from intra-
ascular to extravascular compartments and is
est described by volume of distribution (V_d).
Depending on the pharmacodynamic target, antimicrobial dosing may increase synchronously
with V_d, and in such situations can be conceptu-
lly oversimplified as Dose = $C_{desired} \times V_d$. During
he ebb phase or other instances of high resusci-
ation volumes, patients with burn injuries may
equire larger than normal doses as V_d in-
reases.[105] The chemical structure of the medica-
on best defines the extent of distribution within
he body. In general, highly lipophilic drugs, like
oriconazole, will have a higher V_d.[106] With signif-
cant interplay with structure, the V_d is dependent
n several physiologic factors that impact
diposity or total body water: age, sex, and hy-
ration status.[107] As an example, amikacin is
ighly hydrophilic, with a very small volume of dis-
ribution. Small fluctuations in fluid status can
ave a great impact on the required dose. Dosing
will be significantly reduced in dehydrated or
lderly patients, whereas higher doses are
eeded in edematous patients.

Distribution also plays a key role in delivery of
antimicrobials to the target sites, as most sites of
infection are extravascular. It is important to
remember that therapeutic drug monitoring of
plasma concentrations does not always reflect tissue concentrations. Lipophilic antimicrobials, like
triazole antifungals or fluoroquinolones, penetrate
a variety of compartments and tissues with
adequate concentrations that often exceed
plasma.[108] Vancomycin and aminoglycosides are
hydrophilic, and appropriate concentrations at
the site of infection require adequate vascularity
and perfusion. For example, vancomycin penetration into the lungs has been shown to be approximately 20% that of the plasma, but maintain
concentrations well above the minimum inhibitory
concentration (MIC).[109] Lung concentrations
significantly increase in states of increased pulmonary vascular permeability, edema, and albumin
translocation, such as sepsis or burns.[109,110] A
theoretic disadvantage to using systemic medications in extensive full-thickness burns or peripheral
vascular disease is the difficult penetration into the
potential site of infection. In absence of systemic
signs of infections, local application may offer better delivery of antimicrobials. In addition to topical
agents, other examples of local therapy are the
use of inhaled antimicrobials and bladder irriga-
tions.[111-115] Consideration should be given to
chemical structure, disease state alterations in
V_d, and target site to aid selection and dosing of
antimicrobials.

Metabolism can be in the form of breaking down
medications into biologically inactive components
for preparation for elimination, such as linezolid
oxidation.[112] Rarely, metabolic reactions can
result in antimicrobial prodrugs being converted
into their active moieties.[104] Colistimethate sodium requires activation via hydrolysis to the
active antimicrobial colistin. Oxidation, reduction,
and hydrolysis are examples of phase I metabolic
processes. Phase II processes involve conjugation
of drugs to increase hydrophilicity in preparation
for excretion by bile or urine. Enterohepatic circulation may be lessened in the presence of significant antimicrobial exposure due to reduced gut
flora. Complicating matters, metabolism is also
affected by disease states, comorbid conditions,
and concomitant medications. Generally, metabolism is significantly augmented in patients with
burn injuries secondary to increased cardiac
output and subsequent delivery of medications
to sites of metabolic activity. The hypermetabolic
nature is highly dependent on age, comorbidities,
extent of injury, organ dysfunction, and concomi-
tantly administered medications with duration
starting as early as 24 hours and lasting for

years.[105] The significant hypermetabolism warrants attention from the burn practitioner, as medications frequently require dosing augmentations that can make inexperienced practitioners quite uncomfortable.

Elimination is the process by which medications are removed from the body. The primary pharmacokinetic principles that can be used to best describe elimination are rate elimination constant (k_e), half-life ($T_{1/2}$), and clearance (CL). $T_{1/2}$ (= $0.693/k_e$) of a drug is defined as the amount of time it takes for the plasma concentration to decrease by 50%. By definition, it takes 5 half-lives to eliminate 96.8% of a single dose of medication.[107] CL (= $k_e \times V_d$) is often reported as total clearance but also can be broken down into hepatic-specific or renal-specific clearances.

Much like metabolism, elimination is dramatically expedited in patients with burn injuries, but also heavily reliant on age, TBSA, comorbidities, time since injury, presence of organ dysfunction, and renal replacement therapies.[89,116] For drugs that are primarily renally eliminated, most studies attempt to correlate dosing regimens with CrCl. CrCl is traditionally calculated using the Cockcroft-Gault equation, which has inherent issues when applying to the current critical care patient. The equation was derived in subjects with comparatively low body weights and muscle mass.[117] Admittedly, the investigators also arbitrarily selected the female correction factor, as they were underrepresented in the landmark study. Although dose adjusting to CrCl is effective in some cases, other medications have shown poor correlation. Creatinine is primarily filtered by the kidneys, like most renally eliminated medications. However, some medications, like vancomycin, are also eliminated via renal tubular secretion, which limits but does not negate the equation's applicability.[118] Understanding the limitations of CrCl, the value is still useful for many medications, as glomerular filtration remains the primary mode of elimination for most renally cleared medications. Sticking with the current example, vancomycin clearance is significantly enhanced in patients with burn injuries and a CrCl as low as 80 mL/min has been shown as an indicator that a more frequent administration (15–20 mg/kg every 8 hours) may be warranted.[89]

Pharmacodynamics

To best optimize outcomes, treatments should be individualized through the integration of pharmacokinetics and pharmacodynamics. Pharmacodynamics has been defined as the resultant biologic effect from the interactions of drugs and biologic systems.[119] Biologic response can be from direct receptor binding or indirectly through inhibitory mechanisms. Some antimicrobials can directly bind to membranes, causing damage or preventing cross-linking (amphotericin B, β-lactams, colistin, and vancomycin). Others can cause deleterious effects by inhibiting vital sterol or protein synthesis required for membrane and DNA formation (macrolides, tetracyclines, and azoles). Antibacterials can be bacteriostatic (relying on host immune function for efficacy) or bactericidal. Linezolid, tigecycline, macrolides, and sulfonamides exhibit mainly bacteriostatic tendencies. Some antibacterials can exhibit both properties and can be dependent on host immune system, concentrations, or target pathogen. As an example, linezolid is bacteriostatic against *Staphylococcus* and *Enterococcus* spp., but bactericidal against *Streptococcus* spp.[120]

Bactericidal antibacterials affect bacterial clearance in a time-dependent or concentration-dependent manner.[110] **Table 2** lists common antibacterials used in patients with burn injuries and their most commonly accepted bactericidal pharmacodynamic principle. Time above the MIC (T>MIC) describes agents with slow bactericidal action, little response to increasing concentrations

Table 2
Principle bactericidal pharmacodynamic parameter

Parameter	Antibacterials
C_{max}/MIC	Aminoglycosides
AUC_{24}/MIC	Fluoroquinolones
	Azithromycin
	Tetracyclines
	Vancomycin
	Colistin
	Daptomycin
	Metronidazole
T>MIC	β-lactams
	Oxazolidinones
	Erythromycin
	Clarithromycin
	Clindamycin
PAE	Aminoglycosides
	Fluoroquinolones
	β-lactams
	Colistin
	Vancomycin
	Metronidazole

Abbreviations: AUC_{24}/MIC, area under the 24-hour concentration curve/minimum inhibitory concentration; C_{max}/MIC, peak concentration/minimum inhibitory concentration; PAE, post antibiotic effect; T>MIC, amount of time the concentration > minimum inhibitory concentration.

beyond the MIC, and little to no post antibiotic effect (PAE). PAE is the phenomenon of continued bacterial reduction or suppression even when antimicrobial concentrations fall below the minimum bactericidal concentration or MIC, respectively.[121] Enhanced PAE theories range from intracellular concentrations exceeding that of plasma, reduced bacterial burden, and host immunologic function.[122] Concentration-dependent antibacterials usually have more significant PAE and may best be described by C_{max}/MIC or AUC_{24}/MIC with higher concentrations (or lower MIC) resulting in greater bacterial kill.

DURATION OF THERAPY

Duration of antimicrobial therapy is another question of frequent debate. Most available clinical guidance lacks definitive data or does not directly address the burn population. The patient with burn injury is frequently subjected to a prolonged hospital course fraught with unique challenges that increase the risk of developing infections, including complex wounds, frequent wound excision and grafting, increased systemic inflammation and vascular permeability, higher central venous device utilization ratios, and prolonged mechanical ventilation. Many studies focus on primary sources other than wounds. Current catheter-related blood stream infection guidelines recommend a duration of at least 2 weeks for uncomplicated and a minimum of 4 weeks for complicated bacteremia.[123] However, the investigators admit the recommendations were made without compelling supportive data from large randomized controlled trials. With adequate source control, shorter courses of fewer than 14 days may suffice for uncomplicated bacteremia. As an example, Chong and colleagues[124] prospectively studied the 14-day treatment threshold of uncomplicated *Staphylococcus aureus*. The group with shorter duration had more relapse of infection (n = 3), but no difference in mortality. On closer examination, 1 of the 3 received only 3 days of cefazolin, 2 required ≥26 days to relapse, and linezolid was chosen in 1 patient who also required chronic hemodialysis. With intentions of decreasing drug toxicity and antibiotic resistance, recent pneumonia guidelines stress the importance of a shorter course of 7 days.[7] The added caveat that treatment duration recommendations depend on clinical improvement must not be overlooked, as some patients and pathogens may require longer treatment durations.

Although most patients will be successfully treated with short courses, it may be prudent to consider patient-specific treatment durations instead of arbitrary assignment of a predetermined discontinuation date. Thorough patient examination and clinical picture should supersede arbitrary stop dates or laboratory values. If resources allow, one solution is implementing a PCT-guided algorithm for assisting determination of patient-specific response to treatment.[38] Use of patient-specific reductions in PCT may be preferred over pre-specified thresholds. Furthermore, drug-specific pharmacodynamic principles also should be considered. If adequately dosed, concentration-dependent antibiotics may require a shorter length of treatment than bacteriostatic or time-dependent antibiotics. Treatment should target a balance between long enough to produce the desired effect, and shorter than the period necessary for growth of MDR organisms.[125]

SUMMARY

Caring for patients with burn injuries presents practitioners with many challenges that, to date, lack adequate evidence-driven recommendations. Interpretation of current guidelines should be applied judiciously to this unique patient population. Antimicrobials are an important ordnance in the burn clinician's armament that can dramatically impact infection-related mortality. Although usage is usually necessary, lack of diligent and responsible prescribing can result in significant patient harm. Optimum prescribing requires integrating the unique pathophysiology, pharmacokinetics, and pharmacodynamics of the patient with burn injury. Individual clinical response should supersede predetermined discontinuation of therapy. With such obvious complexity, the proven multidiscipline team-based model will best ensure optimum patient outcomes. Clinicians should strive to continue investigating and producing high-quality evidence to better serve the patient with burn injury.

REFERENCES

1. Pruitt BA Jr, Wolf SE. An historical perspective on advances in burn care over the past 100 years. Clin Plast Surg 2009;36(4):527–45.
2. Keen EF 3rd, Robinson BJ, Hospenthal DR, et al. Prevalence of multidrug-resistant organisms recovered at a military burn center. Burns 2010;36(6):819–25.
3. Bahemia IA, Muganza A, Moore R, et al. Microbiology and antibiotic resistance in severe burn patients: a 5 year review in an adult burns unit. Burns 2015;41(7):1536–42.
4. Soleymanzadeh-Moghadam S, Azimi L, Amani L, et al. Analysis of antibiotic consumption in burn patients. GMS Hyg Infect Control 2015;10:Doc09.

5. Mann EA, Baun MM, Meininger JC, et al. Comparison of mortality associated with sepsis in the burn, trauma, and general intensive care unit patient: a systematic review of the literature. Shock 2012; 37(1):4–16.

6. Chastre J, Fagon JY. Diagnosis of ventilator-associated pneumonia. N Engl J Med 2007; 356(14):1469 [author reply: 1470–1].

7. Kalil AC, Metersky ML, Klompas M, et al. Management of adults with hospital-acquired and ventilator-associated pneumonia: 2016 clinical practice guidelines by the Infectious Diseases Society of America and the American Thoracic Society. Clin Infect Dis 2016;63(5):e61–111.

8. Pham TN, Neff MJ, Simmons JM, et al. The clinical pulmonary infection score poorly predicts pneumonia in patients with burns. J Burn Care Res 2007;28(1):76–9.

9. Chastre J, Combes A, Luyt CE. The invasive (quantitative) diagnosis of ventilator-associated pneumonia. Respir Care 2005;50(6):797–807 [discussion: 807–12].

10. Kollef MH, Ward S. The influence of mini-BAL cultures on patient outcomes: implications for the antibiotic management of ventilator-associated pneumonia. Chest 1998;113(2):412–20.

11. Wahl WL, Ahrns KS, Brandt MM, et al. Bronchoalveolar lavage in diagnosis of ventilator-associated pneumonia in patients with burns. J Burn Care Rehabil 2005;26(1):57–61.

12. Greenhalgh DG, Saffle JR, Holmes JH, et al. American Burn Association consensus conference to define sepsis and infection in burns. J Burn Care Res 2007;28(6):776–90.

13. Krizek TJ, Robson MC. Evolution of quantitative bacteriology in wound management. Am J Surg 1975;130(5):579–84.

14. Lavrentieva A, Kontakiotis T, Lazaridis L, et al. Inflammatory markers in patients with severe burn injury. What is the best indicator of sepsis? Burns 2007;33(2):189–94.

15. Hogan BK, Wolf SE, Hospenthal DR, et al. Correlation of American Burn Association sepsis criteria with the presence of bacteremia in burned patients admitted to the intensive care unit. J Burn Care Res 2012;33(3):371–8.

16. Mann-Salinas EA, Baun MM, Meininger JC, et al. Novel predictors of sepsis outperform the American Burn Association sepsis criteria in the burn intensive care unit patient. J Burn Care Res 2013; 34(1):31–43.

17. Bone RC, Balk RA, Cerra FB, et al. Definitions for sepsis and organ failure and guidelines for the use of innovative therapies in sepsis. The ACCP/SCCM Consensus Conference Committee. American College of Chest Physicians/Society of Critical Care Medicine. Chest 1992;101(6):1644–55.

18. Demling RH. The burn edema process: current concepts. J Burn Care Rehabil 2005;26(3):207–27.

19. Rivers E, Nguyen B, Havstad S, et al. Early goal-directed therapy in the treatment of severe sepsis and septic shock. N Engl J Med 2001;345(19): 1368–77.

20. Dellinger RP, Levy MM, Rhodes A, et al. Surviving sepsis campaign: international guidelines for management of severe sepsis and septic shock: 2012. Crit Care Med 2013;41(2):580–637.

21. Baxter CR, Shires T. Physiological response to crystalloid resuscitation of severe burns. Ann N Y Acad Sci 1968;150(3):874–94.

22. Pruitt BA Jr, Mason AD Jr, Moncrief JA. Hemodynamic changes in the early postburn patient: the influence of fluid administration and of a vasodilator (hydralazine). J Trauma 1971;11(1):36–46.

23. Schultz L, Walker SA, Elligsen M, et al. Identification of predictors of early infection in acute burn patients. Burns 2013;39(7):1355–66.

24. Murray CK, Hoffmaster RM, Schmit DR, et al. Evaluation of white blood cell count, neutrophil percentage, and elevated temperature as predictors of bloodstream infection in burn patients. Arch Surg 2007;142(7):639–42.

25. Pisarchik AN, Pochepen ON, Pisarchyk LA. Increasing blood glucose variability is a precursor of sepsis and mortality in burned patients. PLoS One 2012;7(10):e46582.

26. Reinhart K, Karzai W, Meisner M. Procalcitonin as a marker of the systemic inflammatory response to infection. Intensive Care Med 2000;26(9): 1193–200.

27. Linscheid P, Seboek D, Schaer DJ, et al. Expression and secretion of procalcitonin and calcitonin gene-related peptide by adherent monocytes and by macrophage-activated adipocytes. Crit Care Med 2004;32(8):1715–21.

28. Meisner M. Update on procalcitonin measurements. Ann Lab Med 2014;34(4):263–73.

29. Brunkhorst FM, Heinz U, Forycki ZF. Kinetics of procalcitonin in iatrogenic sepsis. Intensive Care Med 1998;24(8):888–9.

30. Meisner M, Lohs T, Huettemann E, et al. The plasma elimination rate and urinary secretion of procalcitonin in patients with normal and impaired renal function. Eur J Anaesthesiol 2001;18(2):79–87.

31. Sachse C, Machens HG, Felmerer G, et al. Procalcitonin as a marker for the early diagnosis of severe infection after thermal injury. J Burn Care Rehabil 1999;20(5):354–60.

32. von Heimburg D, Stieghorst W, Khorram-Sefat R, et al. Procalcitonin–a sepsis parameter in severe burn injuries. Burns 1998;24(8):745–50.

33. Ren H, Li Y, Han C, et al. Serum procalcitonin as a diagnostic biomarker for sepsis in burned patients: a meta-analysis. Burns 2015;41(3):502–9.

34. Seoane L, Pertega S, Galeiras R, et al. Procalcitonin in the burn unit and the diagnosis of infection. Burns 2014;40(2):223–9.

35. Lavrentieva A, Papadopoulou S, Kioumis J, et al. PCT as a diagnostic and prognostic tool in burn patients. Whether time course has a role in monitoring sepsis treatment. Burns 2012;38(3):356–63.

36. Kim HS, Yang HT, Hur J, et al. Procalcitonin levels within 48 hours after burn injury as a prognostic factor. Ann Clin Lab Sci 2012;42(1):57–64.

37. Bouadma L, Luyt CE, Tubach F, et al. Use of procalcitonin to reduce patients' exposure to antibiotics in intensive care units (PRORATA trial): a multicentre randomised controlled trial. Lancet 2010; 375(9713):463–74.

38. Lavrentieva A, Kontou P, Soulountsi V, et al. Implementation of a procalcitonin-guided algorithm for antibiotic therapy in the burn intensive care unit. Ann Burns Fire Disasters 2015;28(3):163–70.

39. Shirani KZ, McManus AT, Vaughan GM, et al. Effects of environment on infection in burn patients. Arch Surg 1986;121(1):31–6.

40. Langschmidt J, Caine PL, Wearn CM, et al. Hydrotherapy in burn care: a survey of hydrotherapy practices in the UK and Ireland and literature review. Burns 2014;40(5):860–4.

41. Lee JJ, Marvin JA, Heimbach DM, et al. Infection control in a burn center. J Burn Care Rehabil 1990;11(6):575–80.

42. Kagan RJ, Neely AN, Rieman MT, et al. A performance improvement initiative to determine the impact of increasing the time interval between changing centrally placed intravascular catheters. J Burn Care Res 2014;35(2):143–7.

43. Hemmila MR, Taddonio MA, Arbabi S, et al. Intensive insulin therapy is associated with reduced infectious complications in burn patients. Surgery 2008;144(4):629–35 [discussion: 635–7].

44. Neely AN, Gardner J, Durkee P, et al. Are topical antimicrobials effective against bacteria that are highly resistant to systemic antibiotics? J Burn Care Res 2009;30(1):19–29.

45. Barsoumian A, Sanchez CJ, Mende K, et al. In vitro toxicity and activity of Dakin's solution, mafenide acetate, and amphotericin B on filamentous fungi and human cells. J Orthop Trauma 2013;27(8): 428–36.

46. Atiyeh BS, Costagliola M, Hayek SN, et al. Effect of silver on burn wound infection control and healing: review of the literature. Burns 2007;33(2):139–48.

47. Finley PJ, Norton R, Austin C, et al. Unprecedented silver resistance in clinically isolated Enterobacteriaceae: major implications for burn and wound management. Antimicrob Agents Chemother 2015;59(8):4734–41.

48. Hashemi B, Bayat A, Kazemei T, et al. Comparison between topical honey and mafenide acetate in treatment of auricular burn. Am J Otolaryngol 2011;32(1):28–31.

49. Jull AB, Rodgers A, Walker N. Honey as a topical treatment for wounds. Cochrane Database Syst Rev 2008;(4):CD005083.

50. Heggers JP, Sazy JA, Stenberg BD, et al. Bactericidal and wound-healing properties of sodium hypochlorite solutions: the 1991 Lindberg Award. J Burn Care Rehabil 1991;12(5):420–4.

51. Jung WK, Koo HC, Kim KW, et al. Antibacterial activity and mechanism of action of the silver ion in Staphylococcus aureus and Escherichia coli. Appl Environ Microbiol 2008;74(7):2171–8.

52. Fox CL Jr, Modak SM. Mechanism of silver sulfadiazine action on burn wound infections. Antimicrob Agents Chemother 1974;5(6):582–8.

53. Wang XW, Wang NZ, Zhang OZ, et al. Tissue deposition of silver following topical use of silver sulphadiazine in extensive burns. Burns Incl Therm Inj 1985;11(3):197–201.

54. Fuller FW. The side effects of silver sulfadiazine. J Burn Care Res 2009;30(3):464–70.

55. Tang H, Lv G, Fu J, et al. An open, parallel, randomized, comparative, multicenter investigation evaluating the efficacy and tolerability of Mepilex Ag versus silver sulfadiazine in the treatment of deep partial-thickness burn injuries. J Trauma Acute Care Surg 2015;78(5):1000–7.

56. Toussaint J, Chung WT, Osman N, et al. Topical antibiotic ointment versus silver-containing foam dressing for second-degree burns in swine. Acad Emerg Med 2015;22(8):927–33.

57. Wright JB, Lam K, Hansen D, et al. Efficacy of topical silver against fungal burn wound pathogens. Am J Infect Control 1999;27(4):344–50.

58. Murphy RC, Kucan JO, Robson MC, et al. The effect of 5% mafenide acetate solution on bacterial control in infected rat burns. J Trauma 1983; 23(10):878–81.

59. Lee JJ, Marvin JA, Heimbach DM, et al. Use of 5% sulfamylon (mafenide) solution after excision and grafting of burns. J Burn Care Rehabil 1988;9(6): 602–5.

60. Ibrahim A, Fagan S, Keaney T, et al. A simple cost-saving measure: 2.5% mafenide acetate solution. J Burn Care Res 2014;35(4):349–53.

61. Kirby JP, Mazuski JE. Prevention of surgical site infection. Surg Clin North Am 2009;89(2):365–89, viii.

62. Avni T, Levcovich A, Ad-El DD, et al. Prophylactic antibiotics for burns patients: systematic review and meta-analysis. BMJ 2010;340:c241.

63. Ergun O, Celik A, Ergun G, et al. Prophylactic antibiotic use in pediatric burn units. Eur J Pediatr Surg 2004;14(6):422–6.

64. Ozbek S, Ozgenel Y, Etoz A, et al. The effect of delayed admission in burn centers on wound

contamination and infection rates. Ulus Travma Acil Cerrahi Derg 2005;11(3):230–7.

65. Bracco D, Eggimann P. Prophylaxis with systemic antibiotics in patients with severe burns. BMJ 2010;340:c208.

66. Sasaki TM, Welch GW, Herndon DN, et al. Burn wound manipulation-induced bacteremia. J Trauma 1979;19(1):46–8.

67. Mozingo DW, McManus AT, Kim SH, et al. Incidence of bacteremia after burn wound manipulation in the early postburn period. J Trauma 1997; 42(6):1006–10 [discussion: 1010–1].

68. Vindenes H, Bjerknes R. The frequency of bacteremia and fungemia following wound cleaning and excision in patients with large burns. J Trauma 1993;35(5):742–9.

69. Levine BA, Sirinek KR, Pruitt BA Jr. Wound excision to fascia in burn patients. Arch Surg 1978;113(4): 403–7.

70. Petersen SR, Umphred E, Warden GD. The incidence of bacteremia following burn wound excision. J Trauma 1982;22(4):274–9.

71. Ramos GE, Resta M, Durlach R, et al. Peri-operative bacteraemia in burn patients. What does it mean? Ann Burns Fire Disasters 2006;19(3):130–5.

72. Bratzler DW, Dellinger EP, Olsen KM, et al. Clinical practice guidelines for antimicrobial prophylaxis in surgery. Am J Health Syst Pharm 2013;70(3): 195–283.

73. Dalley AJ, Lipman J, Venkatesh B, et al. Inadequate antimicrobial prophylaxis during surgery: a study of beta-lactam levels during burn debridement. J Antimicrob Chemother 2007;60(1):166–9.

74. Zelenitsky SA, Ariano RE, Harding GKM, et al. Antibiotic pharmacodynamics in surgical prophylaxis: an association between intraoperative antibiotic concentrations and efficacy. Antimicrob Agents Chemother 2002;46(9):3026–30.

75. Clinical and Laboratory Standards Institute. Analysis and presentation of cumulative antimicrobial susceptibility test data; approved guideline. 4th Edition. Wayne (PA): Clinical and Laboratory Standards Institute; 2014. CLSI document M39–A4.

76. Mir MA, Khurram MF, Khan AH. What should be the antibiotic prescription protocol for burn patients admitted in the department of burns, plastic and reconstructive surgery. Int Wound J 2016;14:194–7.

77. Hill DM, Schroeppel TJ, Magnotti LJ, et al. Methicillin-resistant *Staphylococcus aureus* in early ventilator-associated pneumonia: cause for concern? Surg Infect (Larchmt) 2013;14(6):520–4.

78. Hindler JF, Stelling J. Analysis and presentation of cumulative antibiograms: a new consensus guideline from the Clinical and Laboratory Standards Institute. Clin Infect Dis 2007;44(6):867–73.

79. Capoor MR, Gupta S, Sarabahi S, et al. Epidemiological and clinico-mycological profile of fungal

wound infection from largest burn centre in Asia. Mycoses 2012;55(2):181–8.

80. Hill D, Brown E, Hickerson W. Evaluation of fungal incidence, outcomes, and empiric therapy in patients with thermal or inhalation injury. 18th Congress of International Society for Burn Injuries. Miami, FL, September 1, 2016.

81. Ballard J, Edelman L, Saffle J, et al. Positive fungal cultures in burn patients: a multicenter review. J Burn Care Res 2008;29(1):213–21.

82. Brown E, Hill D, Hickerson W. Determination of fungal incidence and outcomes in patients with thermal and inhalation injury. Southern Medical Association, 28th annual Southern Region Burn Conference. Dallas, TX, November 22, 2015.

83. Benedict K, Park BJ. Invasive fungal infections after natural disasters. Emerg Infect Dis 2014;20(3) 349–55.

84. Austin CL, Finley PJ, Mikkelson DR, et al. Mucormycosis: a rare fungal infection in tornado victims. J Burn Care Res 2014;35(3):e164–71.

85. Richardson M. The ecology of the zygomycetes and its impact on environmental exposure. Clin Microbiol Infect 2009;15(Suppl 5):2–9.

86. Struck MF, Gille J. Fungal infections in burns: a comprehensive review. Ann Burns Fire Disasters 2013;26(3):147–53.

87. Becker WK, Cioffi WG Jr, McManus AT, et al. Fungal burn wound infection. A 10-year experience. Arch Surg 1991;126(1):44–8.

88. Hallam MJ, Allen JM, James SE, et al. Potential subtherapeutic linezolid and meropenem antibiotic concentrations in a patient with severe burns and sepsis. J Burn Care Res 2010;31(1):207–9.

89. Elder K, Hill D, Hickerson W. Evaluation of variables for potential impact on vancomycin pharmacokinetics in thermal or inhalational injury. Midsouth Pharmacy Residency Conference. Memphis, TN April 22, 2016.

90. Zaske DE, Sawchuk RJ, Gerding DN, et al. Increased dosage requirements of gentamicin in burn patients. J Trauma 1976;16(10):824–8.

91. Wilkinson R, Hill D, Hickerson W. Outcome analysis of colistin-treated burn center patients. Southern Medical Association, 28th annual Southern Region Burn Conference. Dallas, TX, November 22, 2015

92. Whyatt PL, Slywka GW, Melikian AP, et al. Bioavailability of 17 ampicillin products. J Pharm Sci 1976 65(5):652–6.

93. Nauta EH, Mattie H. Dicloxacillin and cloxacillin pharmacokinetics in healthy and hemodialysis subjects. Clin Pharmacol Ther 1976;20(1):98–108.

94. Sawant KK, Patel MH, Patel K. Cefdinir nanosuspension for improved oral bioavailability by media milling technique: formulation, characterization and in vitro-in vivo evaluations. Drug Dev Ind Pharm 2016;42(5):758–68.

95. Welling PG, Dean S, Selen A, et al. The pharmacokinetics of the oral cephalosporins cefaclor, cephradine and cephalexin. Int J Clin Pharmacol Biopharm 1979;17(9):397–400.

96. Scott LJ, Ormrod D, Goa KL. Cefuroxime axetil: an updated review of its use in the management of bacterial infections. Drugs 2001;61(10):1455–500.

97. Winstanley PA, Orme ML. The effects of food on drug bioavailability. Br J Clin Pharmacol 1989;28(6):621–8.

98. Palma R, Vidon N, Houin G, et al. Influence of bile salts and lipids on intestinal absorption of griseofulvin in man. Eur J Clin Pharmacol 1986;31(3):319–25.

99. Boogaerts M, Maertens J. Clinical experience with itraconazole in systemic fungal infections. Drugs 2001;61(Suppl 1):39–47.

100. Neuvonen PJ, Turakka H. Inhibitory effect of various iron salts on the absorption of tetracycline in man. Eur J Clin Pharmacol 1974;7(5):357–60.

101. Cohen SH, Gerding DN, Johnson S, et al. Clinical practice guidelines for Clostridium difficile infection in adults: 2010 update by the society for healthcare epidemiology of America (SHEA) and the infectious diseases society of America (IDSA). Infect Control Hosp Epidemiol 2010;31(5):431–55.

102. McKinnon PS, Davis SL. Pharmacokinetic and pharmacodynamic issues in the treatment of bacterial infectious diseases. Eur J Clin Microbiol Infect Dis 2004;23(4):271–88.

103. Rosini JM, Laughner J, Levine BJ, et al. A randomized trial of loading vancomycin in the emergency department. Ann Pharmacother 2015;49(1):6–13.

104. Garonzik SM, Li J, Thamlikitkul V, et al. Population pharmacokinetics of colistin methanesulfonate and formed colistin in critically ill patients from a multicenter study provide dosing suggestions for various categories of patients. Antimicrob Agents Chemother 2011;55(7):3284–94.

105. Blanchet B, Jullien V, Vinsonneau C, et al. Influence of burns on pharmacokinetics and pharmacodynamics of drugs used in the care of burn patients. Clin Pharmacokinet 2008;47(10):635–54.

106. Theuretzbacher U, Ihle F, Derendorf H. Pharmacokinetic/pharmacodynamic profile of voriconazole. Clin Pharmacokinet 2006;45(7):649–63.

107. Gibaldi M. Biopharmaceutics and clinical pharmacokinetics. 3rd edition. Philadelphia: Lea & Febiger; 1984.

108. Nix DE, Goodwin SD, Peloquin CA, et al. Antibiotic tissue penetration and its relevance: impact of tissue penetration on infection response. Antimicrob Agents Chemother 1991;35(10):1953–9.

109. Lamer C, de Beco V, Soler P, et al. Analysis of vancomycin entry into pulmonary lining fluid by bronchoalveolar lavage in critically ill patients. Antimicrob Agents Chemother 1993;37(2):281–6.

110. Roberts JA, Lipman J. Antibacterial dosing in intensive care: pharmacokinetics, degree of disease and pharmacodynamics of sepsis. Clin Pharmacokinet 2006;45(8):755–73.

111. Wood GC, Chapman JL, Boucher BA, et al. Tobramycin bladder irrigation for treating a urinary tract infection in a critically ill patient. Ann Pharmacother 2004;38(7–8):1318–9.

112. Hill DM, Wood GC, Hickerson WL. Linezolid bladder irrigation as adjunctive treatment for a vancomycin-resistant Enterococcus faecium catheter-associated urinary tract infection. Ann Pharmacother 2015;49(2):250–3.

113. Volkow-Fernandez P, Rodriguez CF, Cornejo-Juarez P. Intravesical colistin irrigation to treat multidrug-resistant Acinetobacter baumannii urinary tract infection: a case report. J Med case Rep 2012;6:426.

114. Giua R, Pedone C, Cortese L, et al. Colistin bladder instillation, an alternative way of treating multiresistant Acinetobacter urinary tract infection: a case series and review of literature. Infection 2014;42(1):199–202.

115. Wood GC. Aerosolized antibiotics for treating hospital-acquired and ventilator-associated pneumonia. Expert Rev Anti Infect Ther 2011;9(11):993–1000.

116. Steele AN, Grimsrud KN, Sen S, et al. Gap analysis of pharmacokinetics and pharmacodynamics in burn patients: a review. J Burn Care Res 2015;36(3):e194–211.

117. Cockcroft DW, Gault MH. Prediction of creatinine clearance from serum creatinine. Nephron 1976;16(1):31–41.

118. Rybak MJ, Albrecht LM, Berman JR, et al. Vancomycin pharmacokinetics in burn patients and intravenous drug abusers. Antimicrob Agents Chemother 1990;34(5):792–5.

119. Holford NH, Sheiner LB. Understanding the dose-effect relationship: clinical application of pharmacokinetic-pharmacodynamic models. Clin Pharmacokinet 1981;6(6):429–53.

120. Kocher S, Muller W, Resch B. Linezolid treatment of nosocomial bacterial infection with multiresistant gram-positive pathogens in preterm infants: a systematic review. Int J Antimicrob Agents 2010;36(2):106–10.

121. Bozkurt-Guzel C, Gerceker AA. Post-antibiotic effect of colistin, alone and in combination with amikacin, on Pseudomonas aeruginosa strains isolated from cystic fibrosis patients. J Antibiot (Tokyo) 2012;65(2):83–6.

122. Levison ME, Levison JH. Pharmacokinetics and pharmacodynamics of antibacterial agents. Infect Dis Clin North Am 2009;23(4):791–815, vii.

123. Liu C, Bayer A, Cosgrove SE, et al. Clinical practice guidelines by the infectious diseases

society of America for the treatment of methicillin-resistant *Staphylococcus aureus* infections in adults and children. Clin Infect Dis 2011;52(3):e18–55.

124. Chong YP, Moon SM, Bang KM, et al. Treatment duration for uncomplicated *Staphylococcus aureus* bacteremia to prevent relapse: analysis of a prospective observational cohort study. Antimicrob Agents Chemother 2013;57(3):1150–6.

125. Dacso CC, Luterman A, Curreri PW. Systemic antibiotic treatment in burned patients. Surg Clin North Am 1987;67(1):57–68.

Sedation and Pain Management in Burn Patients

Cornelia Griggs, MD[a], Jeremy Goverman, MD[b],
Edward A. Bittner, MD, PhD[c], Benjamin Levi, MD[d],*

KEYWORDS

• Pain management • Sedation • Burn • Anesthesia • Operative management

KEY POINTS

• Pain management in patients with burn injuries, while challenging, is critically important to optimum care of this population.
• Better outcomes in healing, anxiety, and rehabilitation are linked to good pain control in burns.
• Pain assessment requires understanding of acute, chronic, and procedural forms of burn-related pain.
• Multimodal pharmacologic approaches, with opioids as the mainstay of pain control, are ideal for burn-injured patients.
• Perioperative management demands understanding of complex physiology and dynamic pharmacokinetic changes that occur during the acute injury and resuscitation phase, especially in larger burns.

INTRODUCTION

From the moment of injury through rehabilitation and beyond, pain control is a major challenge in the management of patients with burn injuries. In fact, some argue that burn pain is the most difficult to treat among any etiology of acute pain.[1] The therapies used to treat burn injuries may exacerbate the difficulty of pain control because most of these interventions are associated with pain, be it dressing changes, excision and grafting, or physical therapy. These therapies can cause pain that is equivalent to or worse than the pain of an initial burn injury. Therefore, pain management must be a foundation of burn care. Good pain control is linked to better wound healing, sleep, participation in activities of daily living, quality of life, and recovery.[2,3]

Despite profound improvements in modern burn care, suboptimal and inconsistent pain management persists throughout all stages of burn treatment. Without aggressive pain control, patients are likely to suffer not only from the acute experience of pain in itself, but the secondary morbidities of higher pain levels, including long-term anxiety and posttraumatic stress,[4,5] or even delayed wound healing.[6] The unique challenge of burn pain is further complicated by a relative dearth of standardized approaches.[7] Instead, tradition and personal/institutional biases often dictate pain management. The complex interaction of anatomic, physiologic, pharmacologic, psychosocial, and premorbid issues can make the treatment of burn pain particularly difficult. An overview of pain management strategies specific to the treatment of burn injuries is summarized here.

Disclosure statement: Dr B. Levi was supported by funding from National Institutes of Health/National Institute of General Medical Sciences grant K08GM109105-0, American Association of Plastic Surgery Academic Scholarship, and American College of Surgeons Clowes Award. Dr B. Levi collaborates on a project unrelated to this review with Boehringer Ingelheim.
[a] Department of Surgery, Massachusetts General Hospital, Boston, MA, USA; [b] Division of Burn and Plastic and Reconstructive Surgery, Department of Surgery, Massachusetts General Hospital, Boston, MA, USA; [c] Department of Anesthesia, Critical Care and Pain Medicine, Massachusetts General Hospital, Boston, MA, USA; [d] Division of Plastic Surgery, University of Michigan, 1500 East Medical Center Drive, Ann Arbor, MI 48109, USA
* Corresponding author.
E-mail address: blevi@med.umich.edu

MECHANISMS AND TYPES OF PAIN IN BURNS

Although burns are classified according to depth, area, and severity of injury, pain does not necessarily correlate with these measures. The individual experience of pain varies widely between patients and throughout the healing process in burn injuries.[7] Because individuals have varying pain thresholds, coping abilities, and even physiologic responses to injury, patients may experience disparate levels of pain despite having similar injuries.[7] The most immediate and acute form of burn pain is the inflammatory nociceptive pain attributed to burn injury and tissue trauma. Nociceptive pain is often followed by and potentially exacerbated by procedural pain related to the treatment of burn wounds, be it surgical debridement, grafting, staple application and removal, physical therapy, or dressing changes. As burn wounds begin to heal, neuropathic pain, characterized by a throbbing or constant burning sensation potentially adds an additional layer of discomfort.

Although all burns are painful, conventionally, deeper, full-thickness burns are thought to be somewhat less painful than superficial and partial thickness burns because of afferent nerve destruction.[8] However, this does not always play out in clinical practice.[9] Additionally, full-thickness burns eventually require debridement and grafting and subsequent dressing changes that all lead to substantial pain. At the time of burn injury, tissue damage is the primary mechanism of pain. Stimulation of local nociceptors transmits an impulse via Ad and C fibers to the dorsal horn of the spinal cord. Peripheral sensory nerves and descending influences from cortical areas can modulate the magnitude of the pain impulse.[10] Ultimately, conscious perception of pain is regulated by areas of the brain, often named the "pain matrix," which is thought to involve a network of higher cortical areas and the thalamus.[11,12] The conscious perception of pain is affected not only by the burn wound itself but also by context, cognition, pharmacologics, mood, and other predisposing factors.[10] Burn pain also may vary and fluctuate widely over the span of recovery. Therefore, the successful treatment of burn pain should involve a multimodal approach tailored to the patient and scenario.

PAIN ASSESSMENT

The first step in determining a pain treatment plan is assessing the degree of the patient's pain, which, in the case of burn injuries, may be mild to excruciating. Reliable, valid pain assessment tools in form of verbal adjective, numeric, or visual analog scales (VASs) can be useful guides for pain management in burns. In adults, VAS and numeric rating scales (NRSs) are commonly used.[13] Both NRS and VAS have undergone repeated validation and have performed well in different patient populations.[14] Children, especially those who are preverbal, and noncommunicative adults present a more difficult challenge. Observational scales and physiologic indicators, such as heart rate and blood pressure, may be used to gauge pain in these populations.

Second, understanding the type and chronicity of a patient's pain is useful for tailoring pain management strategies. The Patterson burn pain paradigm provides a roadmap for the management of burn pain through 5 different phases of injury treatment, and recovery.[15] (1) Background pain is pain that is present while the patient is at rest, results from the thermal tissue injury itself, and is typically of low to moderate intensity and long duration. (2) Procedural pain is brief but intense pain that is generated by wound debridement and dressing changes and/or rehabilitation activities. (3) Breakthrough pain describes unexpected spikes of pain that occur when background analgesic effects are exceeded, when at rest, during procedures, or with stress. (4) Procedural pain is an expected and temporary increase in pain that occurs after burn excision, donor skin harvesting, grafting, or interventions, such as the placement of central lines due to the creation of new and painful wounds in the process. (5) Chronic pain is pain that lasts longer than 6 months or remains after all burn wounds and skin graft donor sites have healed. The most common form of chronic pain is neuropathic pain, which is the result of damage sustained by the nerve endings in the skin. Each of these 5 phases presents unique challenges in the management of burn pain. Clinicians should be prepared to adjust treatment strategies using both pharmacologic and nonpharmacologic techniques, discussed in further detail in the next sections.

PATHOPHYSIOLOGY AND PHARMACOLOGIC CONSIDERATIONS

Major burns cause massive tissue destruction and activation of a cytokine-mediated inflammatory response leading to dramatic pathophysiologic effects.[16] The inflammatory response is initiated within minutes of burn injury, which results in a cascade of irritants that sensitize and stimulate pain fibers. Burn wounds may become primarily hyperalgesic to mechanical and/or thermal stimuli.[10] Two distinct phases, a burn shock phase followed by a hypermetabolic phase, were first described by Cuthbertson in 1942.[17] Burns involving more than 20% of total body surface area cause generalized edema even in noninjured tissues.[16] Continued loss of plasma into burned tissue can occur up to the first 48 hours or even longer in these larger burns.[16] These profound physiologic changes contribute to altered pharmacokinetic and pharmacodynamic responses to many drugs.[16] Plasma protein loss through burned skin and further dilution of plasma proteins by resuscitation fluids decrease the concentration of albumin.[16] Increase in volume of distribution has been shown in almost every drug studied, including propofol, fentanyl, and muscle relaxants.[18] Burned patients may demonstrate variable or unpredictable responses to drugs, thereby requiring adjustments to dosing or complete exclusion of certain drugs (eg, succinylcholine).[16] Cardiac output goes down in the acute injury phase (0–48 hours) even with aggressive volume resuscitation. As a result, elimination of some drugs by the kidney and liver may be decreased. Next, the hyperdynamic phase leads to increased cardiac output and blood flow to the kidneys and liver, meaning increased clearance of drugs dependent on organ blood flow for elimination.[16]

PHARMACOLOGIC MANAGEMENT

Oral nonsteroidal anti-inflammatory drugs (NSAIDs) and acetaminophen are mild analgesics that exhibit a ceiling effect in their dose-response relationship. Such limitations render these agents unsuitable for the treatment of typical, severe burn pain. Oral NSAIDs and acetaminophen are of benefit in treating minor burns, usually in the outpatient setting. For hospitalized patients with burn injuries, opioids are the cornerstone of pharmacologic pain control.[1] Opioids are inexpensive, widely available, and familiar to most clinicians. Opioid requirements are increased in patients with burn injuries and may far exceed standard dosing recommendations; therefore, tolerance is a challenge throughout burn care.[16] Patient-controlled analgesia (PCA) with intravenous opioids is a safe and efficient method of achieving flexible analgesia in burn-injured patients.[1] Studies comparing PCA with other routes of administration have shown mixed results as to benefit and patient satisfaction.[7] Although opioids delivered via oral and intravenous routes are a mainstay of burn pain treatment, it is important to note that pharmacokinetic changes have been documented for morphine, fentanyl, and propofol throughout the hyperdynamic and

hypermetabolic stages of burn recovery.[19] Animal studies of burn injury have shown changes in spinal cord receptors, including downregulation of μ opioid receptors, and upregulation of protein kinase C (PKC)-γ and N-methyl-D-aspartate (NMDA) receptors.[20] Therefore, ketamine requirements to anesthetize patients with burn injuries also may be increased.[16] For patients with burn injuries who develop extreme tolerance to morphine, treatment with clonidine, dexmedetomidine, ketamine, and methadone has been found to be effective.[21,22] Dexmedetomidine has been used to provide sedation–analgesia for burned patients and to decrease opioid requirements.[23,24] Titration of dexmedetomidine may also allow weaning of benzodiazepine, as patients get close to extubation. Dexmedetomidine has been shown to result in less delirium than benzodiazepines in several critical care studies.

Ketamine has many potential advantages for induction and maintenance of anesthesia in patients with burn injuries.[16] Ketamine is associated with hemodynamic stability, preserving airway patency as well as hypoxic and hypercapnic responses, and decreasing airway resistance; therefore, ketamine may be the agent of choice, particularly in scenarios in which airway manipulation is to be avoided.[16] Intensive dressing changes at the bedside, removal of hundreds of staples, or other procedures requiring conscious sedation are examples in which ketamine might be the agent of choice. Administration of benzodiazepines along with ketamine can reduce dysphoria, and coadministered glycopyrrolate can reduce the severity of increased secretions associated with ketamine. Burned patients receiving ketamine must be closely monitored for myocardial depressant affects, however, because persistently high levels of catecholamines results in desensitization and downregulation of β-adrenoreceptors in these patients.[16] Additionally, patients with prior drug use might experience distressing anxiety with ketamine use.

Anxiety is a common issue for burn-injured patients and may be closely linked to pain. Background pain and the anticipation of procedural pain exacerbates anxiety, which can in turn exacerbate the pain.[7] Anxiolytic drugs have commonly been used in conjunction with opioids in the treatment of burn pain.[1] When administered as an adjunct to opioids, benzodiazepines have been shown to decrease both background pain and pain in those patients with high levels of procedural pain.[1] Furthermore, low-dose benzodiazepine administration may reduce burn wound care pain reports.[1] Patients with high anticipatory procedural anxiety and high levels of pain are most likely to benefit from anxiolytic therapy.[7] However, benzodiazepine use, as in other critical care populations, can lead to short-term and long-term delirium. Antipsychotic medications (eg, haloperidol and quetiapine) also are good options and are increasingly used for management of anxiety and agitation associated with burns. Antidepressants appear to enhance opiate-induced analgesia, especially in patients with chronic (neuropathic) pain.[16]

INTRAOPERATIVE MANAGEMENT AND REGIONAL ANESTHESIA

In addition to anesthetic concerns, intraoperative management of burned patients may demand special attention to airway access, vascular access, monitoring, and ventilator management, all of which may be affected by the severity and location of a patient's burn. Facial burns, increased risk of infection from vascular access, profound fluid shifts, and dynamic pharmacokinetic changes during the acute injury phase make intraoperative management of burned patients particularly challenging. If muscle relaxants are given intraoperatively, succinylcholine should not be administered within the first 48 hours of injury due to the risk of exaggerated hyperkalemic response in burned patients.[25] Decreased sensitivity to the neuromuscular effects of nondepolarizing muscle relaxants (NDMRs) also has been observed in this population; therefore, the dosage of NDMRs needed to achieve desired paralysis may be substantially increased in burned patients.[16] Rocuronium and atracurium also demonstrate somewhat reduced effectiveness in burned patients and may require increased dosing as well.[16] Choice of anesthetic should be determined by the hemodynamics, pulmonary status, and predicted difficulty of securing an airway. The choice of volatile anesthetic is not thought to change outcome in burned patients. However, if propofol is chosen as the agent for induction or sedation, then the operative team must be aware that clearance and volume of distribution may be markedly increased.[16] Therefore, patients with major burn injuries may require larger bolus doses and/or increased infusion rates of propofol intraoperatively.[16]

Regional anesthesia has an important role in the intraoperative management of patients with burn injuries, not only because it provides anesthesia in the operating room, but also because it can offer postoperative pain control and facilitates rehabilitation. Regional anesthesia should be considered for both burn wound pain and donor site pain. If both burn and donor sites are on the same extremity, regional anesthesia can be considered. Lateral femoral cutaneous nerve blocks also can be used to improve thigh donor site pain.

Tumescent local anesthesia injected into a donor site before harvesting, subcutaneous catheter infusions, peripheral nerve, and central neuraxial blocks may all have roles in the regional management of burn pain. The use of epidural analgesia has been limited in the burn population because of the potential for increased risk of infection and colonization that has been associated with indwelling vascular access. Therefore, caution should be exercised in selecting appropriate patients with burn injuries who might benefit from central neuroaxial blockade.[16] Truncal blocks can be very advantageous for donor site harvesting. The lateral femoral cutaneous nerve block is particularly well suited for this approach because it is exclusively a sensory nerve and innervates the lateral thigh, which is a donor site for split-thickness skin grafts.[16]

STRATEGIES FOR WEANING VENTILATOR

Weaning the ventilator while maintaining appropriate pain control is one of the most challenging aspects of burn care. Historically, patients with burn injuries would remain intubated and sedated for weeks to months during their burn care, negating the need to titrate pain medications. With obvious improved outcomes with the push for daily spontaneous breathing trials, early extubation, and ambulation in multiple surgical critical care populations, patients with burn injuries also have benefited from more rapid extubation. Concurrently, transitioning patients with burn injuries off the high doses of pain medications and need for analgesia can be challenging. In general, patients who are expected to be extubated within the first 48 hours of admission might tolerate propofol. However, as mentioned previously, propofol can cause hypotension, and high doses may be required given the high fluid resuscitation in patients with burn injuries. Additionally, triglycerides must be monitored for high doses. If patients are expected to be on the ventilator for longer than 48 hours, as is seen in inhalation injuries, fentanyl and midazolam (Versed) is often titrated. As mentioned previously, dexmedetomidine can be added to help wean Versed as the patient gets closer to extubation. Seroquel also serves as a helpful adjunct when beginning to wean benzodiazepine.

HRONIC PAIN MANAGEMENT

ensitivity to analgesics can fluctuate over the ourse of burn injury and recovery, with periods f increased sensitivity acutely followed by toler- nce in the long term. Opioid-induced hyperalge- ia is a complication that may result from the ontinuous administration of analgesics, there- ore creating a cycle of increased opioid dosing nd tolerance. Methadone is a synthetic opioid rug that has both a long and predictable dura- on of action, making this drug a favorable drug or chronic pain management in the burn patient opulation. Because methadone exerts its anal- esic effect not only through opiate receptor inding but also through a weaker pain modula- on at spinal NMDA receptors, it can be a stra- egic drug choice when making an opioid witch in patients with burn injuries.[10] Neuro- athic pain also is an important consideration in oth healed and unhealed burn wounds. Gaba- entin is an agent that has been studied in both ne acute and chronic management of burn ain. The use of gabapentin as an adjunct to tandard analgesia has shown reduction in the everity of neuropathic pain in limited studies of atients with burn injuries and burn injury nodels.[26,27] However, recent data from a ran- omized, double-blind, placebo-controlled study nowed that the use of gabapentin in acute burn ain management did not decrease pain scores r lessen opioid requirements.[28] Antidepressants nd clonidine also have been proposed as poten- al analgesic options for chronic burn pain, but ave not been studied extensively. Further esearch into long-term opioid management and nonopioid adjuncts for chronic burn pain anal- gesia is needed.

NONPHARMACOLOGIC APPROACHES

Hypnosis, cognitive behavioral techniques, and distraction approaches are examples of nonphar- mocologic strategies that have been studied in burn populations. The use of hypnosis for the treatment of procedural pain and anxiety has growing evidence for its effectiveness.[29] Virtual re- ality systems also have been studied and shown some promise in procedural pain control, but may not be practical in certain clinical set- tings.[30,31] Multidisciplinary interventions from psychologists, physiotherapists, and pain man- agement specialists can contribute greatly to the burn patient's recovery. Early introduction to these support mechanisms alongside multimodal thera- peutic approaches may reduce overall anxiety, thereby mitigating the experience of pain in the re- covery from a burn wound.

STANDARDIZATION AND GUIDELINES

Standardized pain and anxiety guidelines are used in many burn centers to ensure appropriate and consistent patient comfort. Ideally, pain manage- ment guidelines should ensure safety and efficacy over a broad range of burn severities while providing clear recommendations for drug selection, dosing, and titration. Frequent reassessment of pain and anxiety levels can safeguard against inadequate treatment of pain in the burn unit. Bittner and colleagues[16] have proposed the following guidelines for sedation and analgesia in acute burns:

Stage of Injury	Background Anxiety	Background Pain	Procedural Anxiety	Procedural Pain
Acute burn ventilated	#1 Midazolam infusion	Morphine infusion	Midazolam boluses	Morphine boluses
	#2 Dexmedetomidine infusion	Morphine infusion	Dexmedetomidine higher infusion rate	Morphine boluses
	#3 Antipsychotics	Morphine infusion	Haloperidol (very slow) boluses	Morphine boluses
	#4 Propofol infusion (<48 h)	Morphine infusion	Propofol boluses	Morphine boluses
Acute burn not ventilated	Dexmedetomidine IV, scheduled lorazepam IV or PO	Morphine IV or PO	Lorazepam IV/PO	Morphine IV/PO or ketamine IV
Chronic acute burn	Scheduled lorazepam or antipsychotics (PO)	Scheduled morphine or methadone	Lorazepam or antipsychotics (PO)	Morphine PO or oxycodone

entanyl infusions could be substituted for morphine infusions. In view of the increased incidence of delirium with ben- odiazepines, minimal use of them is advocated.
Abbreviations: IV, intravenous; PO, per oram (by mouth).

SUMMARY

Although pain management is a major challenge for clinicians, good pain control is the foundation of efficacious burn care from initial injury to long-term recovery. The very treatments designed to treat burn wounds may inflict more pain that the initial injury itself, making it the clinician's duty to embrace a multimodal treatment approach to burn pain. Vigilant pain assessment, meaningful understanding of the pathophysiology and pharmacologic considerations across different phases of burn injury, and compassionate attention to anxiety and other psychosocial contributors to pain will enhance the clinician's ability to provide excellent pain management.

REFERENCES

1. Patterson DR, Hofland HW, Espey K, et al. Pain management. Burns 2004;30:A10–5.
2. Raymond I, Ancoli-Israel S, Choiniere M. Sleep disturbances, pain and analgesia in adults hospitalized for burn injuries. Sleep Med 2004;5:551–9.
3. Christian LM, Graham JE, Padgett DA, et al. Stress and wound healing. Neuroimmunomodulation 2006; 13:337–46.
4. Patterson DR, Carrigan K, Questad KA, et al. Posttraumatic stress disorder in hospitalized patients with burn injuries. J Burn Care Rehabil 1990;11:181–4.
5. Saxe GN, Stoddard F, Hall E, et al. Pathways to PTSD, part 1: children with burns. Am J Psychiatry 2005;162:1299–304.
6. Brown NJ, Kimble RM, Gramotnev G, et al. Predictors of re-epithelialization in pediatric burn. Burns 2014;40(4):751–8.
7. Faucher LD, Furukawa K. Practice guidelines for the management of pain. J Burn Care Rehabil 2006;27:659–68.
8. Meyer WJ III, Wiechman SA, Woodson L, et al. Chapter 64. Management of pain and other discomforts in burned patients. In: Herndon DN, editor. Total burn care. 4th edtion. Philadelphia: Saunders Elsevier; 2012. p. 715.
9. Choiniere M, Melzack R, Rondeau J, et al. The pain of burns: characteristics and correlates. J Trauma 1989;29:1531–9.
10. Richardson P, Mustard L. The management of pain in the burns unit. Burns 2009;35(7):921–36.
11. Tracey I. Imaging pain. Br J Anaesth 2008;101:32–9.
12. Patterson DR, Sharar SR. Burn pain. In: Fishman SM, Ballantyne JC, Rathmell JP, editors. Bonica's management of pain. 4th edition. Philadelphia: Lippincott Williams and Wilkins; 2010. p. 754.
13. Wibbenmeyer L, Sevier A, Liao J, et al. Evaluation of the usefulness of two established pain assessment tools in a burn population. J Burn Care Res 2011;32:52.
14. Williamson A, Hoggart B. Pain: a review of three commonly used pain rating scales. J Clin Nurs 2005;14:798–804.
15. Fishman SM, Ballantyne JC, Rathmell JP, editors. Bonica's management of pain, 4th edition. Philadelphia: Lippincott Williams and Wilkins; 2010. p. 754.
16. Bittner EA, Shank E, Woodson L, et al. Acute and perioperative care of the burn-injured patient. Anesthesiology 2015;122(2):448–64.
17. Cuthbertson DP. Postshock metabolic response. Lancet 1942;239:433–7.
18. Blancet B, Jullien V, Vinsonneau C, et al. Influence of burns on pharmacokinetics and pharmacodynamics of drugs used in the care of burn patients. Clin Pharmacokinet 2008;47:635–54.
19. Han T, Harmatz JS, Greenblatt DJ, et al. Fentanyl clearance and volume of distribution are increased in patients with major burns. J Clin Pharmaco 2009;47:674–80.
20. Wang S, Zhang L, Ma Y, et al. Nociceptive behavior following hindpaw burn injury in young rats: response to systemic morphine. Pain Med 2011;12:87–98.
21. Kariya N, Shindoh M, Nishi S, et al. Oral clonidine for sedation and analgesia in a burn patient. J Clin Anesth 1998;10:514–7.
22. Williams PI, Sarginson RE, Ratcliffe JM. Use of methadone in the morphine-tolerant burned paediatric patient. Br J Anaesth 1998;80:92–5.
23. Walker J, MacCallum M, Fischer C, et al. Sedation using dexmedetomidine in pediatric burn patients. J Burn Care Res 2006;27:206–10.
24. Lin H, Faraklas I, Sampson C, et al. Use of dexmedetomidine for sedation in critically ill mechanically ventilated pediatric burn patients. J Burn Care Res 2001;32:98–103.
25. Martyn JA, Richtsfeld M. Succinylcholine induced hyperkalemia in acquired pathologic states. Anesthesiology 2006;1004:158–69.
26. Gray P, Williams B, Cramon T. Successful use of gabapentin in acute pain management following burn injury: a case series. Pain Med 2008;9(3):371–6.
27. Dirks J, Petersen KL, Rowbotham MC, et al. Gabapentin suppresses cutaneous hyperalgesia following heat-capsaicin sensitization. Anesthesiology 2002;97(1):102–7.
28. Wibbenmeyer L, Eid A, Liao J, et al. Gabapentin is ineffective as an analgesic adjunct in the immediate postburn period. J Burn Care Res 2014;35(2):136–42.
29. Lynn SJ. Hypnosis and the treatment of posttraumatic conditions: an evidence-based approach. Int J Clin Exp Hypn 2007;55(2):167–88.
30. Hoffman HG, Patterson DR, Carrougher GJ. Use of virtual reality for adjunctive treatment of adult burn pain during physical therapy. Clin J Pain 2000;16(3):244–50.
31. Hoffman HG, Patterson DR, Seibel E, et al. Virtual reality pain control during burn wound debridement in the hydrotank. Clin J Pain 2008;24(4):299–304.

Metabolic and Endocrine Considerations After Burn Injury

Felicia N. Williams, MD[a], David N. Herndon, MD[b],*

KEYWORDS

- Hypermetabolism • Hypercatabolism • Insulin resistance • Propranolol • Oxandrolone • Nutrition
- Catecholamines

KEY POINTS

- Severe burn injury results in a significant and persistent hypermetabolic response.
- The hypermetabolic, hypercatabolic response is mediated by catecholamines, glucagon, and cortisol.
- Patients have supraphysiologic metabolic rates, heart rates, and full-body catabolism that persist for years postburn.
- There are multiple pharmacologic and nonpharmacologic modalities that help mitigate the postburn response and prevent physiologic exhaustion.

INTRODUCTION

Severe thermal injury, defined as burns encompassing more than 30% of a patient's total body surface area (TBSA), is followed by a marked and persistent hypermetabolic response. The response is propagated by plasma catecholamines, glucagon, cortisol, and proinflammatory mediators. Physiologic changes are seen with these injuries for years postburn.[1–3] The response is characterized by full-body catabolism, muscle protein degradation, increased metabolic rates, stunted growth, insulin resistance, increased risk for infection, and multiorgan dysfunction.[2–6]

Following any significant injury, there is a compensatory decrease in tissue perfusion and a decrease in metabolic rate: the ebb state. Subsequently, there is a hyperdynamic state characterized by increases in metabolism, and hyperdynamic circulation: the flow state. In severe burns, the "ebb" phase lasts up to 72 hours after injury.

The subsequent magnified "flow" phase in severe burns can be limitless in time and physiologic consequence. When left untreated, physiologic exhaustion ensues, and the injury becomes fatal.[7–10]

Understanding of this response to severe burn injury, advances in critical care management, and infection control in the last two decades has significantly improved morbidity for burn survivors. This article comprehensively describes the gamut of physiologic changes after major burn injury and discusses the effects of various pharmacologic and nonpharmacologic interventions discovered to mitigate the hypermetabolic response (**Table 1**). Numerous therapies imparted to modify this catastrophic response and improve care, quality of life and survival have emerged in the past 50 years, including early excision and grafting; thermoregulation; early continuous enteral feeding with a high-carbohydrate high-protein diet; the use of anabolic agents, such as growth

[a] Department of Surgery, North Carolina Jaycee Burn Center, University of North Carolina, Chapel Hill, 3007D Burnett Womack Building, CB 7206, Chapel Hill, NC 27599-7206, USA; [b] Department of Surgery, Shriners Hospital of Children, University of Texas Medical Branch, 815 Market Street, Galveston, TX 77550, USA
* Corresponding author.
E-mail address: dherndon@utmb.edu

Clin Plastic Surg 44 (2017) 541–553
http://dx.doi.org/10.1016/j.cps.2017.02.013
0094-1298/17/© 2017 Elsevier Inc. All rights reserved.

Table 1
Summary of the main effects of various pharmacologic interventions to alter the hypermetabolic response to burn injury

Drug	Inflammatory Response	Stress Hormones	Body Composition	Net Protein Balance	Insulin Resistance	Hyperdynamic Circulation	Metabolic Rate
Recombinant growth hormone	Improved	No difference	Improved	No difference	Hyperglycemia	No difference	Improved
Insulinlike growth factor-1	Improved	No difference	Improved	Improved	Improved	No difference	Unknown
Oxandrolone	Improved	No difference	Improved	Improved	No difference	No difference	Improved
Insulin	Improved	No difference	Improved	Improved	Improved	No difference	Improved
Fenofibrate	No difference	No difference	No difference	No difference	Improved	No difference	Unknown
Glucagonlike peptide-1	Unknown	Unknown	Unknown	Unknown	Improved (indirect)	Unknown	Unknown
Propranolol	Improved	Improved	Improved	Improved	Improved	Improved	Improved
Ketoconazole	Unknown	Improved	Unknown	Unknown	Unknown	Unknown	No difference
Recombinant growth hormone + propranolol	Improved	Improved	Improved	Improved	Improved	Improved	Improved
Oxandrolone + propranolol	Improved (preliminary)	Improved (preliminary)	Improved (preliminary)	Improved (preliminary)	Improved (preliminary)	Improved (preliminary)	Improved

The data summarized in the table are extrapolated from previously published data.[1,5,11,16,17,25,80–103,116–122,129–165] ormone, insulinlike growth factor-1 (IGF-1), insulnlike growth factor binding protein-3 (IGFBP-3), insulin, oxandrolone, and propranolol; and these of therapeutic exercise.

Mediators of the Hypermetabolic Response

Catecholamines and corticosteroids are the primary mediators of the hypermetabolic response following burns greater than 30% TBSA.[11,12] There is up to a 50-fold surge of plasma catecholamine and corticosteroid levels that last up to months postburn.[13,14] Burn patients have increased cardiac work, increased resting energy expenditures, increased myocardial oxygen consumption, marked tachycardia, severe lipolysis, hepatic dysfunction, full-body catabolism, increased protein degradation, insulin resistance, and growth retardation.[15–18]

Genomic and Proteomic Changes to Burn Injury

After severe burn injury, considerable changes occur in every aspect of the human genome. These changes are immediate and persistent. The genetic response to this injury is so massive, there is no discrimination between desirable or undesirable effects of change. There is significant up-regulation of the innate immune response and down-regulation of the adaptive immune response.[19,20]

Acute Phase Proteins (Cytokines and Hormonal Changes)

Proinflammatory cytokine levels peak immediately after burn, approaching normal levels only at 90 to 180 days postburn.[13] Serum hormones, constitutive, and acute phase proteins are significantly deranged throughout acute hospital stay. Serum IGF-1, IGFBP-3, parathyroid hormone, and osteocalcin drop immediately after the injury and remain decreased compared with normal levels until 0 days postburn.[13] Sex hormones and endogenous growth hormone levels decrease around 1 days postburn and remain low.[13] Larger burn injuries are characterized by more pronounced and persistent inflammatory responses indicated by higher concentrations of proinflammatory cytokines that promote more severe catabolism.[21]

Changes in Resting Energy Expenditures

Past studies showed metabolic rates of burn patients approaching 180% of that of predicted based on the Harris-Benedict equation.[22] The resting metabolic rate of patients with large burns increases from normal predicted levels for TBSA less than 10% to twice that of normal predicted levels at 40% TBSA and higher. For severely burned patients, the resting metabolic rate at thermal neutral temperature (30°C) tops 140% of predicted basal rate on admission, reduces to 130% once the wounds are fully healed, then to 120% at 180 days after injury.[13] Even 1 year postburn, the resting energy expenditures for burn patients are persistently elevated from predicted, based on the Harris-Benedict equation.[2] The persistent muscle protein wasting from increases in catabolism result in decreased immune defenses, decreased wound healing, increased risk for pneumonia and other infections, and risk of death.[2,23]

Multiorgan Dysfunction

Multiorgan dysfunction is a trademark of the acute phase response postburn.[13] Immediately postburn, patients have low cardiac outputs, and low contractility, characteristic of early shock.[24] However, 3 days postburn, cardiac outputs and heart rates are greater than 150% compared with non-burned patients.[13,17] Postburn, patients have increased cardiac work that lasts well into the convalescence.[25,26] Myocardial oxygen consumption values are significantly increased well after discharge.[25] The liver increases significantly in size by 2 weeks postburn and remains increased twice normal.[13]

Whole-Body Catabolism

Postburn, muscle protein is degraded much faster than it is synthesized.[13,17] This leads to loss of lean body mass, and severe muscle wasting leading to decreased strength and failure to fully rehabilitate.[2,27] Profound degradation of lean body mass secondary to chronic illness or hypermetabolism, hypercatabolic states, leads to immune dysfunction, decreased wound healing, pressure sores, pneumonia, and death.[23] Severely burned, catabolic patients can lose up to 25% of total body mass after acute burn injury.[28] The persistent and pervasive muscle wasting persists up to 9 months after burn injury resulting in significant negative whole-body catabolism,[26,29,30] and is directly related to increases in metabolic rate.[29] Severely burned patients have a daily nitrogen loss of 20 to 25 g/m² of burned skin.[26,31] At this rate, a fatal loss is reached in less than 30 days.[31] This protein catabolism leads to significant growth retardation for up to 24 months postinjury.[4]

Changes in Glucose Metabolism

Elevated circulating levels of catecholamines, glucagon, and cortisol in response to severe thermal injury perpetuate inefficient glucose production in the liver.[32] This inefficiency is supported by stable isotope data demonstrating significant derangements in major ATP consumption pathways including urea production, increased protein turnover, and gluconeogenesis.[6] Glycolytic-gluconeogenetic cycling is increased 2.5 times during the postburn hypermetabolic response coupled with an increase of 4.5 times in triglyceride–fatty acid cycling.[6] All of these changes cumulate into impaired insulin sensitivity and severe hyperglycemia related to postreceptor insulin resistance.[6,13] After injury, there are significantly elevated levels of fasting glucose, insulin, and significant reductions in glucose clearance.[5] Despite having restricted glucose oxidation, glucose delivery to peripheral tissues is increased up to three-fold, leading to the elevated levels of fasting glucose. Increased glucose production is directed to support anaerobic metabolism of endothelial cells, fibroblasts, and inflammatory cells in the burn wound.[33,34] Lactate, the end-product of the aforementioned anaerobic glucose oxidation pathway, is inefficient in providing glucose to the liver to produce more via the gluconeogenic pathway.[26] Serum glucose and serum insulin remain significantly increased through the entire acute hospital stay.[13] Insulin resistance appears during the first week postburn and persists for up to 3 years after injury.[1,13]

Sepsis

Complications and/or physiologic derangements, such as sepsis, further increase resting energy expenditures and protein catabolism up to 40% compared with those with like-size burns that do not develop sepsis.[2,35] The immediate and persistent changes in the innate and adaptive immune system postinjury make them more susceptible to sepsis, and thus at increased risk of further muscle and protein catabolism, propagating a vicious cycle.[2,11,20] The emergence of multiresistant organisms has led to increases in sepsis-related infections and death overall.[36,37] In combination, these responses lead to an increase in morbidity and mortality for victims of severe burn injury, compelling health care providers to secure therapeutic strategies to temper the often catastrophic response.

MODULATION OF THE HYPERMETABOLIC RESPONSE IN SEVERE BURNS
Early Excision and Grafting

The body's response to severe burn injury is unlike any other disease state and far exceeds other catabolic, physiologic, and immunologic changes seen.[38] One of the most innovative and constructive modifications of burn care was the institution of early excision and grafting of the burn eschar postburn injury.[39,40] As a testament to the physiologic consequence of large burns, burns larger than 50% TBSA have a subsequent 40% decrease in metabolic rate if excised completely and grafted within 3 days of injury compared with those patients with like-size burns excised and grafted 7 days after injury.[29] The process prevents further net muscle protein degradation and full-body catabolism. By waiting 3 weeks for full excision, patients had more than double the net muscle protein loss measured by stable isotope and 140% increase in log bacterial counts in quantitative tissue cultures. The incidence of sepsis in the "traditional" 3-week group was 2.5 times higher than the early excision and grafting group.[29,41] The ramifications of this modification are enormous: it mitigates exorbitant resting energy expenditures and limits muscle protein catabolism improving morbidity and mortality.[2,23,29,36,3]

Thermoregulation

Thermoregulation is the natural ability of the body to maintain core body temperature independent of environmental temperature and is mediated via metabolic activity and sweating.[42] The ability to regulate core body temperatures is lost in severely burned patients. To complicate matters, there is an exhaustive loss of heat and fluid loss secondary to large burns. Metabolic rates are significantly increased in severe burns to compensate for this loss, nearly 4000 mL/m^2 burn area per day.[43–4] This response is propagated by increased ATP consumption and substrate oxidation. This action and response is analogous to cold acclimatization and raises core and skin temperatures 2°C higher than normal compared with unburned patients.[4] Patients that do not and cannot mount this response likely have sepsis and/or have exhausted physiologic capabilities to maintain needed body temperature.[48] To mitigate fluid and heat losses and the metabolic response, by increasing ambient temperatures to 33°C (a thermal neutral temperature) the energy required for vaporization is derived from the environment rather than from the patient.[49,50] This decreases resting energy expenditures, and muscle protein catabolism, and improves outcomes.

Nutrition

Another important modulator of the hypermetabolic response is early enteral feeding.[51,52] If left with only oral alimentation, patients with severe burns lose 25% of their preadmission weight by 3 weeks postinjury.[28] Nutritional replacement using 25 kcal/kg body weight in addition to 40 kcal per percent TBSA burn per day can maintain body weight in burned adults.[53,54] In general, children require 1800 kcal/m² plus 2200 kcal/m² of burn area per day.[55]

Enteral nutrition reduces bacterial translocation and sepsis. It maintains gut motility, and preserves first pass nutrient delivery to the liver.[52] Parenteral nutrition alone or even in combination with enteral nutrition leads to liver failure, overfeeding, impaired immune response, and increased mortality.[56–58] Parenteral nutrition should be reserved for those with prolonged ileus and or enteral feeding intolerance.

Analogous to resuscitative formulas, formulas used to predict total caloric requirements often provide about 40% more calories than actually needed.[53–55,59] Actual caloric requirements are determined by measuring resting energy expenditures.[60,61] Appropriate nutrient delivery is accomplished by feeding 1.4 times measured resting energy expenditures measured by indirect calorimetry using bedside carts. Feeding patients 1.2 times measured resting energy expenditures resulted in a loss of 10% of lean body mass, but maintained body weight.[60] This increases risks for immune dysfunction.[23] Feeding patients more than 1.4 times the resting energy expenditure there were gains in body weight but they were in fat deposition, not lean body mass.[61,62] Specifically, by overfeeding carbohydrates in burn patients, there is increased fat synthesis, elevated respiratory quotients, and increased elimination of carbon dioxide. Management of ventilated patients becomes more arduous[63]; there is steatosis[64] and hyperglycemia.[12,65]

Burn patients have essential protein requirements 50% greater than healthy individuals in a fasting state[66–68]: 1.5 to 2 g/kg body weight per day.[69–71] The increased protein requirement is to maintain or even increase lean body mass. Higher supplementation of protein leads to increased urea production without improvements in lean body mass or muscle protein synthesis.[72]

The nutritional needs of burn patients are extensive because of the insufficient glycogen stores, increased metabolic rates, and increased muscle protein catabolism. Research has led to dramatic improvements in net protein balance and metabolic rates. In general, diets high in fat demonstrated elevated protein degradation and poor lean body mass gains in comparison with high-carbohydrate diets, which did show the diet increased endogenous insulin production and improved lean body mass, and increased muscle protein synthesis.[17,55,59,73] No studies have shown improvement in survival.[74]

Exercise

The postburn hypermetabolic, hypercatabolic response persists long after the acute hospitalization. Early exicision and grafting, thermoregulation, and early enteral nutrition attenuate the response during the acute phase. Some patients have elevated metabolic rates and sustained muscle and protein catabolism up to 1 year after the original insult.[17,32,75] Growth retardation lasts long into the rehabilitative phase.[4] Burn survivors can often have significant functional limitations and deficits for years. Exercise training is an essential adjunct to any and all metabolic treatments. It increases endurance, strength, and lean body mass, and improves overall cardiopulmonary capacity.[76,77] Resistance and aerobic exercise training programs profoundly improve power, muscle strength, and lean body mass.[78,79]

MODIFYING THE HORMONAL RESPONSE IN SEVERE BURNS

Nonpharmacologic techniques are incapable of reversing hypermetabolic response after severe burn injury. The response is prolonged, the gravity of which is directly related to the size of the original injury.[29] Catecholamines, cortisol, proinflammatory cytokines, and hormones perpetuate the profound changes in metabolic rates, growth, and physiology seen in severely burned patients. Thus, pharmacologic agents to block or reverse mediators of the hypermetabolic response are required to halt the hypercatabolic state.

Recombinant Human Growth Hormone

Full-body catabolism is one of the hallmarks of the hypermetabolic response to severe burn injury. The underlying mechanisms responsible for severe muscle atrophy are not fully understood. One established mechanism is a decrease in the endogenous hormone IGF-1, which is responsible for anabolic properties in adults and growth in children. Levels of IGF-1 are significantly reduced after severe burn injury.[11,80] Growth hormone, which used to be extracted from pituitary glands of corpses to treat children with growth retardation, has been found to be beneficial in mitigating the reduction of IGF-1 in catabolic patients. The genetically engineered recombinant growth hormone (rhGH) in use today increases the release of IGF-1. Other anabolic effects consist of increasing nitrogen retention, increasing cellular uptake of amino acids, and increasing protein synthesis. Because there are growth hormone receptors on epidermal cells, rhGH has beneficial effects directly on skin.[81] When administered intramuscularly to severely burned pediatric burn patients at a dose of 0.2 mg/kg/day, rhGH significantly increased endogenous levels of IGF-1 and lean body mass, and reduced donor site healing times, total cost of care, and scarring.[81–87] Larger, more adequately powered studies need to be done before this can be become standard of care.

rhGH significantly improved the immune response postinjury. It significantly decreased serum tumor necrosis factor-α, interleukin-1, serum amyloid-A, and C-reactive protein. It enhanced T-helper-1 and reduced T-helper-2 cytokine production, a consequence of burn injury that is potentially fatal in severely burned patients.[88–91] It improved the hepatic acute-phase response and increased albumin production.[88,89,92–94] There were significant improvements in weight gain, bone mineral content, height velocities, and cardiac function.[95,96] These effects were seen up to 3 years postinjury.[97,98]

The most notable side effect from the use of rhGH was hyperglycemia.[94,99] The most updated Cochrane Database analysis found no increase in mortality or sepsis. Admittedly the collective studies are not powered enough to find statistically significant results in these categories; it would be prudent for a larger more powered study to be done to comprehensively study this potential modulator.[81,94] rhGH may safely be used in pediatric burn patients to attenuate the hypermetabolic response with close monitoring to prevent adverse outcomes.

Insulinlike Growth Factor-1 and Insulinlike Growth Factor Binding Protein-3

A primary mediator of the effects of rhGH is IGF-1. Infusion of IGF-1 alone led to significant improvements in muscle protein synthesis, but also episodes of hypoglycemia.[100] In combination with equimolar doses of IGFBP-3, severely burned catabolic patients had improved protein synthesis with fewer episodes of hyperglycemia than the use of rhGH alone, and less hypoglycemia than the use of IGF-1 alone.[100–102] The combination reduced muscle and protein degradation, and improved immune function and gut mucosal integrity.[93,101,103] The combination increased serum constitutive proteins and allowed for more efficient use of whole-body protein.[93,103] The risk of side effects of hypoglycemia and peripheral neuropathies with the use of IGF-1 was noteworthy but there were none noted with the combination of modulators.[93,101,103]

Oxandrolone

Under normal circumstances protein synthesis and protein degradation are in homeostasis. When that balance is lost, as in times of exhaustive stress, there is a deluge of amino acids from skeletal muscle to provide substrate for immune function, wound healing, and hepatic protein synthesis.[12,104–107] Unabated, this leads to further breakdown of lean body mass, worsening immune suppression, growth retardation, and increased risk of death.[4,108,109] Prolonged muscle protein loss is a hallmark of the hypermetabolic postburn response. The severe burn also perpetuates an environment with decreased androgen hormone available. Testicular steroid production is substantially decreased in severely burned male patients and is prolonged.[110–112] The elevated levels of cortisol coupled with the decreased levels of testosterone further contribute to the loss of lean body mass.[113] Testosterone is a known anabolic steroid that increases lean body mass and stimulates muscle protein synthesis by increasing the efficiency of amino acids derived from muscle protein breakdown, making testosterone an ideal modulator for this response.[114,115] However, side effects of hepatotoxicity and virilizing effects make it prohibitive. An analogue (oxandrolone) has been approved to use in chronic wasting syndromes and has minimal side effects, making it safe for both genders.[116] Oxandrolone therapy improved net muscle protein synthesis and protein metabolism in severely burned patients.[117,118] It increases lean body mass gains, bone mineral content, bone mineral density, and muscle strength, and improved height velocity.[116,118–120] Oxandrolone therapy increases gene expression for functional muscle proteins.[119,121] Specifically, it increased anabolic gene expression in skeletal muscle and enhanced the efficacy of net protein synthesis.[119] Follow-up studies published this year are showing sustained improvements in body composition when oxandrolone was administered up to 2 years after injury.[120] Improvements in gene expression, body composition, and protein synthesis, outweigh the 1% risk of hirsutism and potential hepatic dysfunction that are seen with treatment.[116,118,119,122]

Insulin

There is enhanced glycogenolysis, proteolysis, and lipolysis after severe burn. Mediated by catecholamines, glucagon and glucocorticoid surges after injury glycogenolysis and protein breakdown occur in the liver and skeletal muscle.[70] There is a subsequent increase in triglycerides, urea, and glucose (gluconeogenesis) leading to hyperglycemia. Hyperglycemia in the severely burned patient leads to further muscle protein catabolism; reduced graft take; and increased risk for fection, morbidity, and mortality.[123,124] Catecholamines alter glucose disposal via derangements of the insulin signaling pathway and glucose transporter-4 translocation in muscle. This results in peripheral insulin resistance.[1] Insulin resistance postburn lasts 3 years and significantly contributes to devastating inefficient substrate use, immunosuppression, hyperglycemia, and worsening full-body catabolism.[1,125,126] For all critically ill patients, hyperglycemia leads to poorer outcomes. The optimal blood glucose levels and how to achieve those levels are still being evaluated in the literature. The landmark study by van den Berghe and colleagues[127] showed that intensive insulin therapy to achieve blood glucose levels between 80 and 110 mL/dL in the critically ill reduces morbidity and mortality in the patient population studied. When attempts were made to duplicate this study for other patient populations, specifically for burned patients, results were different. Although improving body composition, hypoglycemic episodes increased length of stay and mortality.[128] By infusing insulin therapy to maintain blood glucose levels less than 140 mL/dL outcomes were significantly improved including lean body mass, bone mineral density, decreased donor site healing time, and decreased length of hospital stay.[126,128–132] Insulin exerts its anabolic effect by increasing glucose uptake in tissues by activating the sodium-dependent transport systems, increasing amino acid use, and regulating proteolysis and initiation of protein translation.[127] Mechanisms by which one can accomplish these goals without episodes of hypoglycemia need to be researched to further improve outcomes and decrease insulin-resistance in this patient population.

Fenofibrate

One of the attempts to mitigate postburn hyperglycemia was to use fenofibrate, a peroxisome proliferator-activated receptor-α agonist,[133] without causing hypoglycemia. Fenofibrate treatment significantly decreased plasma glucose levels, decreased hepatic gluconeogenesis, and improved mitochondrial oxidative capacity.[134] By weeks of treatment, fenofibrate improved hepatic and muscle insulin resistance in pediatric burn patients without any notable side effects.[134]

Metformin

The use of metformin, a biguanide, has also been used to reverse the detrimental effects of hyperglycemia. It suppresses hepatic gluconeogenesis and glucose absorption by the intestines, and increases glucose use by peripheral muscles by activating AMP-activated protein kinase.[135] It does not cause hypoglycemia.[135] When given to burn patients, metformin did successfully decrease endogenous glucose production and improve glucose use, but it did not reduce muscle protein breakdown. Although there was some improvement in protein synthesis, the overall effect was minimal because it did not significantly improve muscle protein breakdown.[136–138] Its effect is primarily on improving the response of peripheral tissues to insulin, but by not reversing protein breakdown, metformin treatment may not be enough of an anabolic agent for severe burns. The side effect of lactic acidosis is also concerning for this critically ill patient population, although no studies have documented adverse outcomes.[136–138]

Glucagonlike Peptide-1 (Exenatide)

Exogenous glucagonlike peptide-1 (exenatide) reduces glucose concentration, activates incretin receptors on β-islet cells and increases insulin release in response to glucose. Its use in burn patients was to try to minimize the amount of exogenous insulin used to treat hyperglycemia in severely burned patients compared with those receiving standard of care alone to prevent hypoglycemic episodes.[139–142] Exenatide did not reverse insulin resistance but its treatment in burn patients did improve the efficiency of insulin production in response to glucose levels.[141]

β-Antagonists

The 50-fold increase in catecholamine levels after severe burn injury increases myocardial oxygen consumption, increases resting energy expenditures, and contributes greatly to the profound catabolism after severe burn injury.[12,13,38] Mitigating the effects of β-adrenergic stimulation decreases cardiac work, tachycardia, metabolic rates, and thermogenesis, allowing for gains in body composition and physiologic reserve.[25,143–145] β-Antagonist treatment reduces morbidity and mortality after severe trauma.[146] Propranolol, a nonselective β_1 and β_2 receptor antagonist, impedes the increased peripheral lipolysis in severely burned patients by blocking the activation of the β_2-adrenergic receptor.[18,144,147] It reverses hepatic dysfunction by impairing fatty infiltration of the liver postburn by inhibiting the release of free fatty acids from adipose tissue, rate of oxidation, and secretion of triacylglycerol.[148–151] Stable isotope and body composition studies showed propranolol treatment increases lean body mass and decreases skeletal muscle wasting.[17] Propranolol increased the efficiency of muscle protein synthesis by enhancing the availability of free amino acids.[17] Propranolol treatment is associated with the up-regulation of genes involved with muscle protein metabolism and down-regulation of genes involved with gluconeogenesis and insulin resistance.[152] Currently there are multicenter trials looking at the efficacy of this modulator in children and adults after severe burn injury. In the literature, there are no documented cases of bronchospasm, or cardiovascular collapse when propranolol is used in severely burned patients.

Ketoconazole

Elevated levels of cortisol contribute greatly to the immunosuppression and hypercatabolic muscle wasting subsequent to severe burn injury.[153,154] Ketoconazole, an imidazole antifungal agent, reduces the production of cortisol by inhibiting cytochrome P-450 14a-demethylase, an enzyme in the sterol biosynthesis pathway that leads from lanosterol to ergosterol.[155] It functions as a glucocorticoid receptor antagonist by inhibiting the 11β-hydroxylation and 18-hydroxylation reactions in the final steps during the synthesis of adrenocorticosteroids.[156–158] When administered to severely burned patients, there was a statistically significant decrease in urine cortisol levels, but no difference in muscle protein synthesis and breakdown compared with standard of care alone.[159] There were no changes in cathecolamines or proinflammatory cytokine levels between cohorts, which underscores the possibility that cortisol may not drive the devastating catabolism seen postburn.

A ROLE FOR COMBINATION THERAPY

The anticatabolic effect of propranolol and the potent anabolic effects of rhGH and/or oxandrolone potentiate an ideal combination for attenuating the postburn response. Although improving donor site healing, growth, and the inflammatory cascade, rhGH treatment leads to hyperglycemia, increased free fatty acids, and triglycerides. Propranolol treatment demonstrated improved fat metabolism and improvements in insulin sensitivity. In combination, improvements may be limitless in the immune response, metabolic response, and body composition without significant adverse side effects.[160,161] There are ongoing studies looking at the potential synergistic effects of any of the previously mentioned modulators of the postburn response.

SUMMARY

Because of the gains made by the interventions discussed in this article, severely burned, catabolic patients with greater than or equal to 30%

TBSA on average lose up to 10% of lean body mass, compared with 25%.[13,21] This still leads to increased morbidity. The response to injury is pervasive and prolonged and cannot be completely abolished despite pharmacologic and nonpharmacologic interventions. Alone, these interventions have helped improve morbidity and mortality, but it is the combination of nonpharmacologic and certain pharmacologic strategies that continues to advance the standard of care of severely burned patients.

REFERENCES

1. Gauglitz GG, Herndon DN, Kulp GA, et al. Abnormal insulin sensitivity persists up to three years in pediatric patients post-burn. J Clin Endocrinol Metab 2009;94:1656–64.
2. Hart DW, Wolf SE, Mlcak R, et al. Persistence of muscle catabolism after severe burn. Surgery 2000;128:312–9.
3. Reiss E, Pearson E, Artz CP. The metabolic response to burns. J Clin Invest 1956;35:62–77.
4. Rutan RL, Herndon DN. Growth delay in postburn pediatric patients. Arch Surg 1990;125:392–5.
5. Wilmore DW, Mason AD Jr, Pruitt BA Jr. Insulin response to glucose in hypermetabolic burn patients. Ann Surg 1976;183:314–20.
6. Yu YM, Tompkins RG, Ryan CM, et al. The metabolic basis of the increase of the increase in energy expenditure in severely burned patients. JPEN J Parenter Enteral Nutr 1999;23:160–8.
7. Goldstein DS, Kopin IJ. Evolution of concepts of stress. Stress 2007;10:109–20.
8. Selye H. Stress and the general adaptation syndrome. Br Med J 1950;1:1383–92.
9. Selye H. An extra-adrenal action of adrenotropic hormone. Nature 1951;168:149–50.
10. Selye H, Fortier C. Adaptive reaction to stress. Psychosom Med 1950;12:149–57.
11. Williams FN, Jeschke MG, Chinkes DL, et al. Modulation of the hypermetabolic response to trauma: temperature, nutrition, and drugs. J Am Coll Surg 2009;208:489–502.
12. Wilmore DW, Long JM, Mason AD Jr, et al. Catecholamines: mediator of the hypermetabolic response to thermal injury. Ann Surg 1974;180:653–69.
13. Jeschke MG, Chinkes DL, Finnerty CC, et al. Pathophysiologic response to severe burn injury. Ann Surg 2008;248:387–401.
14. Wilmore DW, Aulick LH. Metabolic changes in burned patients. Surg Clin North Am 1978;58:1173–87.
15. Barrow RE, Hawkins HK, Aarsland A, et al. Identification of factors contributing to hepatomegaly in severely burned children. Shock 2005;24:523–8.

16. Barrow RE, Wolfe RR, Dasu MR, et al. The use of beta-adrenergic blockade in preventing trauma-induced hepatomegaly. Ann Surg 2006;243:115–20.

17. Herndon DN, Hart DW, Wolf SE, et al. Reversal of catabolism by beta-blockade after severe burns. N Engl J Med 2001;345:1223–9.

18. Wolfe RR, Herndon DN, Peters EJ, et al. Regulation of lipolysis in severely burned children. Ann Surg 1987;206:214–21.

19. Wolf SE, Tompkins RG, Herndon DN. On the horizon: research priorities in burns for the next decade. Surg Clin North Am 2014;94:917–30.

20. Xiao W, Mindrinos MN, Seok J, et al. A genomic storm in critically injured humans. J Exp Med 2011;208:2581–90.

21. Jeschke MG, Mlcak RP, Finnerty CC, et al. Burn size determines the inflammatory and hypermetabolic response. Crit Care 2007;11:R90.

22. Dickerson RN, Gervasio JM, Riley ML, et al. Accuracy of predictive methods to estimate resting energy expenditure of thermally-injured patients. JPEN J Parenter Enteral Nutr 2002;26:17–29.

23. Chang DW, DeSanti L, Demling RH. Anticatabolic and anabolic strategies in critical illness: a review of current treatment modalities. Shock 1998;10:155–60.

24. Cuthbertson D. Post-shock metabolic response. Lancet 1942;1:433–6.

25. Baron PW, Barrow RE, Pierre EJ, et al. Prolonged use of propranolol safely decreases cardiac work in burned children. J Burn Care Rehabil 1997;18:223–7.

26. Herndon DN, Tompkins RG. Support of the metabolic response to burn injury. Lancet 2004;363:1895–902.

27. Bessey PQ, Jiang ZM, Johnson DJ, et al. Posttraumatic skeletal muscle proteolysis: the role of the hormonal environment. World J Surg 1989;13:465–71.

28. Newsome TW, Mason AD Jr, Pruitt BA Jr. Weight loss following thermal injury. Ann Surg 1973;178:215–7.

29. Hart DW, Wolf SE, Chinkes DL, et al. Determinants of skeletal muscle catabolism after severe burn. Ann Surg 2000;232:455–65.

30. Jahoor F, Desai M, Herndon DN, et al. Dynamics of the protein metabolic response to burn injury. Metabolism 1988;37:330–7.

31. Kinney JM, Long CL, Gump FE, et al. Tissue composition of weight loss in surgical patients. I. Elective operation. Ann Surg 1968;168:459–74.

32. Wolfe RR. Review: acute versus chronic response to burn injury. Circ Shock 1981;8:105–15.

33. Carter EA, Tompkins RG, Babich JW, et al. Thermal injury in rats alters glucose utilization by skin, wound, and small intestine, but not by skeletal muscle. Metabolism 1996;45:1161–7.

34. Wilmore DW, Aulick LH, Mason AD, et al. Influence of the burn wound on local and systemic responses to injury. Ann Surg 1977;186:444–58.

35. Greenhalgh DG, Saffle JR, Holmes JH, et al. American Burn Association consensus conference to define sepsis and infection in burns. J Burn Care Res 2007;28:776–90.

36. Murray CK, Loo FL, Hospenthal DR, et al. Incidence of systemic fungal infection and related mortality following severe burns. Burns 2008;34:1108–12.

37. Pruitt BA Jr, McManus AT, Kim SH, et al. Burn wound infections: current status. World J Surg 1998;22:135–45.

38. Goodall M, Stone C, Haynes BW Jr. Urinary output of adrenaline and noradrenaline in severe thermal burns. Ann Surg 1957;145:479–87.

39. Cope O, Langohr JL, Moore FD, et al. Expeditious care of full-thickness burn wounds by surgical excision and grafting. Ann Surg 1947;125:1–22.

40. Janzekovic Z. A new concept in the early excision and immediate grafting of burns. J Trauma 1970;10:1103–8.

41. Hart DW, Wolf SE, Chinkes DL, et al. Effects of early excision and aggressive enteral feeding on hypermetabolism, catabolism, and sepsis after severe burn. J Trauma 2003;54:755–64.

42. Thermoregulation. 2009. Available at: http://dictionary.reference.com/browse/thermoregulation Accessed January 13, 2009.

43. Barr PO, Birke G, Liliedal SO. The treatment of thermal burns with dry, warm air. Eksp Khir Anesteziol 1968;13:39–43 [in Russian].

44. Barr PO, Birke G, Liljedahl SO, et al. Studies on burns. X. Changes in BMR and evaporative water loss in the treatment of severe burns with warm dry air. Scand J Plast Reconstr Surg 1969;3:30–8.

45. Caldwell FT. Metabolic response to thermal trauma: II. Nutritional studies with rats at two environmental temperatures. Ann Surg 1962;155:119–26.

46. Zawacki BE, Spitzer KW, Mason AD Jr, et al. Does increased evaporative water loss cause hypermetabolism in burned patients? Ann Surg 1970;171:236–40.

47. Wolfe RR, Herndon DN, Jahoor F, et al. Effect of severe burn injury on substrate cycling by glucose and fatty acids. N Engl J Med 1987;317:403–8.

48. Lee J, Herndon DN. The pediatric burned patient. In: Herndon DN, editor. Total burn care. 3rd edition. Philadelphia: Saunders Elsevier; 2007. p. 485–93.

49. Herndon DN. Mediators of metabolism. J Trauma 1981;21:701–5.

50. Wilmore DW, Mason AD Jr, Johnson DW, et al. Effect of ambient temperature on heat production and heat loss in burn patients. J Appl Physiol 1975;38:593–7.

51. Dominioni L, Trocki O, Fang CH, et al. Enteral feeding in burn hypermetabolism: nutritional and

metabolic effects of different levels of calorie and protein intake. JPEN J Parenter Enteral Nutr 1985; 9:269–79.

52. Mochizuki H, Trocki O, Dominioni L, et al. Mechanism of prevention of postburn hypermetabolism and catabolism by early enteral feeding. Ann Surg 1984;200:297–310.

53. Curreri PW, Richmond D, Marvin J, et al. Dietary requirements of patients with major burns. J Am Diet Assoc 1974;65:415–7.

54. Wilmore DW, Curreri PW, Spitzer KW, et al. Supranormal dietary intake in thermally injured hypermetabolic patients. Surg Gynecol Obstet 1971;132: 881–6.

55. Hildreth MA, Herndon DN, Desai MH, et al. Reassessing caloric requirements in pediatric burn patients. J Burn Care Rehabil 1988;9:616–8.

56. Herndon DN, Barrow RE, Rutan RL, et al. A comparison of conservative versus early excision. Therapies in severely burned patients. Ann Surg 1989;209:547–53.

57. Herndon DN, Stein MD, Rutan TC, et al. Failure of TPN supplementation to improve liver function, immunity, and mortality in thermally injured patients. J Trauma 1987;27:195–204.

58. Jeejeebhoy KN. Total parenteral nutrition: potion or poison? Am J Clin Nutr 2001;74:160–3.

59. Hildreth MA, Herndon DN, Desai MH, et al. Caloric needs of adolescent patients with burns. J Burn Care Rehabil 1989;10:523–6.

60. Goran MI, Peters EJ, Herndon DN, et al. Total energy expenditure in burned children using the doubly labeled water technique. Am J Physiol 1990;259:E576–85.

61. Gore DC, Rutan RL, Hildreth M, et al. Comparison of resting energy expenditures and caloric intake in children with severe burns. J Burn Care Rehabil 1990;11:400–4.

62. Hart DW, Wolf SE, Herndon DN, et al. Energy expenditure and caloric balance after burn: increased feeding leads to fat rather than lean mass accretion. Ann Surg 2002;235:152–61.

63. Askanazi J, Rosenbaum SH, Hyman AI, et al. Respiratory changes induced by the large glucose loads of total parenteral nutrition. JAMA 1980;243: 1444–7.

64. Klein CJ, Stanek GS, Wiles CE 3rd. Overfeeding macronutrients to critically ill adults: metabolic complications. J Am Diet Assoc 1998;98:795–806.

65. Turina M, Fry DE, Polk HC Jr. Acute hyperglycemia and the innate immune system: clinical, cellular, and molecular aspects. Crit Care Med 2005;33: 1624–33.

66. Wolfe RR, Goodenough RD, Burke JF, et al. Response of protein and urea kinetics in burn patients to different levels of protein intake. Ann Surg 1983;197:163–71.

67. Yu YM, Ryan CM, Burke JF, et al. Relations among arginine, citrulline, ornithine, and leucine kinetics in adult burn patients. Am J Clin Nutr 1995;62:960–8.

68. Yu YM, Young VR, Castillo L, et al. Plasma arginine and leucine kinetics and urea production rates in burn patients. Metabolism 1995;44:659–66.

69. Matthews DE, Marano MA, Campbell RG. Splanchnic bed utilization of leucine and phenylalanine in humans. Am J Physiol 1993;264:E109–18.

70. Norbury WB, Herndon DN. Modulation of the hypermetabolic response after burn injury. In: Herndon DN, editor. Total burn care. 3rd edition. Philadelphia: Saunders Elsevier; 2007. p. 420–33.

71. Saffle JR, Graves C. Nutritional support of the burned patient. In: Herndon DN, editor. Total burn care. 3rd edition. Philadelphia: Saunders Elsevier; 2007. p. 398–419.

72. Patterson BW, Nguyen T, Pierre E, et al. Urea and protein metabolism in burned children: effect of dietary protein intake. Metabolism 1997;46:573–8.

73. Hart DW, Wolf SE, Zhang XJ, et al. Efficacy of a high-carbohydrate diet in catabolic illness. Crit Care Med 2001;29:1318–24.

74. Hall KL, Shahrokhi S, Jeschke MG. Enteral nutrition support in burn care: a review of current recommendations as instituted in the Ross Tilley Burn Centre. Nutrients 2012;4:1554–65.

75. Ferrando AA, Lane HW, Stuart CA, et al. Prolonged bed rest decreases skeletal muscle and whole body protein synthesis. Am J Physiol 1996;270:E627–33.

76. Celis MM, Suman OE, Huang TT, et al. Effect of a supervised exercise and physiotherapy program on surgical interventions in children with thermal injury. J Burn Care Rehabil 2003;24:57–61 [discussion: 56].

77. Cucuzzo NA, Ferrando A, Herndon DN. The effects of exercise programming vs traditional outpatient therapy in the rehabilitation of severely burned children. J Burn Care Rehabil 2001;22:214–20.

78. Neugebauer CT, Serghiou M, Herndon DN, et al. Effects of a 12-week rehabilitation program with music & exercise groups on range of motion in young children with severe burns. J Burn Care Res 2008;29:939–48.

79. Suman OE, Spies RJ, Celis MM, et al. Effects of a 12-wk resistance exercise program on skeletal muscle strength in children with burn injuries. J Appl Physiol 2001;91:1168–75.

80. Heszele MF, Price SR. Insulin-like growth factor I: the yin and yang of muscle atrophy. Endocrinology 2004;145:4803–5.

81. Breederveld RS, Tuinebreijer WE. Recombinant human growth hormone for treating burns and donor sites. Cochrane Database Syst Rev 2014;(9): CD008990.

82. Barret JP, Dziewulski P, Jeschke MG, et al. Effects of recombinant human growth hormone on the

development of burn scarring. Plast Reconstr Surg 1999;104:726–9.

83. Branski LK, Herndon DN, Barrow RE, et al. Randomized controlled trial to determine the efficacy of long-term growth hormone treatment in severely burned children. Ann Surg 2009;250:514–23.

84. Herndon DN. Nutritional and pharmacological support of the metabolic response to injury. Minerva Anestesiol 2003;69:264–74.

85. Herndon DN, Barrow RE, Kunkel KR, et al. Effects of recombinant human growth hormone on donor-site healing in severely burned children. Ann Surg 1990;212:424–31.

86. Herndon DN, Hawkins HK, Nguyen TT, et al. Characterization of growth hormone enhanced donor site healing in patients with large cutaneous burns. Ann Surg 1995;221:649–59.

87. Klein GL, Wolf SE, Langman CB, et al. Effects of therapy with recombinant human growth hormone on insulin-like growth factor system components and serum levels of biochemical markers of bone formation in children after severe burn injury. J Clin Endocrinol Metab 1998;83:21–4.

88. Jeschke MG, Chrysopoulo MT, Herndon DN, et al. Increased expression of insulin-like growth factor-I in serum and liver after recombinant human growth hormone administration in thermally injured rats. J Surg Res 1999;85:171–7.

89. Jeschke MG, Herndon DN, Wolf SE, et al. Recombinant human growth hormone alters acute phase reactant proteins, cytokine expression, and liver morphology in burned rats. J Surg Res 1999;83: 122–9.

90. Takagi K, Suzuki F, Barrow RE, et al. Recombinant human growth hormone modulates Th1 and Th2 cytokine response in burned mice. Ann Surg 1998;228:106–11.

91. Takagi K, Suzuki F, Barrow RE, et al. Growth hormone improves immune function and survival in burned mice infected with herpes simplex virus type 1. J Surg Res 1997;69:166–70.

92. Jeschke MG, Barrow RE, Herndon DN. Recombinant human growth hormone treatment in pediatric burn patients and its role during the hepatic acute phase response. Crit Care Med 2000;28:1578–84.

93. Jeschke MG, Herndon DN, Barrow RE. Insulin-like growth factor I in combination with insulin-like growth factor binding protein 3 affects the hepatic acute phase response and hepatic morphology in thermally injured rats. Ann Surg 2000;231:408–16.

94. Ramirez RJ, Wolf SE, Barrow RE, et al. Growth hormone treatment in pediatric burns: a safe therapeutic approach. Ann Surg 1998;228:439–48.

95. Hart DW, Herndon DN, Klein G, et al. Attenuation of posttraumatic muscle catabolism and osteopenia by long-term growth hormone therapy. Ann Surg 2001;233:827–34.

96. Mlcak RP, Suman OE, Murphy K, et al. Effects of growth hormone on anthropometric measurements and cardiac function in children with thermal injury. Burns 2005;31:60–6.

97. Aili Low JF, Barrow RE, Mittendorfer B, et al. The effect of short-term growth hormone treatment on growth and energy expenditure in burned children. Burns 2001;27:447–52.

98. Low JF, Herndon DN, Barrow RE. Effect of growth hormone on growth delay in burned children: a 3-year follow-up study. Lancet 1999;354:1789.

99. Singh KP, Prasad R, Chari PS, et al. Effect of growth hormone therapy in burn patients on conservative treatment. Burns 1998;24:733–8.

100. Cioffi WG, Gore DC, Rue LW 3rd, et al. Insulin-like growth factor-1 lowers protein oxidation in patients with thermal injury. Ann Surg 1994;220:310–9.

101. Herndon DN, Ramzy PI, DebRoy MA, et al. Muscle protein catabolism after severe burn: effects of IGF-1/IGFBP-3 treatment. Ann Surg 1999;229: 713–22.

102. Moller S, Jensen M, Svensson P, et al. Insulin-like growth factor 1 (IGF-1) in burn patients. Burns 1991;17:279–81.

103. Spies M, Wolf SE, Barrow RE, et al. Modulation of types I and II acute phase reactants with insulin-like growth factor-1/binding protein-3 complex in severely burned children. Crit Care Med 2002;30:83–8.

104. Biolo G, Maggi SP, Williams BD, et al. Increased rates of muscle protein turnover and amino acid transport after resistance exercise in humans. Am J Physiol 1995;268:E514–20.

105. Gore DC, Chinkes DL, Wolf SE, et al. Quantification of protein metabolism in vivo for skin, wound, and muscle in severe burn patients. JPEN J Parenter Enteral Nutr 2006;30:331–8.

106. Kien CL, Young VR, Rohrbaugh DK, et al. Increased rates of whole body protein synthesis and breakdown in children recovering from burns. Ann Surg 1978;187:383–91.

107. Wolfe RR. Regulation of skeletal muscle protein metabolism in catabolic states. Curr Opin Clin Nutr Metab Care 2005;8:61–5.

108. Pereira C, Murphy K, Jeschke M, et al. Post burn muscle wasting and the effects of treatments. Int J Biochem Cell Biol 2005;37:1948–61.

109. Pereira CT, Barrow RE, Sterns AM, et al. Age-dependent differences in survival after severe burns: a unicentric review of 1,674 patients and 179 autopsies over 15 years. J Am Coll Surg 2006;202:536–48.

110. Ferrando AA, Sheffield-Moore M, Wolf SE, et al. Testosterone administration in severe burns ameliorates muscle catabolism. Crit Care Med 2001; 29:1936–42.

111. Lephart ED, Baxter CR, Parker CR Jr. Effect of burn trauma on adrenal and testicular steroid

hormone production. J Clin Endocrinol Metab 1987;64:842–8.

112. Woolf PD. Hormonal responses to trauma. Crit Care Med 1992;20:216–26.

113. Parker CR Jr, Baxter CR. Divergence in adrenal steroid secretory pattern after thermal injury in adult patients. J Trauma 1985;25:508–10.

114. Ferrando AA, Tipton KD, Doyle D, et al. Testosterone injection stimulates net protein synthesis but not tissue amino acid transport. Am J Physiol 1998;275:E864–71.

115. Sinha-Hikim I, Artaza J, Woodhouse L, et al. Testosterone-induced increase in muscle size in healthy young men is associated with muscle fiber hypertrophy. Am J Physiol Endocrinol Metab 2002;283: E154–64.

116. Demling RH, DeSanti L. Oxandrolone, an anabolic steroid, significantly increases the rate of weight gain in the recovery phase after major burns. J Trauma 1997;43:47–51.

117. Hart DW, Wolf SE, Ramzy PI, et al. Anabolic effects of oxandrolone after severe burn. Ann Surg 2001; 233:556–64.

118. Jeschke MG, Finnerty CC, Suman OE, et al. The effect of oxandrolone on the endocrinologic, inflammatory, and hypermetabolic responses during the acute phase postburn. Ann Surg 2007;246:351–62.

119. Barrow RE, Dasu MR, Ferrando AA, et al. Gene expression patterns in skeletal muscle of thermally injured children treated with oxandrolone. Ann Surg 2003;237:422–8.

120. Reeves PT, Herndon DN, Tanksley JD, et al. Five-year outcomes after long-term oxandrolone administration in severely burned children: a randomized clinical trial. Shock 2016;45:367–74.

121. Wolf SE, Thomas SJ, Dasu MR, et al. Improved net protein balance, lean mass, and gene expression changes with oxandrolone treatment in the severely burned. Ann Surg 2003;237:801–10 [discussion: 810–1].

122. Przkora R, Jeschke MG, Barrow RE, et al. Metabolic and hormonal changes of severely burned children receiving long-term oxandrolone treatment. Ann Surg 2005;242:384–91.

123. Gore DC, Chinkes D, Heggers J, et al. Association of hyperglycemia with increased mortality after severe burn injury. J Trauma 2001;51:540–4.

124. Gore DC, Chinkes DL, Hart DW, et al. Hyperglycemia exacerbates muscle protein catabolism in burn-injured patients. Crit Care Med 2002;30: 2438–42.

125. Jeschke MG, Kraft R, Emdad F, et al. Glucose control in severely thermally injured pediatric patients: what glucose range should be the target? Ann Surg 2010;252:521–7 [discussion: 527–8].

126. Kraft R, Herndon DN, Mlcak RP, et al. Bacterial respiratory tract infections are promoted by systemic hyperglycemia after severe burn injury in pediatric patients. Burns 2014;40:428–35.

127. van den Berghe G, Wouters P, Weekers F, et al. Intensive insulin therapy in the critically ill patients. N Engl J Med 2001;345:1359–67.

128. Finnerty CC, Ali A, McLean J, et al. Impact of stress-induced diabetes on outcomes in severely burned children. J Am Coll Surg 2014;218:783–95.

129. Jeschke MG, Kraft R, Song J, et al. Insulin protects against hepatic damage postburn. Mol Med 2011; 17:516–22.

130. Jeschke MG, Kulp GA, Kraft R, et al. Intensive insulin therapy in severely burned pediatric patients: a prospective randomized trial. Am J Respir Crit Care Med 2010;182:351–9.

131. Pierre EJ, Barrow RE, Hawkins HK, et al. Effects of insulin on wound healing. J Trauma 1998;44:342–5.

132. Thomas SJ, Morimoto K, Herndon DN, et al. The effect of prolonged euglycemic hyperinsulinemia on lean body mass after severe burn. Surgery 2002; 132:341–7.

133. Minnich A, Tian N, Byan L, et al. A potent PPARalpha agonist stimulates mitochondrial fatty acid beta-oxidation in liver and skeletal muscle. Am J Physiol Endocrinol Metab 2001;280:E270–9.

134. Cree MG, Zwetsloot JJ, Herndon DN, et al. Insulin sensitivity and mitochondrial function are improved in children with burn injury during a randomized controlled trial of fenofibrate. Ann Surg 2007;245: 214–21.

135. Tornio A, Niemi M, Neuvonen PJ, et al. Drug interactions with oral antidiabetic agents: pharmacokinetic mechanisms and clinical implications. Trends Pharmacol Sci 2012;33:312–22.

136. Gore DC, Herndon DN, Wolfe RR. Comparison of peripheral metabolic effects of insulin and metformin following severe burn injury. J Trauma 2005; 59:316–22 [discussion: 322–3].

137. Gore DC, Wolf SE, Sanford A, et al. Influence of metformin on glucose intolerance and muscle catabolism following severe burn injury. Ann Surg 2005;241:334–42.

138. Gore DC, Wolf SE, Herndon DN, et al. Metformin blunts stress-induced hyperglycemia after thermal injury. J Trauma 2003;54:555–61.

139. Deane AM, Chapman MJ, Fraser RJ, et al. Effects of exogenous glucagon-like peptide-1 on gastric emptying and glucose absorption in the critically ill: relationship to glycemia. Crit Care Med 2010; 38:1261–9.

140. Drucker DJ, Philippe J, Mojsov S, et al. Glucagon-like peptide I stimulates insulin gene expression and increases cyclic AMP levels in a rat islet cell line. Proc Natl Acad Sci U S A 1987;84:3434–8.

141. Mecott GA, Herndon DN, Kulp GA, et al. The use of exenatide in severely burned pediatric patients. Crit Care 2010;14:R153.

142. Meier JJ, Weyhe D, Michaely M, et al. Intravenous glucagon-like peptide 1 normalizes blood glucose after major surgery in patients with type 2 diabetes. Crit Care Med 2004;32:848–51.

143. Breitenstein E, Chiolero RL, Jequier E, et al. Effects of beta-blockade on energy metabolism following burns. Burns 1990;16:259–64.

144. Herndon DN, Barrow RE, Rutan TC, et al. Effect of propranolol administration on hemodynamic and metabolic responses of burned pediatric patients. Ann Surg 1988;208:484–92.

145. Minifee PK, Barrow RE, Abston S, et al. Improved myocardial oxygen utilization following propranolol infusion in adolescents with postburn hypermetabolism. J Pediatr Surg 1989;24:806–11.

146. Mangano DT, Layug EL, Wallace A, et al. Effect of atenolol on mortality and cardiovascular morbidity after noncardiac surgery. Multicenter Study of Perioperative Ischemia Research Group. N Engl J Med 1996;335:1713–20.

147. Herndon DN, Nguyen TT, Wolfe RR, et al. Lipolysis in burned patients is stimulated by the beta 2-receptor for catecholamines. Arch Surg 1994;129:1301–5.

148. Aarsland A, Chinkes D, Wolfe RR, et al. Beta-blockade lowers peripheral lipolysis in burn patients receiving growth hormone. Rate of hepatic very low density lipoprotein triglyceride secretion remains unchanged. Ann Surg 1996;223:777–89.

149. Barret JP, Jeschke MG, Herndon DN. Fatty infiltration of the liver in severely burned pediatric patients: autopsy findings and clinical implications. J Trauma 2001;51:736–9.

150. Gore DC, Honeycutt D, Jahoor F, et al. Propranolol diminishes extremity blood flow in burned patients. Ann Surg 1991;213:568–74.

151. Morio B, Irtun O, Herndon DN, et al. Propranolol decreases splanchnic triacylglycerol storage in burn patients receiving a high-carbohydrate diet. Ann Surg 2002;236:218–25.

152. Herndon DN, Dasu MR, Wolfe RR, et al. Gene expression profiles and protein balance in skeletal muscle of burned children after beta-adrenergic blockade. Am J Physiol Endocrinol Metab 2003;285:E783–9.

153. Vaughan GM, Becker RA, Allen JP, et al. Cortisol and corticotrophin in burned patients. J Trauma 1982;22:263–73.

154. Wise L, Margraf HW, Ballinger WF. Adrenal cortical function in severe burns. Arch Surg 1972;105:213–20.

155. Lyman CA, Walsh TJ. Systemically administered antifungal agents. A review of their clinical pharmacology and therapeutic applications. Drugs 1992;44:9–35.

156. Engelhardt D, Dorr G, Jaspers C, et al. Ketoconazole blocks cortisol secretion in man by inhibition of adrenal 11 beta-hydroxylase. Klin Wochenschr 1985;63:607–12.

157. Engelhardt D, Mann K, Hormann R, et al. Ketoconazole inhibits cortisol secretion of an adrenal adenoma in vivo and in vitro. Klin Wochenschr 1983;61:373–5.

158. Loose DS, Stover EP, Feldman D. Ketoconazole binds to glucocorticoid receptors and exhibits glucocorticoid antagonist activity in cultured cells. J Clin Invest 1983;72:404–8.

159. Jeschke MG, Williams FN, Finnerty CC, et al. The effect of ketoconazole on post-burn inflammation, hypermetabolism and clinical outcomes. PLoS One 2012;7:e35465.

160. Hart DW, Wolf SE, Chinkes DL, et al. Beta-blockade and growth hormone after burn. Ann Surg 2002;236:450–7.

161. Jeschke MG, Finnerty CC, Kulp GA, et al. Combination of recombinant human growth hormone and propranolol decreases hypermetabolism and inflammation in severely burned children. Pediatr Crit Care Med 2008;9:209–16.

162. Aarsland A, Chinkes DL, Sakurai Y, et al. Insulin therapy in burn patients does not contribute to hepatic triglyceride production. J Clin Invest 1998;101:2233–9.

163. Debroy MA, Wolf SE, Zhang XJ, et al. Anabolic effects of insulin-like growth factor in combination with insulin-like growth factor binding protein-3 in severely burned adults. J Trauma 1999;47:904–11.

164. Ferrando AA, Chinkes DL, Wolf SE, et al. A submaximal dose of insulin promotes net skeletal muscle protein synthesis in patients with severe burns. Ann Surg 1999;229:11–8.

165. Schnabel CA, Wintle M, Kolterman O. Metabolic effects of the incretin mimetic exenatide in the treatment of type 2 diabetes. Vasc Health Risk Manag 2006;2:69–77.

Clinician's Guide to Nutritional Therapy Following Major Burn Injury

Christina Rollins, RD, CNSC[a], Franziska Huettner, MD, PhD[b],
Michael W. Neumeister, MD, FRCSC[b],*

KEYWORDS

- Nutritional therapy • Enteral and parenteral nutrition support • Burn recovery • Wound healing

KEY POINTS

- Nutrition assessment and intervention are vital components of the burn recovery process.
- Hypermetabolic state and increased caloric needs are dependent on burn severity and may remain elevated up to 2 years following injury.
- Supplemental nutrition therapy and pharmacologic support may expedite recovery.

INTRODUCTION

Burn injury is a serious and life-threatening condition. Approximately 486,000 people in the United States undergo treatment of burn injuries each year, with about 40,000 of those injured requiring hospitalization and roughly 3275 cases resulting in death.[1] Major burn patients are arguably the sickest population in the hospital, characterized by a severe inflammatory response, high oxidative stress, and a prolonged hypermetabolic and catabolic response.[2]

Nutrition is vital to the health and recovery of burn patients. Massive fluid shifts immediately following injury, hypermetabolism as early as 24 hours postburn (lasting for up to 2 years), increased risk for loss of lean body mass, and potentially damaging free radial production all indicate the need for targeted and often aggressive medical nutrition therapy to improve clinical outcomes following major burns. Although underfeeding can lead to muscle wasting and delays in wound healing, overfeeding can have equally serious complications, such as hyperglycemia, fatty liver, and prolonged ventilator dependency.[3]

Understanding the physiologic response to burn stress, recognizing the increased risk for nutritional deficit, and applying evidence-based medical and nutritional treatment guidelines are key factors in supporting the recovery of patients postburn injury.

OVERVIEW OF BURNS

Burns are characterized 1 of 3 ways: superficial (first degree), partial thickness, divided into superficial and deep (second degree), and full thickness (third degree). Superficial burns involve only the epidermis and can heal without intervention in about 3 to 4 days. Topical treatments like aloe lotion can be of benefit for symptomatic relieve. Partial-thickness burns involve damage to both the epidermal and the dermal layers of the skin, with superficial burns involving papillary dermis with sparing the skin appendages and deep burns involving the reticular dermis with loss of the skin appendages. They can be very painful (superficial) and typically require 3 or more weeks to heal. Supportive measures like bacitracin and petroleum-based dressing application are beneficial for

[a] Food and Nutrition Services, Memorial Medical Center, 701 North 1st Street, Springfield, IL 62781, USA;
[b] Department of Surgery, Institute for Plastic Surgery, Southern Illinois University School of Medicine, Baylis Medical Building, P.O. Box 19653, 747 North Rutledge Street, 3rd Floor, Springfield, IL 62794-9653, USA
* Corresponding author.
E-mail address: mneumeister@siumed.edu

Clin Plastic Surg 44 (2017) 555–566
http://dx.doi.org/10.1016/j.cps.2017.02.014
0094-1298/17/© 2017 Elsevier Inc. All rights reserved.

superficial, whereas deep second-degree burns benefit from excision and grafting. Full-thickness burns involve damage to the epidermis and dermis, including the skin appendages and free nerve endings and are therefore not painful to the touch. Full-thickness burns require surgical intervention, such as wound debridement and skin grafting, to heal.[2]

Major burn injuries can be defined as injuries with greater than 20% burned total body surface area (TBSA),[4] and severe burns can be defined as greater than 40% TBSA. Early massive capillary leaks and fluid shifts can lead to hypovolemic shock and need for aggressive resuscitation in these patients.[5] Physiologic changes can include a 10- to 50-fold increase in catecholamines and corticosteroids, which can last up to up to 9 months postburn[6,7]; an increase in energy expenditure and metabolic rate,[6] which can still be at 120% 6 months postburn; an increase in cardiac work with an increase in myocardial consumption, which can be increased into the rehabilitation phase.[8,9] Other changes can include lipolysis, liver dysfunction, severe muscle catabolism with net protein loss, insulin resistance, increase in cytokine levels, and decrease in sex hormones and endogenous growth hormone release. The increased metabolism and hyperdynamic circulation can lead to fatality if untreated.

Severity of the physical response to burns depends on many factors, including burn size and depth, gender, age, presence of inhalation injury, timeliness of medical treatment, and other comorbid conditions present.[10] Complications following burn injury vary in severity. Negative outcomes are also associated with inadequate nutritional care. Insufficient intake of calories and protein can lead to a loss of lean muscle mass, which can induce immune dysfunction, impair wound healing, and increase mortality at 10%, 20%, and 40% loss, respectively.[11]

LABORATORY TESTING

There has been a historic link between low serum hepatic proteins, including serum albumin (A), serum prealbumin (PA), and transferrin (T) and the presence of malnutrition. However, current evidence shows that, in hospitalized patients, serum levels of these proteins have a more positive correlation with inflammation, stress, and mortality. Levels may be falsely increased by dehydration, blood, and intravenous A infusion, severe renal failure, corticosteroid and oral contraceptive use, and falsely low with fluid resuscitation, hepatitis and hepatic failure, dialysis, hyperthyroidism, pregnancy, hyperglycemia, infection, inflammation, and generalized stress.[12] A, PA, and T alone poorly reflect malnutrition or the adequacy of calorie/protein intake[12,13] and should alone not be used as indicators of nutritional status or adequacy of nutrition support therapy.[14] Using other laboratory values such C-reactive protein in addition to serum protein values will help assess the inflammatory impact on serum protein levels.[12,13,15]

CALORIES

Calculating precise energy (calorie) requirements can be challenging for clinicians. An ebb-and-flow response is often seen in burn injuries, where an initial reduction of metabolic rate occurs followed by hypermetabolism that can last for weeks. Energy expenditure typically begins to increase about 72 hours postburn, peaks in 5 to 7 days, and can remain elevated for up to 2 years.[16] Factors that may impact energy expenditure postburn include wound closure, surgical procedures, initiation of nutrition support, physical therapy, certain medications,[2] sepsis, and ambient temperature.[17] Size of the burn is also a key determinant of caloric need. For burns greater than 10% TBSA, resting metabolic rate will likely be close to or at the normal range. However, patients with major burn injury are as much as double baseline, with a subsequent rate decline.

The 2 most common methods used to estimate calorie needs are IC and mathematical calculations. Both methods have pros and cons that must be considered.

Indirect calorimetry (IC) is a respiratory test that calculates actual resting energy expenditure (REE) by measuring the exchange of oxygen and carbon dioxide by the lungs by using IC to measure calorie needs, factors that may impact energy expenditure measured, resulting in a more reliable estimation of calorie needs.[18] It is important to note that IC only provides a measurement of energy expenditure for the time frame testing was completed, which is typically at rest. To compensate, measured REE should be multiplied by 1.2 to 1.3.[19] Although IC has long been coined the "gold standard" in estimating energy needs,[20] financial cost often prohibits its use. IC adds cost to both the facility and the patient, including an upfront cost to purchase the machine and employ trained staff as well as a procedural cost to the patient.[21]

Mathematical calculations are a lower-cost alternative to IC and more readily available, although multiple studies have indicated that mathematical equations are less accurate in estimating caloric need because burn patients have highly variable energy expenditure. Inaccuracy can lead to underfeeding as well as massive over-feeding,[22] which can lead to fatty liver infiltration and increased rate of infection.[19,21] Numerous static equations exist and are used to calculate needs based on height, weight, stress, activity, and variety of other variables (**Table 1**).[2,19,23]

PROTEIN

According to the American Society of Parenteral and Enteral Nutrition (ASPEN), critically ill patients are at an increased risk for protein loss related to increases in protein turnover rates, synthesis, breakdown, and oxidation.[3] Current literature recommends providing protein at 1.5 to 2 g per kilogram of body weight per day in the critically ill adult burn population.[14] Higher protein intakes (>2.2 g/kg) do not result in a higher net protein synthesis.[24] For morbidly obese critically ill patients, ideal body weight should be used to calculate protein requirements.[14] To ensure optimal protein utilization, calorie intake should also be adequate, with protein comprising no more than 20% to 25% of estimated caloric needs.[2]

CARBOHYDRATES

Sufficient carbohydrate intake is similar to that of non-burned individuals at 55% to 60% of total energy requirements. Because burn patients have higher than usual energy needs, precaution should be taken to avoid excessive carbohydrate load, which can induce hyperglycemia and shock liver. Although excessive carbohydrate is unlikely via oral or enteral route due to digestive limitations and capacity, it is likely to occur via the parenteral route. The maximum intravenous carbohydrate infusion rate for adults is 5 to 7 mg/kg/d, with excess of 7 mg/kg/d increasing risk of shock liver and hyperglycemia.[22]

Calculating Carbohydrate Infusion Rate = (Carbohydrate grams × 1000)/weight kg/24 hours per day/60 minutes per hour

LIPID

Nonburned individuals require a maximum of 30% of energy from lipid, with less than 10% of lipid calories from saturated fatty acids for cardiovascular health. There is no evidence to support increasing lipid consumption postburn injury.[2] Total lipid intake from all sources should be accounted for to avoid overfeeding, including lipid emulsions included with intravenous medications such as propofol.

FLUID

Adequate fluid resuscitation is an important part of the postburn recovery process. Localized edema is common in smaller burns, and patients with larger burns may experience whole body edema. Although total body water may remain unchanged, circulating fluid is reduced and requires replacement. The Parkland Formula recommends 4 mL lactated Ringers/kg per % TBSA burned, with half of total volume given over the first 8 hours, and the remaining half of total volume given over the next 16 hours. Fluid intake should always be titrated to maintain adequate urine output, which has been shown the best measurement available for adequate tissue perfusion in burns.[2] The use and titration of lactated Ringers solution according to the urine output for burns up to 40% without inhalation injury is a safe and well-tested method. In patients with larger burns (>40%), inhalation injuries, or preexisting heart disease, and in geriatric patients, the use of a lower volume aided by colloid can be beneficial.[24]

NUTRITION THERAPY

Three options exist for route of nutrition therapy: oral, enteral, and parenteral. Oral route with high protein foods and small, frequent feedings is always preferred, if the patient is able to consume adequate intake per the aforementioned guidelines. For instance, when the patient

---

Table 1
Mathematical calculations to estimate energy needs after burns

Harris Benedict equation[19]	Men: [66.47 + (13.75 × W) + (5 × H) − (6.76 × A)] × AF × IF Women: [655.1 + (9.56 × W) + (1.85 × H) − (4.68 × A)] × AF × IF
Calories per kilogram[19]	Non obese population: 25 to 35 kcal/kg body weight Obese, critically ill population: 21 kcal/kg body weight
Curreri[19]	(25 × W) + (40 × %TBSA burn)

Abbreviations: A, age in years; AF, activity factor; H, height in centimeters; IF, injury factor; TBSA, total body surface area burned; W, weight in kilograms.

is unable to eat or unable to consume adequate intake (defined as at least 60% of estimated energy requirement), enteral (EN) and/or parenteral nutrition (PN) should be considered (**Fig. 1**).

Enteral Nutrition

Early EN is the recommended feeding route in patients with major burns.[4,25] EN maintains gut integrity, supports a healthy immune system, and is generally tolerated in most patients. Infusion initiation as early as 4 to 6 hours postburn helps to achieve a positive nitrogen balance, increases insulin levels to support healing, reduces catecholamine levels,[26] and lowers levels of tumor necrosis factor and serum endotoxins.[27] EN in burn patients has also been associated with improved structure and function of the gastrointestinal tract, increased contractility, less ischemia, and reduced intestinal permeability.[28] A decrease in bacterial translocation, support of functional integrity of gut by maintaining tight junctions, and providing stress and ulcer prophylaxis[29–31] as well as a reduction in mortality have also been associated with early EN.[32] This is in accordance with current recommendations by the Society of Critical Care Medicine and ASPEN, who recommend the initiation of EN within 48 hours in critically ill patients, with titration to goal as tolerated by day 7 of hospitalization.[14]

Although gastric feeding is recommended in critically ill, nonburn patients, small bowel (SB) feeding tube placement is suggested for burn patients. SB feedings have been associated with reductions in pneumonia and sepsis rates[25] and also may improve tolerance despite gastric stasis, a common complication of major burns. To further reduce risk of aforementioned complications, SB feeding tubes can be paired with gastric suction via nasogastric or orogastric tubes. In cases when SB access cannot be obtained, gastric feeding can be initiated. Regardless of tube type, efforts should be made to reach goal EN prescription rate by postburn day 5.

EN products are commercially available to meet the needs of a variety of patient types. Standard therapy postburn consists of a low-residue, 1-kcal/mL product with supplemental protein flushes to meet estimated nutritional needs. Routine free water flushes should also be given to meet maintenance fluid requirements following initial fluid resuscitation and also to prevent tube occlusions. Unless contraindicated, begin EN via SB tube at a rate of 40 mL/h and

increase by 20 mL every 2 hours as tolerated to goal. For gastric access, consider a more conservative advancement rate and monitor for tolerance.

Continued feeds are preferred over bolus feeds, because of a lesser risk of aspirations and a trend to decreased mortality.[33] Continued SB feedings during procedures are recommended and have been shown to decrease the infection rate.[34] In fact, stopping the feeding for procedures decreased the chances of meeting the daily nutritional goal and carries the risk of developing an ileus,[35] which then can further delay the administration of EN. However, if the patient is also consuming oral intake, consider transitioning to a nocturnal feeding pattern to stimulate appetite while still meeting estimated needs. Discontinue EN when the patient is able to consistently meet at least 60% of estimated energy needs by mouth.[14]

Although receiving EN, patients should be monitored with each nursing assessment for signs of EN intolerance including but not limited to nausea, vomiting, diarrhea, abdominal pain, and distention. Gastric residual volume (GRV), a marker once considered standard of care, is no longer thought to be a valid marker for EN tolerance. It does not correlate with incidence of pneumonia, regurgitation, or aspiration and should not be monitored unless other signs of intolerance are present.

The use of vasopressor agents is not a contraindication for the use of EN. Ischemic bowel is a rare complication of EN in the setting of low doses of vasopressor use and has shown a decrease in intensive care unit and hospital mortality.[36] EN are recommended to be held in patients with a mean arterial blood pressure <50 mmHg or in patients for whom catecholamine agents are started.[14]

The need for long-term EN support (>4 weeks) is unlikely to occur postburn, but certainly can if the patient develops complications such as dysphasia following prolonged aspiration. In this case, standard guidelines should be followed for placement of long-term enteral access (such as a percutaneous endoscopic gastrostomy or PEG [percutaneous endoscopic gastrostomy] tube).

Parenteral Nutrition

For patients who are unable to begin EN (such as with traumatic bowel perforation or very high-dose vasopressor support), unable to reach EN goal rate by day 8 of admission, or malnourished at admission (ie, pre-existing condition), PN

Nutrition Support Decision Tree

Consider nutrition support options as early as 4–6 h post-burn injury. Re-evaluate daily and adjust nutrition treatment plan according to patient medical condition.

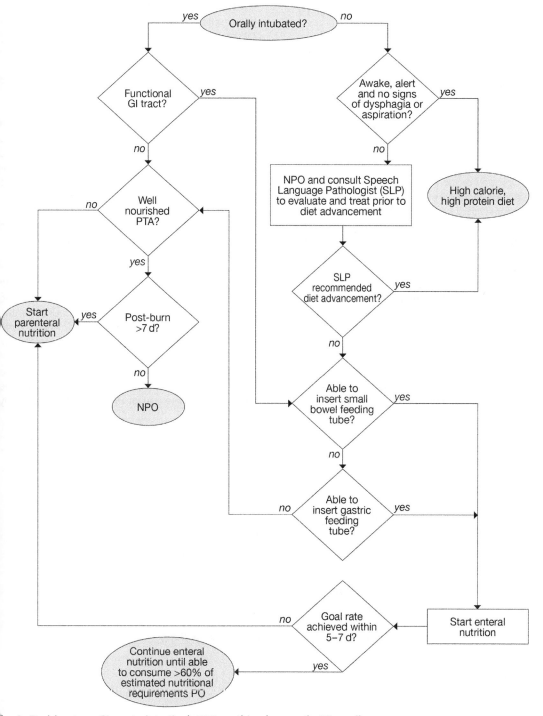

Fig. 1. Decision tree. GI, gastrointestinal; NPO, nothing by mouth; PO, orally.

should be initiated. Initiating PN before day 8 in well-nourished individuals has shown little functional benefit.[37]

COMPLICATIONS OF ENTERAL NUTRITION AND PARENTERAL NUTRITION

Although both EN and PN have functional benefits postburn injury, each presents with its own risk for complications. EN is often associated with nausea, vomiting, abdominal distention, diarrhea, constipation, and aspiration. Using measures such as the use of chlorhexidine mouthwash twice per day in orally intubated patients,[14] elevating the head of the bed to 30 to 45°,[38,39] and the use of prokinetic agents (metoclopramide or erythromycin) may reduce the risk of some gastrointestinal upset and even aspiration of stomach contents with subsequent decreased risk of pneumonia. However, the routine use of prokinetic agents must be cautioned because of the potential side effects, like cardiac toxicity and tachyphylaxis for erythromycin use, tardive dyskinesia for the use of Reglan, and potential QT prolongation for both of these agents.[40,41] Although both have shown an improvement in the GRV, no decrease in length of stay or mortality was associated with their use.[42]

Laboratory imbalances are also common with both EN and PN, including but not limited to electrolytes, acid/base balance, and glucose levels. Although early aggressive feeding is recommended in postburn injury, this does increase the risk of refeeding syndrome, a condition characterized by very low levels of potassium, magnesium, and phosphorus, which may become lethal if left untreated. In addition, PN formulations with insufficient lipid content can lead to essential fatty acid deficiency. Aggressive treatment is warranted following standard treatment guidelines following a comprehensive medical and nutritional assessment.

Hepatobiliary complications, also known as parenteral nutrition associated liver disease (PNALD), have also been associated with PN including steatosis, cholestasis, and gallbladder sludge/stones. Overfeeding of calories, dextrose infusion greater than 5 to 7 mg/kg/min and lipid infusion greater than 1 g/kg/d have been associated with the onset of PNALD. Care should be taken to not only assess but also routinely reassess nutritional requirements to support burn recovery without exceeding the body's need to metabolize and digest these nutrients.[43]

Also, the use of PN is to be done with caution because it carries an increased risk of infection,[44] specifically, pneumonia rate,[45] compared with EN therapy alone. PN does carry an increased risk of bloodstream infections because central venous access is required for PN infusion sufficient to meet estimated nutritional requirements. PN infusion can also lead to atrophy of the gastrointestinal tract and carries an increased risk of bacterial translocation. Care should be taken to limit the use of PN to what is medically

Table 2
Micronutrient repletion and laboratory monitoring

	Oral Dose	Intravenous Dose	Laboratory Monitoring
Multivitamin with minerals	One tablet per day	Multivitamin 10 mL per day	None
Vitamin C	Vitamin C 500 mg twice a day	Vitamin C 500 mg per day	Plasma or serum ascorbic acid
Zinc	Zinc sulfate 110 mg per day, up to 220 mg per day if confirmed zinc deficiency	Zinc (elemental) 10 mg per day	Serum, plasma, or whole blood zinc
Copper	Copper gluconate 2–4 mg per day if on prolonged zinc supplementation	Cuperic chloride 9 mg daily	Ceruloplasmin
Vitamin A	10,000 IU per day × 10 d, up to 25,000 IU per day × 10 d if on steroids or confirmed vitamin A deficiency	None	Serum or plasma retinol

Data from Refs.[12–16]

(to be considered in addition to standard admission orders and according to individual hospital guidelines)

Expected Length of Stay: _____ days

% TBSA _____

Nursing

□ Ambient room temperature 82–91 degrees Fahrenheit burns >20% TBSA

Diet

□ NPO

□ NPO except medications

□ Clear Liquid

□ High protein, high calorie with milkshakes between meals

Consider additional diet restrictions as medically indicated.

□ Continuous calorie count

□ L-Glutamine 15 g PO daily

□ L-Glutamine 15 g mixed with 60 mL free water and flushed via feeding tube

□ Insert nasogastric/orogastric tube to low intermittent suction

□ Small bowel tube insertion per ICU nursing/dietitian

Tube feeding

□ Low residue, 1 cal/mL product □ _____

□ Nasogastric   □ Orogastric   □ Nasoduodenal / NasoJejunal □ PEG

Initiate continues tube feeding □ at 40 mL /h   □ at ___ mL/h

Increase feedings by □ 20 mL □ ___mL every □ 2 h □____h until goal of ____ mL

□ Do not advance tube feeding rate until ordered

□ other:_____

Consider general recommendations regarding hospital wide hypoglycemia protocol

□ Keep head of patient elevated 30 degrees at all times,

□ Bed 30 degrees reverse Trendelenburg position

□ hold if SBP <50 mm/HG continuously

Fig. 2. Initial burn admission order guidelines example (to be considered in addition to standard admission orders and according to individual hospital guidelines). BID, twice a day; IV, intravenously; PEG, percutaneous endoscopic gastrostomy; PRN, as needed; TID, 3 times a day.

Vitamins

☐ Multivitamin with minerals 1 tablet PO daily

☐ Multivitamin with minerals liquid 15 mL PO daily

☐ Thiamine 100 mg PO daily

☐ Zinc Sulfate 110 mg PO daily

☐ Ascorbic Acid (Vitamin C) 500 mg PO BID

☐ Ascorbic Acid (Vitamin C) 500 mg/5 mL oral solution 500 mg PO BID

☐ Copper gluconate 2 mg PO every evening

☐ Selenium 200 mcg PO daily

Stress Ulcer Prophylaxis

☐ Pantoprazole (Protonix) 40 mg IV Push daily

☐ Pantoprazole (Protonix) 40 mg PO daily

Nausea/Vomiting

☐ Ondansetron (Zofran) 4 mg IV Push every 6 h PRN nausea/vomiting

☐ Ondansetron (Zofran) 4 mg PO every 6 h PRN nausea/vomiting

Prokinetic / Nausea (caution in cardiac arrhythmias, bowel obstruction)

☐ Metoclopramide (Reglan) 10 mg IV Push every 6 h PRN nausea/vomiting

☐ Metoclopramide (Reglan) 10 mg PO every 6 h PRN nausea/vomiting

☐ Erythromycin 250 mg TID daily before meals. (Limit duration of therapy, tachyphylaxis
  may occur after 4 wk)

☐ Erythromycin IV: 3 mg/kg IV administered over 45 min Q8h

Appetite stimulant

☐ Oxandralone (Oxandrin) 5 mg tablet PO BID

☐ Megestrol (Megace) 800 mg Suspension Oral PO daily

Cardiovascular / Hypermetabolic State

☐ Propranolol 10 mg PO BID (hold if heart rate less than 80 beats per minute, systolic blood
  pressure less than 120 mm Hg)

☐ Propranolol 20 mg PO BID (hold if heart rate less than 80 beats per minute, systolic blood
  pressure less than 120 mm Hg)

☐ Propranolol 40 mg PO BID (hold if heart rate less than 80 beats per minute, systolic blood
  pressure less than 120 mm Hg)

Fig. 2. (*continued*)

❏ Propranolol 60mg PO BID (hold if heart rate less than 80 beats per minute, systolic blood pressure less than 120 mm Hg)

❏ Propranolol 80 mg PO BID (hold if heart rate less than 80 beats per minute, systolic blood pressure less than 120 mm Hg)

Consultations:

❏ Registered Dietitian for:

❏ Nutrition Assessment

❏ Manage tube feeding

❏ Diet instruction

❏ Speech Therapy to evaluate and treat

Fig. 2. *(continued)*

necessary, with the introduction of EN as soon as possible to avoid further and possibly long-term complications.

MICRONUTRIENT SUPPLEMENTATION

The increased inflammatory response paired with burn-induced oxidative stress leads to depletion of the endogenous antioxidant defense mechanism.[4] For this reason, burn patients have much higher vitamin and trace element requirements when compared with other patient populations. Low plasma levels of micronutrients have been associated with exudative losses, hypoalbuminemia, and induced oxidative stress.[2,20] Zinc and copper in particular have been reported as significantly lower than healthy controls at postburn days 3, 7, and 14.[46] Similar findings were also reported by Berger,[47] who correlated copper, selenium, and zinc supplementation with improved clinical outcomes, namely fewer pulmonary infections and improved burn wound healing.

Commercially available EN and PN products are not sufficient to provide adequate amounts of micronutrients to meet the increased micronutrient demand. In addition, because of antagonist mechanisms and competing forces, additional enteral substitution is not enough,[4] and intravenous supplementation is indicated. The exception to this statement is glutamine. Enteral glutamine has been shown to have a tropic effect in maintaining gut integrity postburn, and sufficient intake of glutamine can be obtained via enteral formula infusion alone.[48] Although literature is mixed regarding the effectiveness of glutamine postburn, glutamine supplementation has been associated with a

decrease in gram-negative bacteremia and hospital mortality.[49,50]

To support adequate wound healing postburn, the following supplementation regimen should be considered in addition to EN formula infusion: multivitamin with minerals, vitamin C, zinc, copper, vitamin A, and thiamine.[51–53] Administration of very high doses of vitamin C in first 24 hours helps to stabilize the cell membrane and can reduce the fluid resuscitation needs by 30%.[54] **Table 2** provides dosing information and laboratory monitoring. The supplementation has to be used with caution in patients with renal and hepatic failure.

OTHER PHARMACOLOGIC AGENTS

One potentially beneficial pharmacologic agent often used postburn is propranolol. In a recent systematic review, propranolol was associated with significant decreases in REE and insulin resistance.[55] Treatment recommendations include initiation of propranolol as early as 24 hours postburn.

Following initial resuscitation and achievement of hemodynamic stability, propranolol is often given in combination with oxandrolone.[4] A synthetic analogue to testosterone, oxandrolone improves muscle protein synthesis and protein metabolism leading to increases lean body mass, bone mineral content, and muscle strength. In a recent meta-analysis and systematic review, oxandrolone was shown to be significantly effective without obvious side effects, including decreased length of stay, decreased donor site healing time, reduced weight and nitrogen loss, decreased time between surgeries, gain in lean body mass,[56,57] and decreased mortality.[58] With close monitoring of liver function, oxandrolone is safe for both genders. Side effects are rare, and the risk of masculinization effect and hirsutism are low at 5% and 1%, respectively.

Intensive insulin therapy to achieve blood sugar levels of 80 to 110 mg/dL has also been linked to a decreased mortality as well as sepsis rates post-burn.[46] Tight glycemic control with insulin therapy stimulates muscle protein synthesis and increased lean body mass. However, current critical care nutrition guidelines recommend more liberal blood sugar control at target range of 140 to 180 mg/dL. Care must be taken to avoid hypoglycemic events with tight blood sugar control.

ADDITIONAL CONSIDERATIONS

In addition to pharmacologic agents, maintaining an ambient temperature of 28°C to 33°C[17] has been shown to reduce energy requirements, decrease protein and muscle catabolism, and improve overall survival. Early excision and coverage[59] of burned tissue has also been shown to improve survival rate by reducing infectious complications and overall inflammatory response.

SUMMARY

Adequate nutritional intake is crucial to the burn recovery process. Care of the burn patient should be individualized to include adequate calorie, protein, and fluid intake. Nutrition therapy, vitamin and mineral supplementation, and other pharmacologic agents should also be considered to support wound healing. For a comprehensive list of nutrition-related order options, see **Fig. 2**.

REFERENCES

1. American Burn Association. Burn Incidence Fact Sheet. Available at: http://www.ameriburn.org/resources_factsheet.php. Accessed July 14, 2016.
2. Herndon D. Total burn care. Philadelphia: Saunders Elsevier; 2007.
3. Merritt R. The A.S.P.E.N. Nutrition support practice manual. 2nd edition. Silver Springs (MD): A.S.P.E.N; 2005.
4. Rousseau AF, Losser MR, Ichai C, et al. ESPEN endorsed recommendations: nutritional therapy in major burns. Clin Nutr 2013;32(4):497–502.
5. Deitch EA. Intestinal permeability is increased in burn patients shortly after injury. Surgery 1990; 107(4):411–6.
6. Jeschke MG, Chinkes DL, Finnerty CC, et al. Pathophysiologic response to severe burn injury. Ann Surg 2008;248(3):387–401.
7. Wilmore DW, Aulick LH. Metabolic changes in burned patients. Surg Clin North Am 1978;58(6):1173–87.
8. Cuthbertson DP, Angeles Valero Zanuy MA, Leon Sanz ML. Post-shock metabolic response. 1942. Nutr Hosp 2001;16(5):176–82 [discussion: 175–6].
9. Baron PW, Barrow RE, Pierre EJ, et al. Prolonged use of propranolol safely decreases cardiac work in burned children. J Burn Care Rehabil 1997; 18(3):223–7.
10. Graves C, Saffle J, Cochran A. Actual burn nutrition care practices: an update. Presented at the American Burn Association conference in Chicago, IL April 29 – May 2, 2008.
11. Chang DW, DeSanti L, Demling RH. Anticatabolic and anabolic strategies in critical illness: a review of current treatment modalities. Shock 1998;10(3) 155–60.
12. Davis CJ, Sowa D, Keim KS, et al. The use of prealbumin and C-reactive protein for monitoring nutrition support in adult patients receiving enteral nutrition in an urban medical center. JPEN J Parenter Enteral Nutr 2012;36(2):197–204.
13. Jensen GL, Hsiao PY, Wheeler D. Adult nutrition assessment tutorial. JPEN J Parenter Enteral Nutr 2012;36(3):267–74.
14. McClave SA, Taylor BE, Martindale RG, et al. Guidelines for the provision and assessment of nutrition support therapy in the adult critically ill patient: Society of Critical Care Medicine (SCCM) and American Society for Parenteral and Enteral Nutrition (A.S.P.E.N. JPEN J Parenter Enteral Nutr 2016 40(2):159–211.
15. Ferrie S, Allman-Farinelli M. Commonly used "nutrition" indicators do not predict outcome in the critically ill: a systemic review. Nutr Clin Pract 2013 28(4):463–84.
16. A.S.P.E.N. Board of Directors and the Clinical Guidelines Task Force. Guidelines for the use of parenteral and EN in adult and pediatric patients. JPEN J Parenter Enteral Nutr 2002;26S:88SA–90SA.
17. Wilmore DW, Mason AD Jr, Johnson DW, et al. Effect of ambient temperature on heat production and heat loss in burn patients. J Appl Physiol 1975 38(4):593–7.
18. Prelack K, Dylewski M, Sheridan R. Practical guidelines for nutritional management of burn injury and recovery. Burns 2007;33:14–24.
19. Academy of Nutrition and Dietetics Nutrition Care Manual. Burns Nutrition Prescription. 2011. Available at: www.nutritioncaremanual.com. Accessed May 26 2016.
20. Turza K, Krenitsky J, Sawyer R. Enteral feedings and vasoactive agents: suggested guidelines for clinicians. Pract Gastroenterol 2009;78:11–22.
21. Davis K. Nutritional gain versus financial gain: the role of metabolic carts in the surgical ICU J Trauma 2006;61:1436–40.

22. Cresci G, Gottschlich M, Mayes T, et al. Trauma, surgery, and burns. The A.S.P.E.N. nutrition support core curriculum: a case-based approach – the adult patient. Silver Springs (MD): A.S.P.E.N; 2007. p. 455–72.

23. Dickerson R, Gervasio JM, Riley ML, et al. Accuracy of predictive methods to estimate resting energy expenditure of thermally-injured patients. J Parenter Enteral Nutr 2002;26:17–29.

24. Wolfe RR, Goodenough RD, Wolfe MH. Isotopic approaches to the estimation of protein requirements in burn patients. Adv Shock Res 1983;9:81–98.

25. Vicic VK, Radman M, Kovacic V. Early initiation of enteral nutrition improves outcomes in burn disease. Asia Pac J Clin Nutr 2013;22(4):543–7.

26. Chiarelli A, Enzi G, Casadei A, et al. Very early nutrition supplementation in burned patients. Am J Clin Nutr 1990;51(6):1035–9.

27. Peng YZ, Yuan ZQ, Xiao GX. Effects of early enteral feeding on the prevention of enterogenic infection in severely burned patients. Burns 2001;27(2):145–9.

28. Chen Z, Wang S, Yu B, et al. A comparison study between early enteral nutrition and parenteral nutrition in severe burn patients. Burns 2007;33(6):708–12.

29. Jabbar A, Chang WK, Dryden GW, et al. Gut immunology and the differential response to feeding and starvation. Nutr Clin Pract 2003;18(6):461–82.

30. Windsor AC, Kanwar S, Li AG, et al. Compared with parenteral nutrition,enteral feeding attenuates the acute phase response and improves disease severity in acute pancreatitis. Gut 1998;42(3):431–5.

31. Ammori BJ. Importance of the early increase in intestinal permeability in critically ill patients. Eur J Surg 2002;168(11):660–1.

32. Lewis SJ, Andersen HK, Thomas S. Early enteral nutrition within 24 h of intestinal surgery versus later commencement of feeding: a systematic review and meta-analysis. J Gastrointest Surg 2009;13(3): 569–75.

33. MacLeod JB, Lefton J, Houghton D, et al. Prospective randomized control trial of intermittent versus continuous gastric feeds for critically ill trauma patients. J Trauma 2007;63(1):57–61.

34. Jenkins ME, Gottschlich MM, Warden GD. Enteral feeding during operative procedures in thermal injuries. J Burn Care Rehabil 1994;15(2):199–205.

35. Caddell KA, Martindale R, McClave SA, et al. Can the intestinal dysmotility of critical illness be differentiated from postoperative ileus? Curr Gastroenterol Rep 2011;13(4):358–67.

36. Khalid I, Doshi P, DiGiovine B. Early enteral nutrition and outcomes of critically ill patients treated with vasopressors and mechanical ventilation. Am J Crit Care 2010;19(3):261–8.

37. Casaer MP, Mesotten D, Hermans G, et al. Early versus late parenteral nutrition in critically ill adults. N Engl J Med 2011;365(6):506–17.

38. Drakulovic MB, Torres A, Bauer TT, et al. Supine body position as a risk factor for nosocomial pneumonia in mechanically ventilated patients: a randomised trial. Lancet 1999;354(9193):1851–8.

39. van Nieuwenhoven CA, Vandenbroucke-Grauls C, van Tiel FH, et al. Feasibility and effects of the semi-recumbent position to prevent ventilator-associated pneumonia: a randomized study. Crit Care Med 2006;34(2):396–402.

40. Al-Khatib SM, LaPointe NM, Kramer JM, et al. What clinicians should know about the QT interval. JAMA 2003;289(16):2120–7.

41. Li EC, Esterly JS, Pohl S, et al. Drug-induced QT-interval prolongation: considerations for clinicians. Pharmacotherapy 2010;30(7):684–701.

42. Nguyen NQ, Chapman M, Fraser RJ, et al. Prokinetic therapy for feed intolerance in critical illness: one drug ortwo? Crit Care Med 2007; 35(11):2561–7.

43. Gottschlich MM. The APSEN nutrition support core curriculum: a case based approach – the adult patient. 2007. Available at: https://www.valorebooks.com/textbooks/aspen-nutrition-support-core-curriculum-a-case-based-approach-the-adult-patient-1st-edition/9781889622088.

44. Herndon DN, Barrow RE, Stein M. Increased mortality with intravenous supplemental feeding in severely burned patients. J Burn Care Rehabil 1989;10(4):309–13.

45. Lam NN, Tien NG, Khoa CM. Early enteral feeding for burned patients–an effective method which should be encouraged in developing countries. Burns 2008;34(2):192–6.

46. van den Berghe G, Wouters P, Weekers F, et al. Intensive insulin therapy in critically ill patients. N Engl J Med 2001;345(19):1359–67.

47. Berger M. Trace element supplementation modulates pulmonary infection rates after major burns: a double-blind, placebo controlled trial. Am J Clin Nutr 1998;68:365–71.

48. Garrel D, Patenaude J, Nedelec B, et al. Decreased mortality and infectious morbidity in adult burn patients given enteral glutamine supplements: a prospective, controlled, randomized clinical trial. Crit Care Med 2003;31(10):2444–9.

49. Lin JJ, Chung XJ, Yang CY, et al. A meta-analysis of trials using the intention to treat principle for glutamine supplementation in critically ill patients with burn. Burns 2013;39(4):565–70.

50. van Zanten AR, Dhaliwal R, Garrel D, et al. Enteral glutamine supplementation in critically ill patients: a systematic review and meta-analysis. Crit Care 2015;19:294.

51. Falder S, Silla R, Phillips M, et al. Thiamine supplementation increases serum thiamine and reduces pyruvate and lactate levels in burn patients. Burns 2010;36(2):261–9.

52. Al-Jawad FH, Sahib AS, Al-Kaisy AA. Role of antioxidants in the treatment of burn lesions. Ann Burns Fire Disasters 2008;21(4):186–91.

53. Barbosa E, Faintuch J, Machado Moreira EA, et al. Supplementation of vitamin E, vitamin C, and zinc attenuates oxidative stress in burned children: a randomized, double-blind, placebo-controlled pilot study. J Burn Care Res 2009;30(5):859–66.

54. Tanaka H, Matsuda T, Miyagantani Y, et al. Reduction of resuscitation fluid volumes in severely burned patients using ascorbic acid administration: a randomized, prospective study. Arch Surg 2000; 135(3):326–31.

55. Flores O, Stockton K, Roberts JA, et al. The efficacy and safety of adrenergic blockade after burn injury: a systematic review and meta-analysis. J Trauma Acute Care Surg 2016;80(1):146–55.

56. Li H, Guo Y, Yang Z, et al. The efficacy and safety of oxandrolone treatment for patients with severe burns: a systematic review and meta-analysis. Burns 2016;42(4):717–27.

57. Wolf SE, Edelman LS, Kemalyan N, et al. Effects of oxandrolone on outcome measures in the severely burned: a multicenter prospective randomized double-blind trial. J Burn Care Res 2006;27(2):131–9 [discussion: 140–1].

58. Pham TN, Klein MB, Gibran NS, et al. Impact of oxandrolone treatment on acute outcomes after severe burn injury. J Burn Care Res 2008;29(6):902–6.

59. Hart DW, Wolf SE, Chinkes DL, et al. Effects of early excision and aggressive enteral feeding on hypermetabolism, catabolism, and sepsis after severe burn. J Trauma 2003;54(4):755–61 [discussion: 761–4].

Acalculous Cholecystitis in Burn Patients

Is There a Role for Percutaneous Cholecystostomy?

Steven J. Hermiz, MD[a], Paul Diegidio, MD[b],
Roja Garimella, BS[c], Shiara Ortiz-Pujols, MD[b],
Hyeon Yu, MD[d], Ari Isaacson, MD[d],
Matthew A. Mauro, MD[d], Bruce A. Cairns, MD[b],
Charles Scott Hultman, MD, MBA[e],*

KEYWORDS

- Acalculous cholecystitis • Sepsis • Percutaneous cholecystostomy

KEY POINTS

- Plastic surgeons who take care of burn patients must be able to diagnose and treat sepsis, which can include acute acalculous cholecystitis (AAC).
- AAC is uncommon in burn patients but is associated with high mortality, especially when there is a delay in diagnosis and treatment.
- Percutaneous cholecystostomy can be performed for both diagnostic and therapeutic indications, with minimal morbidity, in burn patients.
- Improved survival in burn patients with acute acalculous cholecytitis requires treatment of the underlying conditions that contribute to end-organ hypoperfusion.

INTRODUCTION

AAC is an acute, necrotic inflammation of the gallbladder in the absence of gallstones.[1] It is a rare cause of acute cholecystitis, ranging from 2% to 14% of all cases of acute cholecystitis, and AAC affects 0.2% to 0.4% of critically ill patients.[1–3] Incidence of AAC is higher among burn patients (0.4%–3.5%) and is associated with complications, such as gangrene, perforation, and empyema.[1]

Clinical findings of AAC are indistinguishable from calculous cholecystitis. The clinical signs and laboratory values are nonspecific, especially in burn patients, but include right upper quadrant pain, leukocytosis, fever, and abnormal liver function tests.[1,2,4,5] Further factors complicating the diagnosis include overlying burn, intubation, narcotics, and sedation.[1,4] Therefore, the diagnosis becomes difficult and often delayed, leading to high mortality ranging from 10% to 90%.[2,6,7]

As a follow-up to the authors' previous study examining the efficacy of percutaneous cholecystostomy tube (PCT) placement in critically ill patients, published in 1996, the authors noted that

[a] Department of Surgery, University of South Carolina School of Medicine, Columbia, SC 29209, USA; [b] Department of Surgery, University of North Carolina School of Medicine, Chapel Hill, NC 27599, USA; [c] Alpert Medical School, Brown University, Providence, RI 02903, USA; [d] Department of Radiology, University of North Carolina School of Medicine, Chapel Hill, NC 27599, USA; [e] Division of Plastic Surgery, Department of Surgery, University of North Carolina School of Medicine, Suite 7038, Burnett Womack, CB#7195, Chapel Hill, NC 27599, USA
* Corresponding author.
E-mail address: cshult@med.unc.edu

Clin Plastic Surg 44 (2017) 567–571
http://dx.doi.org/10.1016/j.cps.2017.02.025

there had been a gradual decrease in PCT placement over the past few years compared with this same patient population in decades past.[8] The authors hypothesized that this was likely explained by advances in critical care and set out to evaluate institutional data to review the trends in placement, indications, and outcomes.

METHODS

An institutional interventional radiology (IR) register was queried to identify all patients who had a percutaneous cholecystostomy tube placed over the last 10 years. Cross-referencing the IR database with the institutional American Burn Association (ABA) registry identified the burn-specific cohort. A post hoc review was performed on individual charts to extrapolate data for analysis.

RESULTS

From 2004 to 2014, 21 critically ill burn patients had percutaneous cholecystostomy tubes placed by IR; 15 of the 21 patients had thermal injury, 4 patients had Stevens-Johnson syndrome/toxic epidermal necrolysis, and 2 patients had traumatic injuries with associated burns/degloving. **Table 1** provides a summary of patient demographics; outcome measures, such as length of stay and mortality; and clinical response to PCT. The average age of the patients was 49 years old. Charleson comorbidity index scores were calculated on admission for all patients; the mean was 8.2. The average length of stay was 102 days. Mean length of stay in the burn center ICU was 97 days, and the average number of ventilator days was 90. Mean total burn surface area was 47.8%; 80% (12 of 15) of the burn patients also had inhalation injury. Baux scores were also calculated, the average being 104.5. Overall mortality

rate was 66.7%. The average length of drainage of the PCT was 70 days. On right upper quadrant ultrasound, all patients had some degree of gallbladder dilation, wall thickening, sludge, and/or pericholecystic fluid; 5 of the 21 patients (23.8%) had incidental gallstones on ultrasound, and there was no obstruction visualized; 4 of the 21 (19.0%) patients had a normal liver function tests prior to PCT placement. The most common abnormal liver function test was gamma-glutamyltransferase (16 patients), followed by alkaline phosphatase (12 patients), aspartate aminotransferase (11 patients) alanine aminotransferase (6 patients), and total bilirubin (6 patients); 13 of the 21 patients (61.9%) had negative bile cultures, 7 patients did not have cultures obtained, and only 1 patient with Stevens-Johnson syndrome/toxic epidermal necrolysis, had a positive culture, for *Enterobacter* and *Pseudomonas*. Two-thirds of the patients, or 7 of 21, had burns/injuries at or near the PCT placement site. Average number of blood transfusions prior to PCT was 18.5 units of packed red blood cells. The average time to defervescence in the 6 patients (28.5%) who responded to PCT placement was 29.6 hours.

Fifteen of 21 patients (71.4%), however, did not respond to PCT placement and did not clinically improve, in contrast to the authors' experience in critically ill patients in the surgery ICU.[8] Defervescence did not predict survival, because 4 of these 6 patients died (66.7%); 12 of the 21 patients were in shock, on vasopressor therapy at the time of PCT placement; 2 of the 21 patients eventually underwent a cholecystectomy; and 14 of the 21 patients died, with 7 surviving to discharge, either to home (n = 5) or rehabilitation (n = 2). The average follow-up time was 14 months, with all 7 patients still alive, more than 1 year from their discharge.

The number of PCTs placed at the authors' institution decreased considerably from 2004 to 2014 (**Fig. 1**), with two-thirds placed in the first half of the study period. One was placed in 2004, 14 placed in 2005, 6 placed in 2006, 1 placed in

Table 1
Inpatient variables

Patient Variables (n = 21)	
Average age	49 y
Percentage total burn surface area	47.8
Length of stay (d)	102
ICU/ventilator days	97/90
Average length of drainage (d)	70
Mortality rate	66.7%
Average number of packed red blood cells transfusions prior to placement	18.5
Shock/vasopressors during placement	57%
Defervescence after placement	28.5%
Culture performed on fluid	66.7%

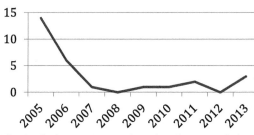

Fig. 1. Cholecystostomy tubes placed per year in burn patients.

2007, 1 placed in 2009, 1 placed in 2010, 2 placed in 2011, 3 placed in 2013, and 1 placed in the first 6 months of 2014.

Technically, placement of PCT in burn patients, by the IR service, was accomplished with a combination of ultrasound and fluoroscopy. No acute or long-term complications occurred in these 21 burn patients, and no long-term sequelae were observed, although 2 patients did undergo semielective cholecystectomy, for the management of cholelithiasis.

DISCUSSION

Throughout the literature, multiple studies have portrayed the mechanism for gallbladder inflammation at the cellular level. Laurila and other authors[2,9,10] revealed histologic evidence leading to gallbladder epithelial damage, including leukocyte margination, increased lymphatic dilation, and bile infiltration in the gallbladder wall. Vakkala and colleagues[11] were able to show that cell proliferation and apoptosis were increased in both AAC and calculous cholecystitis. Caclulous cholecystitis had stronger hypoxia-inducible factor 1-alpha expression (100% vs 57%), which accounts for the local inflammatory response in calculous cholecystitis and systemic inflammation with visceral hypoperfusion seen in acalculous cholecystitis.[11] Nag and colleagues[12] described lysoecithin as the mediator that increases prostanoid and platelet activating factor in mucosal cells, which promotes inflammation.

In the outpatient setting, the diagnosis of acute cholecystitis is based on symptoms, laboratory values, and imaging studies. Hirota and colleagues[13] conveyed the Tokyo guidelines for diagnosis, which include symptoms of right upper quadrant pain, physical examination findings (ie, Murphy sign), imaging findings (ie, thickened gallbladder), and severity (ie, grades I–III). This becomes difficult, however, in intubated and sedated patients. Imaging modalities have been studied throughout the literature and the consensus remains that no one study is the best.[2,14] Ultrasound is usually the first choice of imaging modality, due to its noninvasive nature and ability to be performed at bedside.[2,4] Ultrasonographic findings do not necessarily indicate acute biliary pathology, and the usefulness of ultrasound in evaluating acalculous cholecystitis in critically ill trauma patients has a sensitivity of only 30% and should not be used as a screening tool.[5,15,16] Hepatobiliary iminodiacetic acid and paraisopropylminodiacetic acid scans are used to confirm the diagnosis but have a sensitivity of only 68%.[5] Kaliafas and colleagues[5] showed that morphine cholescintigraphy (MC) had the highest sensitivity (90%) for diagnosis followed by CT (67%) and then ultrasonography (29%). Mariat and colleagues[16] had similar outcomes with MC compared with ultrasound, with a higher sensitivity (67% vs 50%) and specificity (100% vs 94%) in the former. The investigators concluded that MC is superior to ultrasound in confirming acalculous cholecystitis and the combination of the 2 improves diagnostic accuracy.[16]

The authors' retrospective review of 21 cases reports that 15 of 21 patients (71.4%) did not respond to or improve after PCT placement. The mortality rate was high at 66.7%, despite PCT placement. Defervescence did not predict survival because 4 of the 6 patients who initially responded eventually died.

Acalculous cholecystitis is a potentially life-threatening complication of critical illness and carries a high mortality rate.[3,5,17,18] Risk factors associated with acalculous cholecystitis include trauma, recent surgery, shock, burns, sepsis, critical illness, total parenteral nutrition, prolonged fasting, duration of ventilator support, positive end-expiratory pressure, and activation of factor XII.[1,2,4] The suggested common pathways leading to the pathogenesis of acalculous cholecystitis include bile stasis and ischemia.[3]

Laurila and colleagues[19] found that AAC was associated with severe illness, long ICU stay, and multisystem organ failure, with a high mortality rate of 44%. Multiple studies suggest ease and low complication rate of PCT placement; however, mortality remains high despite lack of procedural morbidity, suggesting other causes of these poor outcomes.[20] Multiple reports suggest that organ dysfunction should improve on the third postoperative/drainage day if the gallbladder is the cause of the patient's sepsis or hemodynamic instability.[21] Unfortunately, mortality rates are similar compared with emergency cholecystectomy, as reported by Melloul and colleagues.[21]

Percutaneous drainage and emergency cholecystectomy are efficacious in resolution of sepsis; however, some advocate that the drainage alone requires a secondary cholecystectomy.[22,23] The timing for subsequent cholecystectomy was investigated by Morse and colleagues,[18] who noted a high incidence of recurrence and complications without the secondary procedure. They concluded that although the morbidity associated with PCT is low (4%), the in-hospital morbidity and mortality rates remained high, at 62% and 50%, respectively.[18]

Alternative therapies to treat AAC have been proposed. Xu and colleagues[23] prospectively studied 34 high-risk patients in a 13-year period who underwent minicholecystectomy followed by ethanol chemical ablation. The patients were followed by ultrasound for 2 years to 14 years, with a long-term success rate of 85.3% and a 15% complication rate. This treatment method is unconventional, however, and will not likely replace PCT placement.

Some patients do not require cholecystectomy after placement, and in older or critically ill patients, PTC may be the definitive treatment.[24] Simorov and colleagues[25] showed decreased morbidity, fewer ICU admissions, decreased length of stay, and lower costs compared with operative intervention; however, perioperative outcomes were statistically similar. The best choice of treatment of AAC is cholecystectomy, in an otherwise clinically stable patient.[5,19] Clinicians should be wary of older patients with severe leukocytosis, which is a clinical predictor of severe gallbladder complications.[26] Recurrence of disease also has been documented, however, at 22% to 41% in some studies, suggesting that patients suffer recurrent attacks after PCT placement, and elective cholecystectomy should be considered.[27–29] Kalliafas and colleagues[5] reported a high incidence of gangrene (63%), 15% incidence of perforation, and 4% incidence of abscesses. An uncommon complication of acute cholecystitis that has been reported is cholecystocutaneous/cholecystoduodenal fistulas resulting from perforation.[8,30]

Patients are most susceptible within 20 days to 30 days postburn.[4] Arnoldo and colleagues[17] conducted a retrospective review at their institution over a 21-year period and concluded that 21 of 10,762 burn patients (0.18%) developed acute cholecystitis, with a 25% mortality rate. Burn patients having PCT placed for suspected cholecystitis have a higher mortality rate than general critical care patients with a PCT,[8,30] ranging from 25% to 53.3%.[1,3,5,8,17] Theodorou and colleagues[1] identified 3 independent risk factors for developing acalculous cholecystitis in burn patients, which included age, units of packed red blood cells administered, and length of ventilatory support.

Percutaneous cholecystostomy placement is a minimally invasive procedure and was first described in 1980 by Radder and colleagues.[24] PCT is a common procedure used to treat acute cholecystitis in patients with severe comorbid disease or in patients with severe sepsis.[27] Throughout the literature, multiple studies have examined the efficacy and complication rate of PCT placement. Boland and colleagues[31,32] concluded diagnosing acute cholecystitis in critically ill patients is difficult secondary to nonspecific findings. The study concluded that PCT is warranted for unexplained sepsis given its high rate of success, low rate of complications, and ability to rule out the gallbladder as the source. Hultman and colleagues[8] reported the successful placement of PCT in critically ill patients with no direct mortality or major complications. They determined that PCT is a safe, cost-effective, minimally invasive procedure that has diagnostic as well as therapeutic value. Atar and colleagues[33] had similar outcomes with successful drain placement with no immediate major procedural complications, albeit an 18.5% mortality rate within 30 days. Dabus Gde and colleagues[6] concluded that PCT is efficacious, with a 56% to 100% clinical response rate, 98% to 100% technical success rate, and 12% complication rate, and should be considered a definitive treatment in patients unfit for surgery with acalculous cholecystitis. Similarly, Sanjay and colleagues[27] reported a 13% complication rate, which included bile leaks, hemorrhage, and duodenal fistula formation.

SUMMARY

Cholecystitis in critically ill patients remains a diagnostic dilemma and is associated with high in-hospital mortality. Clinicians should maintain a high index of suspicion in burn patients with sepsis of an unknown source. Even with prompt diagnosis and external drainage, however, there is no guarantee of response to treatment or impact on survival. Because a majority of the patients in the authors' study did not respond to decompression, we concluded that some degree of hepatic insufficiency, perhaps due to end-organ hypoperfusion, contributed to both the diagnostic challenges and to the failure to have a positive impact on survival. Individual patients may selectively benefit from PCT, but this does not preclude the need for an exhaustive search for the source of sepsis. Biliary dysfunction may occur as a primary event, but, more likely than not, AAC is a secondary response to underlying systemic pathology—which must be successfully treated to improve survival in critically ill burn patients.

REFERENCES

1. Theodorou P, Maurer CA, Spanholtz TA, et al. Acalculous cholecystitis in severely burned patients: incidence and predisposing factors. Burns 2009; 35(3):405–11.
2. Huffman JL, Schenker S. Acute acalculous cholecystitis: a review. Clin Gastroenterol Hepatol 2010; 8:15–22.

3. Ganpathi IS, Diddapur RK, Eugene H, et al. Acute acalculous cholecystitis: challenging the myths. HPB (Oxford) 2007;9:131–4.

4. Castana O, Rempelos G, Anagiotos G, et al. Acute acalculous cholecystitis: a rare complication of burn injury. Ann Burns Fire Disasters 2009;22(1): 48–50.

5. Kalliafas S, Ziegler DW, Flancbaum L, et al. Acute acalculous cholecystitis: incidence, risk factors, diagnosis, and outcome. Am Surg 1998;64(5):471–5.

6. Dabus Gde C, Dertkigil SS, Baracat J. Percutaneous cholecystostomy: a nonsurgical therapeutic option for acute cholecystitis in high-risk and critically ill patients. Sao Paulo Med J 2003;121(6):260–2.

7. Lee SB, Ryu KH, Ryu JK, et al. Acute acalculous cholecystitis associated with cholecystoduodenal fistula and duodenal bleeding. Korean J Intern Med 2003;18:109–14.

8. Hultman CS, Herbst CA, McCall JM, et al. The efficacy of percutaneous cholecystostomy in critically ill patients. Am Surg 1996;62(4):263–9.

9. Laurila JJ, Karttunen T, Koivukangas V, et al. Tight junction proteins in gallbladder epithelium: different expression in acute acalculous and calculous cholecystitis. J Histochem Cytochem 2007;55(6):567–73.

10. Laurila JJ, Ala-Kokko TI, Laurila PA, et al. Histopathology of acute acalculous cholecystitis in critically Ill patients. Histopathology 2005;47(5):485–92.

11. Vakkala M, Laurila JJ, Saarnio J, et al. Cellular turnover and expression of hypoxic-inducible factor in acute acalculous and calculous cholecystitis. Crit Care 2007;11(5):1–6.

12. Nag MK, Deshpande YG, Beck D, et al. The effect of lysolecithin on prostanoid and platelet-activating factor formation by human gallbladder mucosal cells. Mediators Inflamm 1995;4:90–4.

13. Hirota M, Takada T, Kawarada Y, et al. Diagnostic criteria and severity assessment of acute cholecystitis: Tokyo Guidelines. J Hepatobiliary Pancreat Surg 2007;14:78–82.

14. Sheridan RL, Ryan CM, Lee MJ, et al. Percutaneous cholecystostomy in the critically ill burn patient. J Trauma 1995;38(2):248–51.

15. Puc MM, Tran HS, Wry PW, et al. Ultrasound is not a useful screening tool for acute acalculous cholecystitis in critically ill trauma patients. Am Surg 2002; 68(1):65–9.

16. Mariat G. Contribution of ultrasonography and cholescintigraphy to the diagnosis of acute acalculous cholecystitis in intensive care unit patients. Intensive Care Med 2000;26(11):1658–63.

17. Arnoldo BD, Hunt JL, Purdue GF. Acute cholecystitis in burn patients. J Burn Care Res 2006;27(2):170–3.

18. Morse BC, Smith JB, Lawdahl RB, et al. Management of acute cholecystitis in critically ill patients: contemporary role for cholecystostomy and subsequent cholecystectomy. Am Surg 2010;76(7):708–12.

19. Laurila J, Syrjälä H, Laurila PA, et al. Acute acalculous cholecystitis in critically ill patients. Acta Anaesthesiol Scand 2004;48(8):986–91.

20. Winbladh A, Gullstrand P, Svanvik J, et al. Systematic review of cholecystostomy as a treatment option in acute cholecystitis. HPB (Oxford) 2009;11:183–93.

21. Melloul E, Denys A, Demartines N, et al. Percutaneous drainage versus emergency cholecystectomy for the treatment of acute cholecystitis in critically ill patients: does it matter? World J Surg 2011;35(4):826–33.

22. Koebrugge B, van Leuken M, Ernst MF, et al. Percutaneous cholecystostomy in critically ill patients with a cholecystitis. Dig Surg 2010;27(5):417–21.

23. Xu Z, Wang L, Zhang N, et al. Chemical ablation of the gallbladder: clinical application and long-term observations. Surg Endosc 2005;19(5):693–6.

24. Griniatsos J, Petrou A, Pappas P, et al. Percutaneous cholecystostomy without interval cholecystectomy as definitive treatment of acute cholecystitis in elderly and critically ill patients. South Med J 2008; 101(6):586–90.

25. Simorov A, Ranade A, Parcells J, et al. Emergent cholecystostomy is superior to open cholecystectomy in extremely ill patients with acalculous cholecystitis: a large multicenter outcome study. Am J Surg 2013;206(6):935–40.

26. Wang AJ, Wang TE, Lin CC, et al. Clinical predictors of severe gallbladder complications in acute acalculous cholecystitis. World J Gastroenterol 2003;9(12): 2821–3.

27. Sanjay P, Mittapalli D, Marioud A, et al. Clinical outcomes of a percutaneous cholecystostomy for acute cholecystitis: a multicenter analysis. HPB (Oxford) 2013;15:511–6.

28. McKay A, Abulfaraj M, Lipschitz J. Short and long-term outcomes following percutaneous cholecystostomy for acute cholecystitis in high-risk patients. Surg Endosc 2012;26(5):1343–51.

29. Still J, Scheirer R, Law E. Acute cholecystectomy performed through cultured epithelial autografts in a patient with burn injuries: a case report. J Burn Care Rehabil 1996;17(5):429–31.

30. Pripotnev S, Petrakos A. Cholecystocutaneous fistula after percutaneous gallbladder drainage. Case Rep Gastroenterol 2014;8:119–22.

31. Boland GW, Lee MJ, Leung J, et al. Percutaneous cholecystostomy in critically ill patients: early response and final outcome in 82 patients. AJR Am J Roentgenol 1994;163:339–42.

32. Patel M, Miedema BW, James MA, et al. Percutaneous cholecystostomy is an effective treatment for high-risk patients with acute cholecystitis. Am Surg 2000;66(1):33–7.

33. Atar E, Bachar GN, Berlin S, et al. Percutaneous cholecystostomy in critically ill patients with acute cholecystitis: complications and late outcome. Clin Radiol 2014;69(6):e247–52.

Venous Thromboembolism in Patients with Thermal Injury

A Review of Risk Assessment Tools and Current Knowledge on the Effectiveness and Risks of Mechanical and Chemical Prophylaxis

Christopher J. Pannucci, MD, MS[a],*, Andrea T. Obi, MD[b], Benjamin H. Timmins, MD[c], Amalia L. Cochran, MD, MA[d]

KEYWORDS

- Deep venous thrombosis • Pulmonary embolus • VTE prophylaxis

KEY POINTS

- Venous thromboembolism is an important patient safety issue in patients with thermal injury.
- Large database research is an excellent way to research rare events.
- Further research into the optimal means to provide chemical prophylaxis to burn patients is needed.

INTRODUCTION

Virchow's triad of stasis, hypercoagulability, and intimal damage describes the broad categories of factors that contribute to thrombotic risk. Patients with thermal injury seem to have the ideal physiologic predisposition to the Virchow's triad, and thus should be at high risk for postinjury venous thromboembolism events. Endothelial dysfunction via disruption of junctional proteins and stress fibers results in altered paracellular flow of solutes or capillary leak, manifested by edema and altered fluid balance.[1,2] Alterations in coagulation, including deficiency of natural anticoagulant antithrombin and altered fibrinogen, predispose toward a prothrombotic state.[3–6] In addition, burn dressings and use of split-thickness skin grafts make immobilization and resulting venous stasis inevitable in the current treatment paradigm of major cutaneous burns.

Virchow's triad notwithstanding, venous thromboembolism (VTE) is a rare event (0.6%) in the burn population. However, more than 10-fold variability in postinjury VTE risk exists among the overall population with thermal injury.[7,8] As a rare event, VTE in thermally injured patients cannot rigorously be studied using case series or small, single-center studies. This article reviews the current knowledge of VTE in the thermally injured populations, with a focus on (1) the utility of large-database approaches for VTE research, and (2) an overview of VTE risk stratification and prevention.

[a] Division of Plastic Surgery, University of Utah, 30 North 1900 East 3B400, Salt Lake City, UT 84132, USA;
[b] Department of Surgery, University of Michigan, 1500 East Medical Center Drive, Ann Arbor, MI 48109, USA;
[c] Division of Plastic Surgery, Oregon Health Sciences University, 3181 Southwest Sam Jackson Park Road, Portland, OR 97239, USA; [d] Department of Surgery, University of Utah Burn Center, University of Utah, 30 North 1900 East 3B400, Salt Lake City, UT 84132, USA
* Corresponding author.
E-mail address: christopher.pannucci@hsc.utah.edu

Clin Plastic Surg 44 (2017) 573–581
http://dx.doi.org/10.1016/j.cps.2017.02.002
0094-1298/17/© 2017 Elsevier Inc. All rights reserved.

LARGE-DATABASE APPROACHES TO RISK MODELING
Large-Database Research in Plastic Surgery, with a Focus on Rare Events

In outcomes analysis of dichotomous events (such as a yes/no VTE event), statistical analysis can examine observed differences in event frequency between patients with or without a certain risk factor, or with or without a certain intervention. Sample size calculation for dichotomous outcomes are based on the study's tolerance for type I (alpha) and type II (beta) errors, as well as the expected event rate in the two groups. Large-database research is ideally suited for outcome events that occur infrequently, or for more common outcome events in which the expected difference between 2 interventions is small. Large-database approaches allow the use of regression-based techniques to control for identified confounding variables. This method, in turn, allows more rigorous estimation of risk directly attributable to different factors. Regression is a powerful tool when used correctly but admittedly requires a high number of outcome events. In general, the so-called "rule of 10s" states that, for each additional degree of freedom in the model, 10 outcome events are required. Thus, for a regression model that contains 10 dichotomous independent variables, approximately 100 outcomes events would need to be present in the data set in order for the regression to be valid. The advantage of large-database research for rare events becomes immediately apparent here.

Large-database approaches have been used in the plastic surgery literature to examine many rare but important complications, and to examine small but important differences between two treatment modalities. Examples include use of the National Surgical Quality Improvement Program (NSQIP)[9] and the Tracking Operations and Outcomes in Plastic Surgery[10] databases to examine complications associated with acellular dermal matrix in breast reconstruction, the NSQIP to examine readmission rates after reconstructive surgery,[11,12] Medicare data to examine practice patterns in rheumatoid hand surgery,[13] and the State Inpatient Database of New York to examine the effect of Medicaid expansion on access to reconstructive breast surgery.[14] Several large-database approaches toward VTE risk model generation in surgical patients have been developed using the Veterans' Affairs Patient Safety Study,[15] the NSQIP,[16] and the Michigan Surgical Quality Collaborative,[17] although none are specific to patients with thermal injury. The authors have previously used the American Burn Association's National Burn Repository (NBR) to create a condition-specific VTE risk assessment model for thermally injured patients, as discussed later.

Universal Risk Calculators Versus Condition-Specific Risk Calculators

Bilimoria and colleagues[18] published a universal risk calculator based on more than 1 million cases in the NSQIP. This model uses a 21-point, Web-based, behind-the-scenes calculator to conceptualize and quantify risk for perioperative 30-day morbidity, 30-day mortality, and 6 additional postoperative complications. Their analysis showed that prediction for the universal calculator was similar to condition-specific models. The model was validated in a large cohort of colon surgery patients, in which the universal model and the colon-specific model performed similarly.[18]

The advantage of such a universal risk calculator is that the maximum amount of information can be obtained from a minimum amount of effort. However, this assumes that risk calculation is being performed by a person. As the interface between medicine and technology continues to improve, risk calculators will likely be run behind the scenes by computers, instead of calculated by hand by individual providers. Our prior research has shown that a computer-based VTE risk score calculation, based on administrative data, is more accurate than a physician-reported VTE risk score.[19] In this regard, it is noteworthy that, for examined complications in the study by Bilimoria and colleagues[18] (including mortality, morbidity, pneumonia, cardiac, surgical site infection, urinary tract infection, VTE, and renal failure), the colon-specific model c-statistics were slightly higher and the Brier score slightly lower. These data indicate that the procedure-specific risk assessment tool may have slightly improved calibration and discrimination compared with the universal calculator. VTE risk stratification may evolve to a behind-the-scenes calculation, and, if calculations are being performed behind the scenes by computers (eg, with no additional human effort), then the most accurate model should be used. In this regard, the authors support ongoing development of procedure-specific or injury-specific VTE risk models, if their ability to risk-stratify exceeds that of a universal calculator.

VENOUS THROMBOEMBOLISM INCIDENCE AND RISK FACTORS IN PATIENTS WITH BURNS
Incidence

Single-center studies have a reported VTE incidence as low as 0.25% when only clinically symptomatic VTE is considered, and as high as 23.3%

when patients are routinely surveyed via duplex ultrasonography for asymptomatic thrombosis.[20,21] This wide range of variability is highlighted by other single-center studies reporting VTE incidences of 4.8%, 5.9%, and 6.0%.[22–24] The variation in reported incidence can in some part be explained by the heterogeneity of the thermally injured patient population. This heterogeneity is highlighted by a recent analysis of the American Burn Association's NBR, which was used to examine VTE in a population of more than 33,000 patients.[7] The overall incidence for postburn VTE was low (0.61%), including deep venous thrombosis (DVT) (0.48%) and PE (0.18%). However, a large volume of patients had only minor injuries, biasing the results to represent patients with less severe injuries.

Among patients with total body surface area (TBSA) burns of greater than 10%, VTE rates double to 1.22%, approximating the incidence of VTE in hospitalized general, urologic, and vascular surgery patients (1.44%).[7,25] Independent predictors for VTE included increased total burn size, increased length of intensive care unit (ICU) stay, and increased number of operative procedures. When controlling for other baseline risk and comorbidities, VTE carries a 3-fold increased risk of death.[7] This fact underscores the importance of VTE risk stratification and prevention.

Risk Factors

Previous studies have identified multiple risk factors for VTE among patients with thermal injury. Most of these risk factors are acquired during the patient's inpatient stay. Identified risk factors include increased age,[22] increased body mass index,[22] increased TBSA burned,[7,20,22,26] infected burn wounds,[27] central venous access,[7,24] increased mechanical ventilation days,[7] longer ICU stays,[7,26] and increased number of operative procedures.[7] In addition, patients with thermal injury are known to have normal coagulation parameters at admission but become hypercoagulable during hospitalization, as shown by increased fibrinogen, protein C, protein S, and antithrombin III levels.[28–30]

VENOUS THROMBOEMBOLISM RISK MODELING IN PATIENTS WITH THERMAL INJURY

The Caprini Risk Assessment Model is a widely used and well-validated risk prediction tool.[31] The 2005 Caprini score has been validated to predict perioperative VTE risk in multiple surgical populations, including general, vascular, and urology surgery[25,32]; otolaryngology head and neck surgery[33,34]; plastic and reconstructive surgery[35]; patients in the surgical ICU[36]; gynecology-oncology patients[37]; and general hospitalized patients.[38,39] However, the 2005 Caprini score was designed to be used in the preoperative setting based on a patient's baseline risk factors, and injury severity or extent of surgery are small contributors to the aggregate risk score. Similarly, existing VTE risk-stratification tools derived from large-database research[15–17] are ill-suited to the specifics of patients with thermal injury. Recognizing this fact, the authors previously used a large-database approach to examine VTE risk in thermally injured patients through an analysis of the American Burn Association's NBR.[8] The NBR is a voluntary database that acquires patient-level, deidentified, Health Insurance Portability and Accountability Act–compliant data from participating burn centers in the United States and Canada. The database contains comprehensive information on patient demographics and comorbid conditions; the nature and extent of their thermal injuries; and hospital course, including operative interventions and identified complications. The NBR has previously been described in detail.[40,41]

Potential risk factors incorporated into the regression model included those that were either available or could be derived at the initial patient contact. The risk model specifically excluded risk factors that were acquired after admission (such as central venous line or infectious complications), and this was done for 2 reasons. First, the NBR database does not contain a time-to-event variable for complications or International Classification of Diseases, Ninth Revision, procedural codes. Thus, the authors were unable to ascertain whether complications or procedures that might contribute to VTE risk occurred before or after the VTE event was diagnosed. Second, a risk score that encompasses risk factors acquired in hospital can, by definition, only estimate VTE risk at the end of a patient's hospital stay. At this point, the opportunity for acute prophylaxis has been missed.

The tool was created using statistically rigorous methods, including multivariable regression to control for identified confounders. The tool was derived based on an analysis of 16,581 adult patients with thermal injury, and was subsequently validated in a separate group of 5761 thermally injured patients. Independent risk factors were weighted, or assigned an increasing number of points in the final risk model, based on the adjusted odds ratios in the final regression model.[42] In this analysis, TBSA burned and presence of inhalation injury were the most important predictors of downstream VTE events. The risk prediction tool (**Fig. 1**) explained more than 75% of the variability in patients who did or did not develop VTE during their hospitalizations, and also identified a wide variation

Two-point Risk Factors	Four-point Risk Factors
☐ Inhalation Injury ☐ TBSA 5%–9%	☐ TBSA 10%–19%
Five-point Risk Factors	**Six-point Risk Factors**
☐ TBSA 20%–49% ☐ TBSA>65%	☐ TBSA 50%–65%

TOTAL SCORE _____

Total Score	Inpatient VTE Rate
0–4	<1.0%
5	~2.0%
6	~3.0%
7	~3.5%
8	~5.0%

Fig. 1. Weighted, validated risk scoring model for VTE after thermal injury. (*From* Pannucci CJ, Osborne NH, Wahl WL. Creation and validation of a simple venous thromboembolism risk scoring tool for thermally injured patients: analysis of the National Burn Repository. J Burn Care Res 2012;33:20–5.)

in risk among patients (from <1.0% to >5.0%). Similar trends were seen in both the working and validation data sets (**Fig. 2**). VTE risk increased linearly with risk score. The calculated risk score can identify patients at particularly high VTE risk using risk factors identified at their initial presentation, and may be an appropriate guide to risk-stratify patients for VTE prophylaxis.

The 2005 Caprini Risk Assessment Model has been validated in multiple North American and international studies in a wide variety of surgical and medical patients. However, its utility in patients with thermal injury has never been examined. The Caprini score incorporates many patient-level variables and may be construed as a calculator for general medical fitness. To that end, the 2005 Caprini score has been shown to predict non-VTE complications.[43] However, in patients with burn injury, injury severity, as quantified by TBSA burned and inhalation injury, seems to be the major driver of VTE risk, and trumps the influence of patient-level factors.

VENOUS THROMBOEMBOLISM PREVENTION IN PATIENTS WITH THERMAL INJURY
Sequential Compression Devices

Intermittent pneumatic compression devices recreate the normal action of the calf muscle pump in nonambulatory patients, including those who are paralyzed for operations or critical illness. Venous stasis is known to promote venous dilation with resultant intimal microtears.[44] Operative venodilation is known to be an independent predictor of postoperative VTE.[44] The calf muscle pump action minimizes venous stasis in the lower legs, decreasing the likelihood of venous dilation and increasing endogenous fibrinolytic potential.[45] Thus, intermittent pneumatic compression devices directly address 2 components of the Virchow's triad (stasis and intimal damage) and may indirectly affect the third (hypercoagulable state, via fibrinolysis activation). Prior meta-analyses have shown that intermittent pneumatic compression can substantially reduce risk for DVT, but not necessarily for pulmonary embolus.[46] In other surgical populations, combination prophylaxis, which includes intermittent pneumatic compression and chemoprophylaxis, has been shown to significantly reduce VTE risk compared with intermittent pneumatic compression alone.[47,48] Thus, for high-risk patients, the combination of intermittent pneumatic compression and chemoprophylaxis is desirable, because the addition of chemoprophylaxis is associated with significantly lower VTE risk. However, when a patient's clinical situation precludes chemoprophylaxis, intermittent pneumatic compression alone is of substantial benefit.

Chemoprophylaxis Benefits

At present, no randomized controlled studies have examined chemoprophylaxis effectiveness specific to patients with thermal injury. Of note, recommendations regarding this population have been removed from the latest edition of the widely cited American College of Chest Physicians' (ACCP) evidence-based clinical practice guidelines for the prevention of VTE.[49] The ACCP guidelines are an exhaustively referenced compendium of surgery-specific VTE prophylaxis. It is noteworthy that the 2008 ACCP guidelines make VTE prophylaxis recommendations for patients with thermal injury,[50] but that these were removed from the 2012 version; this omission is likely from a paucity of data specific to the thermally injured population

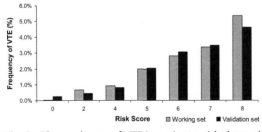

Fig. 2. Observed rates of VTE in patients with thermal injury stratified by risk score from **Fig. 1**. Gray bars represent the working data set and black bars the validation data set. The validation data set was an independent cohort not used to create the model in **Fig. 1**. (*From* Pannucci CJ, Osborne NH, Wahl WL. Creation and validation of a simple venous thromboembolism risk scoring tool for thermally injured patients: analysis of the National Burn Repository. J Burn Care Res 2012;33:20–5.)

Data from retrospective studies suggest a low incidence of VTE when low-dose unfractionated heparin (UFH) or low-molecular-weight heparin (LMWH) are administered as routine thromboprophylaxis in burned patients.[51,52] Survey data from European burn centers found the lowest rates of DVT and heparin-induced thrombocytopenia (HIT) in units using routine LMWH for thromboprophylaxis compared with those without standard protocol or those administering low-dose intravenous UFH.[53] These data have yet to be confirmed in a prospective randomized fashion. Although it is certain that thermally injured patients have a definite risk of VTE, the relative risk reduction by prophylaxis with low-dose UFH or LMWH remains undefined.[50,54]

Anti-Xa Levels in Thermal Injury

Enoxaparin accelerates the activity of antithrombin, which, in turn, accelerates the rate at which factor Xa is inactivated. Factor Xa inactivation results in decreased conversion of prothrombin to thrombin. Inhibition of this critical step in the coagulation cascade decreases the likelihood that clot will form. Anti–factor Xa (aFXa) levels can be used as a marker of enoxaparin activity.[55] Peak aFXa level, drawn at 4 hours after subcutaneous injection, is the most accurate marker of enoxaparin activity and safety.[55]

Established recommendations from both the Plastic Surgery Foundation–funded Venous Thromboembolism Prevention Study (VTEPS) and the American Society of Plastic Surgeons (ASPS) consensus guidelines support the clinical effectiveness of once-daily enoxaparin dosing.[56,57] However, the standard doses of enoxaparin (40 mg subcutaneously daily) supported by the ASPS may be insufficient in patients with thermal injury.[58–60] Our institution has previously studied enoxaparin metabolism in thermally injured patients. Standard dosing has been shown to be inadequate, with only 21% to 34% of patients having an acceptable initial steady-state aFXa level.[52,61,62] Real-time enoxaparin dose adjustment in response to a written protocol can substantially increase the proportion of patients with in-range levels (from 21% to 79%).[61] Our institution has previously created a linear regression–based equation to determine initial enoxaparin prophylaxis dose based on patient-level characteristics in patients with burns.[52,61] The equation ($22.8 + [3.3 \times \%TBSA$ burned/$10] + [1.89 \times$ (weight in kilograms)]/10) can be used to predict the starting dose of subcutaneous enoxaparin in milligrams, and enoxaparin should be provided twice daily. Thermally injured patients dosed based on this equation were significantly

more likely have initial steady-state aFXa levels that were in range (73% vs 32%; $P = .002$) and were significantly more likely to achieve in-range aFXa levels than patients in whom standard dosing was used (85% vs 68%; $P = .006$).[58] In a series of 35 pediatric patients with burns, 60% had an undetectable aFXa level based on initial dosing, and only 34% were in range.[62] Importantly, dose escalation based on aFXa levels does not substantially increase bleeding events.[62]

Case series of thermally injured patients who receive dose adjustment have a low rate of VTE (2.9%),[52] although no controlled studies exist to definitely correlate real-time aFXa monitoring and dose adjustment with decreased VTE. Importantly, inadequate initial peak aFXa levels have been shown to be significantly associated with DVT in the trauma and orthopedic surgery populations.[55,63]

Chemoprophylaxis Risks

Recent survey data suggest that the proportion of North American burn centers that routinely prescribe VTE prophylaxis ranges from 50% to 75%.[64,65] Among those centers that use prophylaxis, 22% use mechanical prophylaxis such as intermittent pneumatic compression but do not use chemoprophylaxis.[65] The primary reason provided by plastic surgeons for not using chemoprophylaxis is risk of postoperative bleeding.[66] Concerns regarding HIT are also present. The reported incidence of HIT as a result of low-dose UFH in this patient population ranges from 0.0% to 3.1%, with some investigators postulating that the severely burned are among the highest-risk patient populations for development of this complication.[51,67,68] HIT diagnosis is complicated by postburn platelet consumption and hemodilution from massive fluid resuscitation, resulting in thrombocytopenia that renders the standard diagnostic criteria largely irrelevant.[68] Episodes of HIT secondary to LMWH are less common in both general postoperative patients (0.68%)[69] and the burn population in particular (0.0%–0.2%).[51,53] HIT is an important issue among thermally injured patients, and patients with a clinical picture concerning for HIT are typically transitioned to a direct thrombin inhibitor such as argatroban. Of note, use of argatroban is an independent predictor of red blood cell and plasma transfusion after thermal injury.[70] LMWH is ideally dosed using real-time dose adjustment and the substantial decreased likelihood of HIT supports LMWH as a first-line agent for VTE prophylaxis in the burn population.

Despite blood conservation techniques and judicious use of blood products, transfusion requirement for patients undergoing major burn excision remains substantial.[71,72] In addition, nonmajor bleeding in this patient population, such as wound hematoma, can be a significant source of morbidity. Graft loss from hematoma can result in repeat operations, thus further increasing VTE risk. In the absence of chemoprophylaxis, baseline risk of hematomas among plastic and reconstructive patients is 0.5% to 2.7%.[73–76] In an analysis of the VTEPS study, including 3681 general plastic and reconstructive surgery patients, receipt of postoperative enoxaparin was not associated with statistically significant increases in 60-day reoperative hematoma; the absolute risk increase in the enoxaparin group was 0.7%.[76] In thermally injured patients, prophylactic anticoagulation does not substantially increase red blood cell transfusion, although therapeutic anticoagulation is an independent predictor.[70] Increased TBSA burned is known to have a linear relationship with red blood cell transfusion requirements, and patients with inhalation injury are known to have higher rates of red blood cell transfusion than patients without.[70]

Existing data support that red blood cell transfusion is not an independent predictor of mortality[70] and that VTE is an independent predictor of mortality.[7] However, based on existing data, the risks of major and nonmajor bleeding complications need to be better defined to identify the subset of patients in whom the benefits of prophylactic anticoagulants outweigh the risks. However, until such data become available, the authors strongly support the opinions voiced by Davison and Massoumi[77] in a 2007 *Plastic and Reconstructive Surgery* editorial. They remind readers that the consequences of hematomas can typically be addressed with hospital admission, transfusion, and/or an additional operative procedure; these usually represent a transient issue for patients that can be completely resolved. In contrast, the consequences of pulmonary embolus, in which 10% of symptomatic patients are dead within 60 minutes, cannot necessarily be fixed.[77,78]

SUMMARY

Large-database research is useful in plastic and reconstructive surgery to examine rare complications or to compare interventions in which the expected difference in outcomes is small. VTE can be a life-threatening or limb-threatening complication of thermal injury. The severity of burn injury, as quantified by TBSA burned and presence of inhalation injury, can be used to predict VTE risk among patients with thermal injury, and a weighted risk-stratification tool has been developed. There is no level I evidence regarding the risks or benefits of chemoprophylaxis after thermal injury, and further

research is necessary in these areas. Real-time aFXa monitoring and enoxaparin dose adjustment may optimize the effectiveness of VTE prophylaxis and minimize the risk of bleeding in patients with thermal injury.

REFERENCES

1. Wu W, Huang Q, He F, et al. Roles of mitogen-activated protein kinases in the modulation of endothelial cell function following thermal injury. Shock 2011;35:618–25.
2. Wang S, Huang Q, Guo X, et al. The P38alpha and P38delta MAP kinases may be gene therapy targets in the future treatment of severe burns. Shock 2010; 34:176–82.
3. Niedermayr M, Schramm W, Kamolz L, et al. Antithrombin deficiency and its relationship to severe burns. Burns 2007;33:173–8.
4. Lavrentieva A, Kontakiotis T, Bitzani M, et al. The efficacy of antithrombin administration in the acute phase of burn injury. Thromb Haemost 2008;100: 286–90.
5. King DR, Namias N, Andrews DM. Coagulation abnormalities following thermal injury. Blood Coagul Fibrinolysis 2010;21:666–9.
6. Schaden E, Hoerburger D, Hacker S, et al. Fibrinogen function after severe burn injury. Burns 2012; 38:77–82.
7. Pannucci CJ, Osborne NH, Wahl WL. Venous thromboembolism in thermally injured patients: analysis of the National Burn Repository. J Burn Care Res 2011; 32:6–12.
8. Pannucci CJ, Osborne NH, Wahl WL. Creation and validation of a simple venous thromboembolism risk scoring tool for thermally injured patients: analysis of the National Burn Repository. J Burn Care Res 2012;33:20–5.
9. Davila AA, Seth AK, Wang E, et al. Human acellular dermis versus submuscular tissue expander breast reconstruction: a multivariate analysis of short-term complications. Arch Plast Surg 2013;40:19–27.
10. Pannucci CJ, Antony AK, Wilkins EG. The impact of acellular dermal matrix on tissue expander/implant loss in breast reconstruction: an analysis of the Tracking Outcomes and Operations in Plastic Surgery database. Plast Reconstr Surg 2013;132:1–10.
11. Nelson JA, Fischer J, Chung CC, et al. Readmission following ventral hernia repair: a model derived from the ACS-NSQIP datasets. Hernia 2015;19: 125–33.
12. Tahiri Y, Fischer JP, Wink JD, et al. Analysis of risk factors associated with 30-day readmissions following pediatric plastic surgery - a review of 5,376 procedures. Plast Reconstr Surg 2014;135(2):521–9.
13. Zhong L, Chung KC, Baser O, et al. Variation in rheumatoid hand and wrist surgery among Medicare

beneficiaries: a population-based cohort study. J Rheumatol 2015;42:429–36.

4. Giladi AM, Chung KC, Aliu O. Changes in use of autologous and prosthetic postmastectomy reconstruction after Medicaid expansion in New York state. Plast Reconstr Surg 2015;135:53–62.

5. Rogers SO Jr, Kilaru RK, Hosokawa P, et al. Multivariable predictors of postoperative venous thromboembolic events after general and vascular surgery: results from the Patient Safety in Surgery study. J Am Coll Surg 2007;204:1211–21.

6. Pannucci CJ, Shanks A, Moote MJ, et al. Identifying patients at high risk for venous thromboembolism requiring treatment after outpatient surgery. Ann Surg 2012;255:1093–9.

7. Pannucci CJ, Laird S, Dimick JB, et al. A validated risk model to predict 90-day VTE events in postsurgical patients. Chest 2014;145:567–73.

8. Bilimoria KY, Liu Y, Paruch JL, et al. Development and evaluation of the universal ACS NSQIP surgical risk calculator: a decision aid and informed consent tool for patients and surgeons. J Am Coll Surg 2013; 217:833–42.e1–3.

9. Pannucci CJ, Obi A, Alvarez R, et al. Inadequate venous thromboembolism risk stratification predicts venous thromboembolic events in surgical intensive care unit patients. J Am Coll Surg 2014;218: 898–904.

20. Fecher AM, O'Mara MS, Goldfarb IW, et al. Analysis of deep vein thrombosis in burn patients. Burns 2004;30:591–3.

21. Wahl WL, Brandt MM, Ahrns KS, et al. Venous thrombosis incidence in burn patients: preliminary results of a prospective study. J Burn Care Rehabil 2002;23: 97–102.

22. Harrington DT, Mozingo DW, Cancio L, et al. Thermally injured patients are at significant risk for thromboembolic complications. J Trauma 2001;50: 495–9.

23. Mullins F, Mian MA, Jenkins D, et al. Thromboembolic complications in burn patients and associated risk factors. J Burn Care Res 2013;34:355–60.

24. Wibbenmeyer LA, Hoballah JJ, Amelon MJ, et al. The prevalence of venous thromboembolism of the lower extremity among thermally injured patients determined by duplex sonography. J Trauma 2003; 55:1162–7.

25. Bahl V, Hu HM, Henke PK, et al. A validation study of a retrospective venous thromboembolism risk scoring method. Ann Surg 2009;251(2):344–50.

26. Chung KK, Blackbourne LH, Renz EM, et al. Global evacuation of burn patients does not increase the incidence of venous thromboembolic complications. J Trauma 2008;65:19–24.

27. Wahl WL, Brandt MM. Potential risk factors for deep venous thrombosis in burn patients. J Burn Care Rehabil 2001;22:128–31.

28. Meizoso JP, Ray JJ, Allen CJ, et al. Hypercoagulability and venous thromboembolism in burn patients. Semin Thromb Hemost 2015;41:43–8.

29. Van Haren RM, Valle EJ, Thorson CM, et al. Hypercoagulability and other risk factors in trauma intensive care unit patients with venous thromboembolism. J Trauma Acute Care Surg 2014;76: 443–9.

30. García-Avello A, Lorente JA, Cesar-Perez J, et al. Degree of hypercoagulability and hyperfibrinolysis is related to organ failure and prognosis after burn trauma. Thromb Res 1998;89:59–64.

31. Caprini JA. Thrombosis risk assessment as a guide to quality patient care. Dis Mon 2005;51:70–8.

32. Cassidy MR, Rosenkranz P, McAneny D. Reducing postoperative venous thromboembolism complications with a standardized risk-stratified prophylaxis protocol and mobilization program. J Am Coll Surg 2014;218:1095–104.

33. Shuman AG, Hu HM, Pannucci CJ, et al. Stratifying the risk of venous thromboembolism in otolaryngology. Otolaryngol Head Neck Surg 2012;146: 719–24.

34. Yarlagadda BB, Brook CD, Stein DJ, et al. Venous thromboembolism in otolaryngology surgical inpatients receiving chemoprophylaxis. Head Neck 2014;36:1087–93.

35. Pannucci CJ, Bailey SH, Dreszer G, et al. Validation of the Caprini risk assessment model in plastic and reconstructive surgery patients. J Am Coll Surg 2011;212:105–12.

36. Chang EY, Pannucci CJ, Wilkins EG. Quality of clinical studies in aesthetic surgery journals: a 10-year review. Aesthet Surg J 2009;29:144–7 [discussion: 147–9].

37. Stroud W, Whitworth JM, Miklic M, et al. Validation of a venous thromboembolism risk assessment model in gynecologic oncology. Gynecol Oncol 2014;134: 160–3.

38. Mokhtari M, Attarian H, Norouzi M, et al. Venous thromboembolism risk assessment, prophylaxis practices and interventions for its improvement (AVAIL-ME Extension Project, Iran). Thromb Res 2014;133:567–73.

39. Zhou H, Wang L, Wu X, et al. Validation of a venous thromboembolism risk assessment model in hospitalized Chinese patients: a case-control study. J Atheroscler Thromb 2014;21:261–72.

40. Latenser BA, Miller SF, Bessey PQ, et al. National burn repository 2006: a ten-year review. J Burn Care Res 2007;28:635–58.

41. Jeng JC, Advisory Committee to the National Burn Repository. "Open for business!" a primer on the scholarly use of the National Burn Repository. J Burn Care Res 2007;28:143–4.

42. Rassi A Jr, Rassi A, Little WC, et al. Development and validation of a risk score for predicting death

in Chagas' heart disease. N Engl J Med 2006;355: 799–808.

43. Jeong HS, Miller TJ, Davis K, et al. Application of the Caprini risk assessment model in evaluation of non-venous thromboembolism complications in plastic and reconstructive surgery patients. Aesthet Surg J 2014;34:87–95.

44. Comerota AJ, Stewart GJ, Alburger PD, et al. Operative venodilation: a previously unsuspected factor in the cause of postoperative deep vein thrombosis. Surgery 1989;106:301–8 [discussion: 308–9].

45. Comerota AJ, Chouhan V, Harada RN, et al. The fibrinolytic effects of intermittent pneumatic compression: mechanism of enhanced fibrinolysis. Ann Surg 1997; 226:306–13 [discussion: 313–4].

46. Vanek VW. Meta-analysis of effectiveness of intermittent pneumatic compression devices with a comparison of thigh-high to knee-high sleeves. Am Surg 1998;64: 1050–8.

47. Henke PK, Arya S, Pannucci C, et al. Procedure-specific venous thromboembolism prophylaxis: a paradigm from colectomy surgery. Surgery 2012; 152:528–34 [discussion: 534–6].

48. Turpie AG, Bauer KA, Caprini JA, et al. Fondaparinux combined with intermittent pneumatic compression vs. intermittent pneumatic compression alone for prevention of venous thromboembolism after abdominal surgery: a randomized, double-blind comparison. J Thromb Haemost 2007;5:1854–61.

49. Gould MK, Garcia DA, Wren SM, et al. Prevention of VTE in nonorthopedic surgical patients: Antithrombotic Therapy and Prevention of Thrombosis, 9th ed: American College of Chest Physicians Evidence-based Clinical Practice Guidelines. Chest 2012;141: e227S–277S.

50. Geerts WH, Bergqvist D, Pineo GF, et al. Prevention of venous thromboembolism: American College of chest physicians evidence-based clinical practice guidelines (8th edition). Chest 2008;133:381S–453S.

51. Bushwitz J, LeClaire A, He J, et al. Clinically significant venous thromboembolic complications in burn patients receiving unfractionated heparin or enoxaparin as prophylaxis. J Burn Care Res 2011;32: 578–82.

52. Lin H, Faraklas I, Saffle J, et al. Enoxaparin dose adjustment is associated with low incidence of venous thromboembolic events in acute burn patients. J Trauma 2011;71:1557–61.

53. Busche MN, Herold C, Kramer R, et al. Evaluation of prophylactic anticoagulation, deep venous thrombosis, and heparin-induced thrombocytopenia in 21 burn centers in Germany, Austria, and Switzerland. Ann Plast Surg 2011;67:17–24.

54. Faucher LD, Conlon KM. Practice guidelines for deep venous thrombosis prophylaxis in burns. J Burn Care Res 2007;28:661–3.

55. Kopelman TR, O'Neill PJ, Pieri PG, et al. Alternative dosing of prophylactic enoxaparin in the trauma patient: is more the answer? Am J Surg 2013;206: 911–5 [discussion: 915–6].

56. Pannucci CJ, Dreszer G, Wachtman CF, et al. Postoperative enoxaparin prevents symptomatic venous thromboembolism in high-risk plastic surgery patients. Plast Reconstr Surg 2011;128:1093–103.

57. Murphy RX, Alderman A, Gutowski K, et al. Evidence based practices for thromboembolism prevention: summary of the ASPS venous thromboembolism task force report. Plast Reconstr Surg 2012;130:168e–75e.

58. Faraklas I, Ghanem M, Brown A, et al. Evaluation of an enoxaparin dosing calculator using burn size and weight. J Burn Care Res 2013;34:621–7.

59. Bickford A, Majercik S, Bledsoe J, et al. Weight-based enoxaparin dosing for venous thromboembolism prophylaxis in the obese trauma patient. Am J Surg 2013; 206:847–51 [discussion: 851–2].

60. Robinson S, Zincuk A, Strøm T, et al. Enoxaparin, effective dosage for intensive care patients: double-blinded randomised clinical trial. Crit Care 2010;14:R41.

61. Lin H, Faraklas I, Cochran A, et al. Enoxaparin and antifactor Xa levels in acute burn patients. J Burn Care Res 2011;32:1–5.

62. Brown A, Faraklas I, Ghanem M, et al. Enoxaparin and antifactor Xa levels in pediatric acute burn patients. J Burn Care Res 2013;34:628–32.

63. Levine MN, Planes A, Hirsh J, et al. The relationship between anti-factor Xa level and clinical outcome in patients receiving enoxaparine low molecular weight heparin to prevent deep vein thrombosis after hip replacement. Thromb Haemost 1989;62:940–4.

64. Abedi N, Papp A. A survey of current practice patterns in prophylaxis against venous thromboembolism (VTE) and gastrointestinal (GI) ulceration among Canadian burn centers. Burns 2011;37: 1182–6.

65. Ferguson RE, Critchfield A, Leclaire A, et al. Current practice of thromboprophylaxis in the burn population: a survey study of 84 US burn centers. Burns 2005;31:964–6.

66. Clavijo-Alvarez JA, Pannucci CJ, Oppenheimer AJ, et al. Prevention of venous thromboembolism in body contouring surgery: a national survey of 596 ASPS surgeons. Ann Plast Surg 2011;66:228–32.

67. Scott JR, Klein MB, Gernsheimer T, et al. Arterial and venous complications of heparin-induced thrombocytopenia in burn patients. J Burn Care Res 2007; 28:71–5.

68. Hejl CG, Leclerc T, Bargues L, et al. Incidence and features of heparin-induced thrombocytopenia (HIT) in burn patients: a retrospective study. Thromb Haemost 2008;99:974–6.

69. Junqueira DR, Perini E, Penholati RR, et al. Unfractionated heparin versus low molecular weight heparin for avoiding heparin-induced thrombocytopenia

in postoperative patients. Cochrane Database Syst Rev 2012;(9):CD007557.

70. Lu RP, Lin FC, Ortiz-Pujols SM, et al. Blood utilization in patients with burn injury and association with clinical outcomes (CME). Transfusion 2013;53:2212–21 [quiz: 2211].

71. Criswell KK, Gamelli RL. Establishing transfusion needs in burn patients. Am J Surg 2005;189: 324–6.

72. Palmieri TL, Caruso DM, Foster KN, et al. Effect of blood transfusion on outcome after major burn injury: a multicenter study. Crit Care Med 2006;34: 1602–7.

73. Hatef DA, Kenkel JM, Nguyen MQ, et al. Thromboembolic risk assessment and the efficacy of enoxaparin prophylaxis in excisional body contouring surgery. Plast Reconstr Surg 2008;122: 269–79.

74. Liao EC, Taghinia AH, Nguyen LP, et al. Incidence of hematoma complication with heparin venous thrombosis prophylaxis after TRAM flap breast reconstruction. Plast Reconstr Surg 2008;121: 1101–7.

75. Kim EK, Eom JS, Ahn SH, et al. The efficacy of prophylactic low-molecular-weight heparin to prevent pulmonary thromboembolism in immediate breast reconstruction using the TRAM flap. Plast Reconstr Surg 2009;123:9–12.

76. Pannucci CJ, Wachtman CF, Dreszer G, et al. The effect of post-operative enoxaparin on risk for re-operative hematoma. Plast Reconstr Surg 2012; 129(1):160–8.

77. Davison SP, Massoumi W. Our complication, your problem. Plast Reconstr Surg 2007;120:1428–9.

78. Kearon C. Natural history of venous thromboembolism. Circulation 2003;107:I22–30.

Burn Center Care of Patients with Stevens-Johnson Syndrome and Toxic Epidermal Necrolysis

Robert Cartotto, MD, FRCS(C)

KEYWORDS

• Toxic epidermal necrolysis • Stevens-Johnson syndrome • Burn center • Exfoliative conditions

KEY POINTS

• Although patients with Stevens-Johnson syndrome (SJS) and toxic epidermal necrolysis (TEN) are now routinely referred to burn centers for definitive care, not all cases of SJS or even SJS-TEN overlap automatically warrant burn center admission. However, the more extensive the degree of exfoliation (especially in TEN), the greater is the need for and benefit from providing care in a burn center setting.

• Diagnosis of SJS and TEN relies on careful documentation of systemic, cutaneous, and mucosal features obtained from a detailed history and physical examination, combined with histologic confirmation by biopsy.

• The treatment bundle in the burn center should include cessation of the causative medication; careful airway assessment and protection, if indicated; directed (rather than routine) fluid replacement for hypovolemia; early enteral nutrition; wound coverage with skin substitutes; urgent ophthalmologic consultation; careful surveillance for infection; avoidance of prophylactic antibiotics; and consideration of a pharmacologic intervention to attempt to halt the disease process.

• Pharmacologic interventions to halt the disease process have not been examined through large high-quality studies and consensus on use of these agents is lacking.

INTRODUCTION

Stevens-Johnson syndrome (SJS) and toxic epidermal necrolysis (TEN) are severe, potentially life-threatening, adverse cutaneous reactions that most commonly are precipitated by the use of a medication. Although these conditions are rare, with only 1.5 to 1.9 cases occurring per million of the population per year, the associated mortality ranges between 9% for SJS to 30% to 50% for TEN.[1] An important feature of these conditions is varying degrees of detachment of the epidermis, which results in wounds that are analogous to superficial partial thickness burns. Consequently, patients with SJS and TEN are frequently referred to specialized burn units for their care, primarily to optimize wound and dressing management but also to garner all of the other beneficial aspects of multidisciplinary care that modern burn treatment facilities can offer for patients with large cutaneous wounds. Not surprisingly, a multicenter review of TEN found that delayed referral of patients with TEN to a burn center was associated with significantly lower odds of survival.[2] This article reviews all aspects of SJS and TEN but

Disclosure statement: The author has nothing to disclose.
Department of Surgery, Ross Tilley Burn Centre, Sunnybrook Health Sciences Centre, University of Toronto, Room D712, 1075 Bayview Avenue, Toronto, Ontario M4N 3M5, Canada
E-mail address: robert.cartotto@sunnybrook.ca

Clin Plastic Surg 44 (2017) 583–595
http://dx.doi.org/10.1016/j.cps.2017.02.016
0094-1298/17/Crown Copyright © 2017 Published by Elsevier Inc. All rights reserved.

primarily focuses on the important principles of management of patients with these conditions.

NOMENCLATURE AND CLASSIFICATION

SJS and TEN likely represent different degrees of severity of the same disease process.[3] In both conditions, there must be a skin rash that features epidermal detachment as well as erosion of mucosal membranes (mucositis) at 2 or more locations. In SJS, epidermal detachment is limited to less than 10% of the total body surface area (TBSA) whereas in TEN, epidermal loss occurs over greater than 30% of the TBSA. When the epidermal detachment involves 10% to 30% of the TBSA, the condition is referred to as SJS-TEN overlap. In SJS, SJS-TEN overlap, and TEN, the rash features spots but not typical target lesions, although flat atypical target lesions can be seen. The spectrum of SJS-TEN should be distinguished from another distinct condition, erythema multiforme major, which occurs following infection with herpes simplex virus or *Mycoplasma pneumoniae*, and which features oral mucositis, a rash consisting of typical target lesions, as well as raised atypical target lesions but minimal to no epidermal detachment. A final entity, TEN without spots, features diffuse erythema but no spots or target lesions and epidermal detachment involving greater than 10% of the TBSA. These points of classification are summarized in **Table 1**.[4]

CAUSES OF STEVENS-JOHNSON SYNDROME AND TOXIC EPIDERMAL NECROLYSIS

Although approximately 75% of cases of SJS-TEN result from the use of a drug, it is recognized that viral illnesses, influenza-like illnesses, and *M*

pneumoniae infections may also be causative.[5] A recent case-control study[6] identified that drugs with the highest risk of inducing SJS-TEN included allopurinol, anti-infective sulfonamides (eg, cotrimoxazole), phenytoin, carbamazepine, phenobarbital, lamotrigine (an antiepileptic drug), nevirapine (an anti–human immunodeficiency virus [HIV] drug), and oxicam-type nonsteroidal anti-inflammatory drugs (NSAIDs) (eg, meloxicam) The latency period between initiation of these high-risk drugs and onset of the cutaneous reaction ranged between 4 and 28 days. Commonly prescribed drugs that carry a moderate risk o inducing SJS-TEN included cephalosporins, macrolide and quinolone antibiotics, tetracycline, and acetic acid–type NSAIDs (eg, diclofenac) Frequently prescribed drugs that had no increased risk of causing SJS-TEN included valproic acid (in contrast to most of the other antiepileptics), angiotensin converting enzyme (ACE)-inhibitors, beta blockers, calcium channel blockers, diuretics and oral hypoglycemic drugs that carry a sulfonamide structure, and propionic type NSAIDs (eg ibuprofen). Although these drugs do not seem to carry a higher risk of causing SJS-TEN, they have been implicated in individual cases of SJS-TEN and, in general, have a much longer latency period than the high-risk drugs (eg, >30 weeks in the case of valproic acid). Unfortunately, there are no reliable in vivo or in vitro tests to identify drug causality in SJS-TEN, although the lymphocyte transformation test and granulysin expression test have been explored.[7,8] Two essential principles to remember with respect to medication use and causes of SJS-TEN are

- All medications should be considered as potential suspects, including intermittently used drugs such as vitamins and analgesics

Table 1
Classification of exfoliative skin reactions

	Erythema Multiforme Major	SJS	SJS-TEN Overlap	TEN	TEN Without Spots
Mucositis	Oral mucositis	≥2 sites	≥2 sites	≥2 sites	≥2 sites
Spots	No	Yes	Yes	Yes	No
Atypical target lesions	Yes, raised	Yes, flat	Yes, flat	Yes, flat	No
Typical target lesions	Yes	No	No	No	No
Epidermal detachment	Negligible	<10% TBSA	10%–30% TBSA	>30% TBSA	>10% TBSA
Mortality	None	10%	—	30%–50%	—

Adapted from Bastuji-Garin S, Rzany B, Stern RS, et al. Clinical classification of cases of toxic epidermal necrolysis, Stevens Johnson syndrome, and erythema multiforme. Arch Dermatol 1993;129:92–6.

and homeopathic, traditional, or natural products.

- Drugs may be started to treat the initial prodromal symptoms of SJS-TEN, and must not be mistaken as the causative agent. A careful history noting the time sequence of medication use and appearance of systemic and cutaneous signs and symptoms is mandatory.

GENETIC SUSCEPTIBILITY

A genetic predisposition to SJS-TEN has long been suspected and, in the last few decades, various relationships between genetic expression of certain human leukocyte antigen (HLA) alleles, specific medications, and racial background have been identified. One of the earliest discovered associations was a weak link between expression of HLA-B*12 and oxicam-induced TEN in patients of European ancestry.[9] More recently, a very strong association between expression of HLA-B*15:02, carbamazepine-induced SJS-TEN, and Han Chinese, Thai, Indian, and Malaysian origin has been observed; as has a very strong association between HLA-B*58:01 expression and allopurinol-induced SJS-TEN, in Han Chinese, Thai, Japanese, Korean, and European populations.[10–13] Although many other associations have been discovered,[8] the US Food and Drug Administration currently only recommends HLA-B*15:02 screening in patients of Asian ancestry before starting carbamazepine.

PATHOGENESIS AND PATHOLOGIC FEATURES

The pathogenesis of SJS-TEN is complex and incompletely understood. Current theories all generally involve activation of keratinocyte apoptosis, which leads to extensive full thickness loss of the epidermal layer, and then separation of the nonviable epidermis at the dermal-epidermal junction. The underlying dermis is viable and usually shows only a mild infiltration of lymphocytes. How a drug elicits this response is unknown but it seems to involve an immune reaction featuring activation of CD 8+ cytotoxic T lymphocytes, natural killer cells, and increased production of the proapoptotic protein, granulysin. Serum levels of granulysin seem to correlate with disease severity, suggesting that granulysin is a critical mediator for keratinocyte death.[14] Activation of T cells seems to involve an interaction between the drug, HLA molecules on antigen-presenting cells, and T cell receptors.[15] In addition, keratinocyte apoptosis also seems to be stimulated by the interaction of the Fas ligand (FasL) binding with the Fas receptor on the keratinocyte cell membrane. Raised serum levels of soluble FasL, arising either from the keratinocytes themselves and/or peripheral blood mononuclear cells, have been identified in patients with SJS-TEN, presumably leading to an interaction with keratinocyte Fas to activate keratinocyte apoptosis.[16,17] Finally, inflammatory cascades involving reactive oxygen species and tumor necrosis factor (TNF)-α also act to intensify stimulation of apoptotic pathways among keratinocytes.[18,19]

CLINICAL PICTURE AND DIAGNOSIS

SJS and TEN appear most commonly between 4 days and 4 weeks after exposure to the drug.[8] There is usually an initial nonspecific prodromal illness lasting 2 or 3 days that may feature malaise and fatigue, fever, sore throat, rhinitis, and irritation or pruritus of the skin and eyes. Patients often take, or are prescribed a medication for these symptoms, which is then erroneously implicated as the causative drug once the cutaneous manifestations appear and the diagnosis of SJS or TEN becomes apparent.

After this prodromal phase, cutaneous lesions start to appear on the central trunk, face, and proximal limbs, eventually spreading to the distal extremities, including the palms and soles. The initial lesions are dusky erythematous, purpuric, and irregularly shaped macules and spots. Some lesions have the appearance of atypical flat target lesions with 2 concentric rings around a necrotic center. These lesions begin to blister and coalesce to form bullae. The epidermis in these involved areas is unstable and tangential digital pressure on the skin causes the epidermis to shear off and detach (the positive but nonspecific Nikolsky sign). Further confluence of the blistered skin and bullae leads formation of larger flaccid bullae and, ultimately, to spontaneous sheet-like detachment of necrotic epidermis, leaving painful raw areas of glistening bright red dermis exposed (Figs. 1 and 2). The percent of the TBSA in which there is imminent or actual epidermal detachment determines where the patient is placed on the SJS-TEN spectrum: less than 10% TBSA in SJS, 10% to 30% TBSA in SJS-TEN overlap, and greater than 30% TBSA in TEN.[4]

Simultaneously, erosions and sloughing of the mucous membranes in at least 2 sites have also been progressing. The lips and oropharynx are the most commonly involved, followed by the conjunctiva, genital mucosa, and anorectal mucosa. Mucosal sloughing may also involve the esophagus, the remainder of the gastrointestinal tract, and the tracheobronchial surfaces. Aggressive involvement of the lips and oropharynx is common, with severe pain, erosions and bleeding,

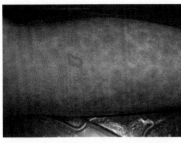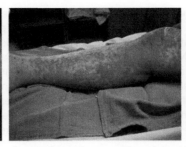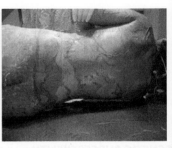

Fig. 1. Initial rash featuring dusky purpuric macules and spots with early vesicle and blister formation (*left*). Initial progression of rash with coalescence of lesions, formation of larger blisters and bullae, and early epidermal detachment (*center*). Final progression to extensive sheet-like epidermal detachment (*right*).

dysphagia, odynophagia, and drooling. The lips typically become crusted with dried blood. Patients usually are unable to eat or drink because of the severity of this mucositis (**Fig. 3**). Similarly, ocular involvement is also usually severe, with photophobia, tearing, conjunctivitis, purulent exudates, crusting, and pseudomembranous conjunctival erosions that result in the formation of synechiae between the lids or between the conjunctiva and the eyelids (**Fig. 4**). Keratitis and corneal ulcerations can occur and may lead to permanent partial or complete visual loss.[8] Erosions involving the glans penis, vulva, or vagina may cause the patient to report pain or burning during micturition.

By the time a patient presents to the burn unit, systemic manifestations may be well advanced. Often the patient is dehydrated and malnourished. Significant upper airway mucositis may compromise the airway and around one-fourth of TEN cases may have early respiratory dysfunction featuring cough, trachea-bronchial mucosal involvement, and dyspnea.[20] Gastrointestinal mucosal involvement is much less common but when it occurs may present with diarrhea, or bleeding or excretion of sloughing bowel mucosal epithelium.[21] Early acute kidney injury may be manifested by elevation in the serum creatinine and oliguria. Hematuria and microalbuminuria may also be present.[22] On presentation, laboratory abnormalities may include anemia, neutropenia, thrombocytopenia, and elevated hepatic enzymes.[23] In cases in which there have been extensive areas of epidermal loss, the patient may develop problems related to fluid loss, hypothermia, and invasive infection. Not uncommonly, hospital-acquired infections related to invasive care with urinary catheters, central lines, and endotracheal intubation eventually appear, leading to sepsis and multiorgan failure, which is the main cause of death in patients with TEN.[2,24,25]

The diagnosis of SJS-TEN rests on 2 factors: (1) presence of systemic, cutaneous, and mucosal features consistent with SJS-TEN based on a detailed history and physical examination and (2) histologic confirmation. A clear identification of the prodromal illness followed by onset of skin and mucosal changes, a positive Nikolsky sign, and a clear documentation of the percent body surface area where there is actual or imminent epidermal slough only, using the rule of nines and/or a Lund and Browder burn diagram are

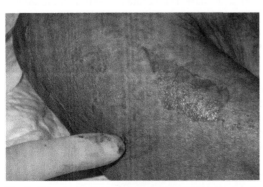

Fig. 2. Demonstration of the positive Nikolsky sign in a patient with TEN.

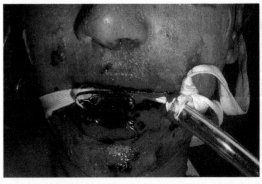

Fig. 3. Severe oral mucositis in a patient with TEN. This patient was intubated because of the severity of the upper airway mucositis and exfoliation of more than 70% TBSA.

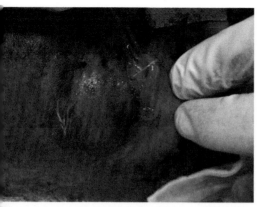

Fig. 4. Florid conjunctivitis with exudate and strands between upper and lower eyelids. A glass rod is inserted into the medial lower conjunctival fornix to be swept across the fornix to break up these bands.

considered the minimum elements needed to make the clinical diagnosis. Several punch biopsies should be obtained from representative areas where the epidermis is still intact for both immediate frozen section and fixed section analysis. Histologic examination will show complete necrosis of all epidermal layers with a cleavage plane separating the epidermis from the dermis.[26] Direct immunofluorescence should be performed to prove that there is no immunoglobulin or complement deposition in the epidermis, which are features more in keeping with other autoimmune blistering disorders, such as paraneoplastic pemphigus and bullous pemphigoid.[26]

The differential diagnosis includes staphylococcal scalded skin syndrome (SSSS), autoimmune blistering diseases (paraneoplastic pemphigus, pemphigus vulgaris, bullous pemphigoid), Acute generalized exanthematous pustulosis (AGEP), and generalized bullous fixed drug eruption (GBFDE).[8,26] Mucositis is absent in SSSS and frozen section biopsy will show that the epidermal separation arises from an intraepidermal cleavage plane rather than a dermoepidermal split as in SJS-TEN. Intraepidermal cleavage is also featured in AGEP. In GBFDE, blistering is limited and mucositis is minimal and there are usually no systemic symptoms.[8] Autoimmune blistering disorders may need to be diagnosed by immunofluorescence testing as previously described. Finally, an acute graft versus host reaction may closely mimic SJS-TEN but would typically be seen within 2 weeks of an allogeneic hematopoietic stem cell transplant.[8]

WHEN TO REFER TO A BURN CENTER

Early referral of patients with TEN to a burn center seems to be beneficial in many respects. The obvious reason to consider burn center transfer is to optimize wound care and dressing application to extensive and complex anatomic areas. Burn centers also may provide availability of skin substitutes for temporary coverage of large wounds. Strict adherence to isolation and barrier precautions, multidisciplinary care involving burn-critical care nurses, dietitians, and rehabilitation therapists, and the capability of environmental temperature regulation and specialty pressure reduction beds make burn units the ideal place to care for patients with SJS-TEN.

However, there has been a recent increasing trend to inappropriately refer patients with rashes, nonexfoliative skin conditions, and patients with mild SJS to burn centers. Clearly, the decision to involve a burn center must be based on an accurate estimation of the extent of epidermal detachment. Detachment of 10% or less of the TBSA does not automatically warrant transfer, whereas cases of TEN with detachment greater than 30% of the TBSA should be transferred as soon as possible. In between these 2 extremes is a gray zone in which referral should be considered on an individual basis.

MANAGEMENT PRINCIPLES IN THE BURN CENTER

This section discusses the details of a treatment bundle for care of SJS-TEN (**Box 1**).

Identify and Withdraw the Inciting Drugs

Ultimately, this step relies on obtaining a careful history and making a timeline showing all medication use, onset of prodromal symptoms, and development of the skin manifestations. In a young healthy patient on few medications this task is relatively easy but becomes much more complex in an elderly patient, with poor memory, who may be taking several medications. The moderate and high-risk drugs have shorter latency periods, generally less than 4 weeks; whereas low-risk drugs have much longer latency periods. In general but not always, more than 8 weeks of use of a drug would suggest a low likelihood that the drug was responsible.[7] There is no reliable in vitro test to identify the culprit drug. Methods used to identify drug allergies, such as patch testing, pin prick, or intradermal injection, are not suitable in identification of the drug responsible for SJS-TEN.[27]

Airway Management

Intubation may be required for upper airway obstruction from excessive secretions, bleeding,

---

Box 1
At-a-glance: burn center treatment bundle for Stevens-Johnson syndrome and toxic epidermal necrolysis

Withdraw inciting drug

Consider airway protection

- Significant oral-pharyngeal or airway involvement
- Extensive exfoliation

Fluid replacement if evidence of dehydration or volume contraction

Enteral nutritional support

Infection surveillance and antibiotics for identified infections, not prophylactic antibiotics.

Wound and mucosal care

- Use of skin substitutes (semisynthetic or biological)
- Dressings
- Separation of adjacent involved mucosal surfaces
- Mouth care

Ophthalmologic consultation

Consider pharmacologic therapy

- Steroids: benefits unknown, generally withdrawn or tapered at burn center admission
- Intravenous immunoglobulin: poor-quality evidence suggests no survival benefit; reasonable safety profile
- Cyclosporine: possible benefit supported by limited poor-quality evidence; significant associated adverse effects
- TNF inhibitors: possible benefit supported by very limited poor-quality evidence; thalidomide should not be used

Other supportive care

- Analgesia (opioid-based)
- Gastrointestinal stress ulcer and venous thromboembolism prophylaxis
- Warm ambient environment
- Pressure reduction bed

---

or edema or when a patient presents with severe dyspnea or hypoxemia from bronchopulmonary desquamation, established bronchopneumonia, or evolving acute respiratory distress syndrome.[20,28] Sometimes, the massive extent of skin exfoliation will dictate the need for intubation and mechanical ventilation to allow appropriate wound care and analgesia. The decision to intubate an SJS-TEN patient should be carefully considered and weighed against the potential risk of causing ventilator-associated pneumonia. Intubation of these patients may be extremely difficult because of mucosal sloughing, swelling, and bleeding in the upper airway, and it is prudent to involve anesthesiologists because of their expertise in dealing with the difficult airway. The airway is best secured with ties around the neck or by wiring the endotracheal tube to the dentition.

Adhesive tape should not be used because it will not securely stick to the skin and may peel off facial and neck epidermis. If the endotracheal tube is secured with wires, a wire cutter must be immediately available at the bedside. It is recommended that TEN patients who are intubated undergo immediate fiberoptic bronchoscopy to assess the state of the tracheobronchial mucosa and to obtain bronchoalveolar lavage specimens for culture and sensitivity testing. Bronchial mucosal detachment identified at early fiberoptic bronchoscopy carries a poor prognosis.[28]

Fluid Therapy

Unlike a burn, patients with SJS-TEN do not require a directed acute fluid resuscitation based on body weight and the extent of epidermal loss

However, fluid replacement may be required for dehydration or hypovolemia. The authors have found that patients with TEN generally require between 1 and 2 mL/kg per percent of TBSA epidermal detachment per day during the first 3 days of burn center admission.[29] This volume should not be viewed as a prescribed resuscitation formula and only represents what was provided to maintain hemodynamic stability and adequate urinary output. In general, balanced salt solutions, such as lactated Ringer solution, may be used. In patients who are severely hypoalbuminemic, provision of human albumin solutions may be considered to improve the plasma colloid osmotic pressure but there is no evidence to support this approach. Similarly, the optimal hemoglobin concentration to trigger blood transfusion in this patient population is unknown. We have followed the approach used for other critically ill populations[30] of transfusing blood to maintain the hemoglobin greater than 70 gm/L (7 gm/dL).

Nutritional Support

In contrast to a burn of similar size, patients with SJS-TEN do not develop a comparable hypermetabolic response. However, almost all patients with SJS do require nutritional support because of their limited ability to eat and the need to replace protein loss from the wounds, optimize wound healing, and maintain immune function. Enteral nutrition is, therefore, a mainstay of treatment and should be initiated as early as possible with a small caliber orogastric or nasogastric feeding tube. The appropriate amounts of calories and proteins to deliver are not known but based on pediatric studies seem to be less than those required for a burn of similar size.[31] Calorie and protein requirements may be initially calculated as for a burn of similar extent but the estimated requirements should be adjusted based on measured resting energy expenditure derived from a metabolic cart. Parenteral nutrition has been associated with increased mortality in TEN[2] and should be avoided whenever possible.

Infection Control

Prophylactic antibiotics are not indicated in SJS-TEN. Frequently, patients with SJS-TEN arrive in the burn center having been started on 1 or more antibiotics to prevent infection. These should be continued only if there is an identified or strongly suspected infection present. Careful infection surveillance with frequent obtainment of microbiological cultures and initiation of antibiotics only for a culture positive infection source is the preferred strategy.

Skin and Wound Management

The overriding principle is to prevent infection and desiccation of the raw exposed dermis. As long as a healthy, moist, and viable dermis is maintained, the dermal appendages will produce a new epidermal layer within 2 weeks, allowing complete spontaneous healing.[32] One approach to achieve this goal is to cover the exfoliated areas with a biological skin substitute (eg, porcine xenograft[24,32,33] or cadaveric allograft[34]) or a biosynthetic skin substitute, such as Biobrane[35–37] (Smith and Nephew, Mississauga, Canada; **Fig. 5**). These materials are left intact until epithelialization occurs underneath, at which point the material lifts off. A topical antimicrobial dressing is usually applied on top of the substitute. The use of a skin substitute necessitates aggressive cleansing and irrigation of the wound and debridement of any loose or imminently detached epidermis before application of the material. This is painful and usually requires liberal analgesia and deep sedation, or full general anesthesia. In some burn centers this procedure is done in the operating room. Critics of this approach maintain that the epidermis should not be disturbed and should be left intact as much as possible, even when imminently detached, to act as a biological dressing, to avoid scar formation. However, in the authors' experience using a more aggressive debridement approach and coverage with Biobrane, we have not seen any scarring from these wounds at long-term follow-up except for punctate scars where staples had been inserted to attach the Biobrane.[38] Conversely, the advantages of a skin substitute in this application are numerous and include reduction in heat and fluid loss from the wound, reduced wound pain, less frequent and less painful dressing changes, and facilitation of movement of the underlying parts due to less pain.

An alternative approach involves the use of dressings alone, with careful preservation of any loose epidermis and blister or bullae roofs, allowing these to act as biological membranes. In fact, the multicenter review of TEN treated in burn centers found that alternatives to skin substitutes were used in almost all cases (80%), including dressing changes with silver nitrate, bacitracin, silver sulfadiazine, Acticoat (Smith and Nephew, United Kingdom), and fine mesh gauze (eg, Xeroform [Medtronic Canada, Brampton, Ontario]).[2] A recent systematic review found that a wide variety of wound care approaches exist, many of which involve dressings with antimicrobial agents such as silver sulfadiazine, Acticoat, or silver nitrate; whereas other approaches use

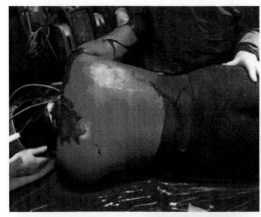
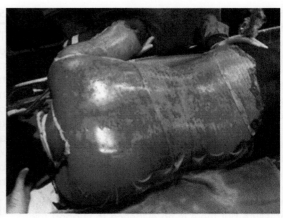
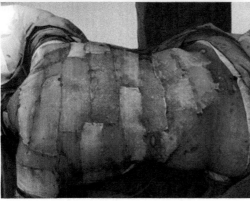

Fig. 5. Extensive actual and imminent epidermal detachment of the entire back in a patient with toxic epidermal necrolysis (*top left*). Removal of all loose epidermis and coverage of the dermis with a biosynthetic skin substitute, Biobrane (Smith and Nephew, Mississauga, Canada) (*top right*). A different case in which cryopreserved allograft was applied to cover the raw exposed dermis on the back (*bottom*).

nonantimicrobial dressings such as greasy tulle gauze.[39] Thus, it is reasonable to conclude that there is no consensus on the optimal dressing strategy for patients with SJS-TEN.

In the absence of any prospective randomized trials comparing skin substitutes to dressings in SJS-TEN, several retrospective studies[40–42] have not shown any difference in time to healing between dressings and skin substitutes, noting that this occurs in around 12 to 14 days with either strategy.

Care of Mucosal Surfaces

The oropharyngeal and genital mucosal surfaces may be involved in SJS-TEN. Erosions of these surfaces lead to pain, bleeding, and eventually adhesion formation if the raw mucosal surfaces are left in contact with each other. In the mouth, frequent mouth care and regular irrigation with an antiseptic solution or plain mouthwash in combination with viscous lidocaine is advisable, and lubricants such as Glaxal Base can be applied the lips. In female patients, we have found it useful to place layered nonadherent Telfa pads lubricated with Vaseline between the vaginal labia if there are erosions present, to keep these mucosal surfaces separated. The goal of this is to prevent adhesion formation. Some investigators have described topical steroids for the vaginal mucosa as well.[8]

Ocular Care

It is imperative to consult ophthalmology for assistance with care of the eyes in patients with SJS-TEN. Late ocular sequelae are the most common and debilitating problems among patients who survive SJS-TEN (see later discussion). Acute management usually includes daily sweeping of the conjunctival fornices with a glass rod to break down mucosal strands and adhesions between the lids or between the lids and the globe, topical antimicrobial drops to prevent infection, topical corticosteroids to reduce inflammation and scarring, and cycloplegic drops to lessen pain and photophobia. Amniotic membrane transplantation has also been adopted in some centers as an effective means to temporarily protect the corneas.[43]

Pharmacologic Therapies

Many studies have examined a wide variety of pharmacologic interventions to halt or slow the SJS-TEN disease process, including steroids, intravenous immunoglobulin (IVIG), cyclosporine, cyclophosphamide, plasmapheresis, and TNF inhibitors, including thalidomide. Unfortunately, nearly all of these studies provide poor-quality evidence due to small subject numbers, absence of control groups or use of historical control groups, and heterogeneity between study populations. In fact, only 1 randomized prospective controlled study of a drug therapy for SJS-TEN has ever been conducted. The trial compared the anti-TNF agent thalidomide with placebo, which was halted because of high mortality in the thalidomide group.[44] Current concepts regarding these agents are discussed in the next section.

Intravenous immunoglobulin

In 1998, Viard and colleagues[16] showed that immunoglobulins within pooled human IVIG blocked the Fas (CD95) receptor on keratinocytes to allow interruption of Fas-FasL-mediated keratinocyte apoptosis in vitro. In an open, uncontrolled pilot study, the same group observed rapid cessation of skin disease and no deaths in 10 subjects with SJS-TEN with epidermal detachment between 9% and 60% of the TBSA who had received a mean total dose of 2.5 gm/kg of IVIG (range 0.8–3.0 gm/kg).[16] These promising findings led to numerous case reports, case series, and a variety of controlled and uncontrolled studies over the ensuing 15 years, which revealed mixed findings regarding benefit from IVIG. In 2012, a systematic review and meta-analysis by Huang and colleagues[45] identified that only 6 controlled trials in adults[46–51] (all retrospective) comparing IVIG to supportive care had been conducted since the initial observations of Viard and colleagues[16] in 1998. These 6 trials involved a total of 243 subjects with SJS-TEN overlap or TEN and the pooled odds ratio (OR) for mortality in subjects treated with IVIG did not show a survival benefit compared with supportive care alone (OR 1.0, 95% CI 0.58–1.75). When only subjects treated with high-dose IVIG (defined as ≥2.0 gm/kg) were considered, there was a slight but statistically significant improvement in the pooled OR for mortality compared with supportive care alone (OR 0.63, 95% CI 0.27–1.44). It is worth noting that the only 2 studies to have been conducted among SJS-TEN treated in North American burn units[46,47] (which arguably might represent patients with the most severe SJS-TEN), were included in this meta-analysis, and neither study showed

benefit to use of IVIG over supportive care alone. Since the meta-analysis by Huang and colleagues,[45] 2 other studies have investigated IVIG. Both were retrospective uncontrolled studies that reported mortality relative to score of TEN (SCORTEN)-predicted mortality. Lee and colleagues[52] reviewed 64 SJS-TEN overlap and TEN subjects who received a mean total IVIG dose of 2.4 gm/kg. The overall standardized mortality ratio (SMR) compared with SCORTEN was 1.1 (95% CI 0.62–1.58), which would indicate that use of IVIG was not associated with a survival benefit. Kirchhof and colleagues[53] evaluated 37 SJS-TEN subjects (mean maximum percent of TBSA detachment 29%) who received 3 gm/kg IVIG. The SMR compared with SCORTEN was 1.43 (95% CI 0.71–2.56), again suggesting no survival improvement from IVIG.

Thus, low-quality evidence suggests that IVIG does not produce a survival benefit in adults with SJS-TEN, leading some experts to recommend that IVIG not be used for this disease.[8] However, in the absence of a definitive randomized controlled trial, and because of inconclusive findings on the effects of use of higher dose IVIG (3 gm/kg), batch-to-batch variation in anti-Fas activity of IVIG, and timing of intervention with IVIG, it is impossible to conclude that IVIG has no role in the treatment of SJS-TEN. IVIG has a relatively good safety profile with infrequently reported significant complications.[45] Conclusions regarding the use of IVIG in pediatric SJS-TEN should be considered separately because there is some evidence that suggests a possible benefit from IVIG in that population.[54]

Cyclosporine

Cyclosporine is a calcineurin inhibitor that inhibits function of cytotoxic T lymphocytes. It has recently gained popularity as a possible therapeutic agent for SJS-TEN. There are no controlled trials comparing cyclosporine to supportive care alone. One study has compared subjects with TEN using cyclosporine (N = 11) with a historical cohort using a regimen of cyclophosphamide and corticosteroids (N = 6). The study found that the cyclosporine-treated subjects had a significantly shorter delay until arrest of the skin progression, along with significantly higher survival.[55] More recently, 2 retrospective uncontrolled studies have evaluated mortality relative to SCORTEN-predicted mortality in SJS-TEN subjects treated with cyclosporine.[53,56] Both studies found actual mortality to be lower than predicted by SCORTEN but it should be noted that the subjects cohorts treated with cyclosporine had relatively mild disease with a high proportion of subjects with only

SJS (34%[56] and 59%[53]), a small average percent of TBSA area of epidermal detachment (23%[56] and 16%[53]), and a low admission SCORTEN (1.3[56] and 1.7[53]).

Hence, the use and positive effect of cyclosporine is supported by relatively poor-quality evidence in SJS-TEN and the decision to use this agent should also take into account the potential adverse effects of this agent, which include nephrotoxicity, hypertension, neutropenia, and immunosuppression. In the study by Valyrie-Allanore and colleagues,[56] an oral dose of 3 mg/kg/day for 10 days followed by weaning over the ensuing 20 days was used. Treatment was prematurely stopped in 10% of the subjects because of significant complications (leukoencephalopathy, neutropenia, severe infection) and other complications, including hypertension, decreased renal function, and neuropathy, were reported.

Corticosteroids

Corticosteroids are immune modulators that suppress inflammation that have been and continue to be frequently used to treat SJS-TEN. Numerous low-quality observational retrospective studies have shown conflicting results with respect to their safety and efficacy in adults with SJS-TEN. At 1 end of the spectrum, some studies involving SJS-TEN treated in burn centers found that steroids were significantly associated with increased mortality,[40,57] higher rates of infection, and more prolonged hospitalization.[40] At the other end of the spectrum, the large retrospective European study on Severe Cutaneous Adverse Reactions (EuroSCAR) study involving 281 SJS-TEN subjects found that corticosteroids had no significant effect on mortality (OR for death was 0.4 [95% CI 0.1–1.7] in French subjects and 0.3 [95% CI 0.1–1.1] in German subjects).[48] In practical terms, when patients with SJS-TEN are admitted into a burn unit, the prevailing approach is to stop or taper steroids if they were in use because of the known risks of infection and delayed wound healing from corticosteroids. This may be the safest approach given that patients with SJS-TEN who are transferred to a burn unit usually have extensive and advanced disease and are probably at higher risk of developing infection and sepsis. This does not suggest that steroids have no role in SJS-TEN and some investigators have recommended a short course of pulse dose steroids in SJS-TEN (1.5 mg/kg/day of intravenous dexamethasone for 3 days).[58]

Tumor necrosis factor inhibitors

TNF-α seems to play an important role in amplifying apoptosis among keratinocytes in SJS-TEN.[18,19] Consequently, there has been recent interest in use of the TNF inhibitors infliximab and etanercept to slow or halt disease progression. The largest study is an uncontrolled case series of 10 subjects with TEN (extent of epidermal detachment unreported, mean admission SCORTEN 3.6), who were administered a single 50 mg subcutaneous injection of etanercept.[59] All subjects survived and healing occurred at a median of 8.5 days, with no reported adverse effects from the medication. These observations are promising but, until more subjects have been studied, these agents cannot be recommended as routine therapy.

General Supportive Care

Many aspects of general supportive care that are used for burn patients can also be applied to patients with SJS-TEN who have been admitted to a burn treatment center. Ideally, a warm ambient environment should be maintained for patients with extensive areas of epidermal loss. Similarly specialized pressure reduction beds are desirable for patients with wide-ranging wounds. Gastric stress ulcer prophylaxis and standard venous thromboembolism prophylaxis are recommended. Provision of analgesia is highly important. It may be necessary to temporarily intubate and mechanically ventilate patients with very large areas of epidermal detachment to allow safe administration of adequate amounts of analgesia in the form of continuous parenteral morphine or hydromorphone infusions. Nonintubated patients may be provided with continuous background analgesia using long-acting opioids with use of short-acting opioids for breakthrough or procedural pain, along with appropriate cardiovascular and respiratory monitoring. Patient-controlled analgesia is a suitable alternative approach for some nonintubated patients.

OUTCOMES

Prediction of survival in patients with SJS is usually done by using SCORTEN, which is a scoring system that uses 7 variables (**Table 2**): age, heart rate, presence of malignancy, extent of epidermal detachment, blood urea nitrogen level, serum bicarbonate level, and the blood glucose level.[6] The predicted mortality rate is then calculated by entering the total SCORTEN score into the predictive equation, which yields the following predicted mortality rates: score 0, 1.2%, score 1, 3.9%; score 2, 12.2%; score 3, 32.4%; score 4, 62.2%; score 5, 85%; score 6, 95.1%; and score 7, 98.5%.[60] The SCORTEN is administered on admission but its predictive accuracy may be

Table 2
Variables used to calculate score of toxic epidermal necrolysis

Variable	SCORTEN
Age >40 y	1
Malignancy present	1
Epidermal detachment >10% of the TBSA	1
Heart rate >120 beats/min	1
Blood urea nitrogen >28 mg/dL (>10 mmol/L)	1
Blood glucose >252 mg/dL (>14 mmol/L)	1
Serum bicarbonate <20 mEq/L	1
Maximum possible score	7

From Bastuji-Garin S, Fouchard N, Bertocchi M, et al, SCORTEN: a severity of illness score for toxic epidermal necrolysis. J Invest Dermatol 2000;115:149–53.

improved by use in a serial fashion by determining scores on days 3 and 5 postadmission.[61] The SCORTEN has been validated among SJS-TEN patients cared for in a burn center setting.[62]

Patients who survive SJS-TEN often are left with a variety of long-term health problems that affect their quality of life.[38] Foremost among these are ocular problems, including chronic dry eye syndrome, chronic photophobia, trichiasis, symblepharon, chronic corneal irritation and inflammation, and (rarely, in very severe cases) permanent loss of visual acuity or even blindness.[63] Although cutaneous scar formation does not seem to be a problem, patients are often left with permanent pigmentation alterations, including hyperpigmentation, hypopigmentation, and spotty or speckled mixed pigmentation. Nail deformities, such as split nails, unstable nails, and missing nails, may be seen. Strictures across mucosal structures, such as the urethra, may lead to voiding difficulties. In female patients, vaginal dryness and or strictures may form, leading to dyspareunia.[38] Some patients develop psychological problems, such as anxiety or depression, related either to the prior critical illness or ongoing associated chronic physical manifestations of the disease process.[8]

REFERENCES

1. Mockenhaupt M. Stevens-Johnson syndrome and toxic epidermal necrolysis: clinical patterns, diagnostic considerations, etiology, and therapeutic management. Semin Cutan Med Surg 2014;33:10–5.
2. Palmieri T, Greenhalgh D, Saffle J, et al. A multicenter review of Toxic Epidermal Necrolysis treated in US burn centers at the end of the twentieth century. J Burn Care Res 2002;23(2):87–96.
3. Auquier-Dunant A, Mockenhaupt M, Naldi L, et al. Correlations between clinical patterns and causes of erythema multiforme majus, Stevens-Johnson Syndrome, and toxic epidermal necrolysis: results of an international prospective study. Arch Dermatol 2002;138:1019–24.
4. Bastuji-Garin S, Rzany B, Stern RS, et al. Clinical classification of cases of toxic epidermal necrolysis, Stevens-Johnson syndrome, and erythema multiforme. Arch Dermatol 1993;129:92–6.
5. Grosber M, Carsin H, Leclerc F. Epidermal necrolysis in association with mycoplasma pneumonia infection. J Invest Dermatol 2006;126(S3):S3–116.
6. Mockenhaupt M, Viboud C, Dunant A, et al. Stevens Johnson syndrome and toxic epidermal necrolysis: assessment of medication risks with emphasis on recently marketed drugs. The Euro-SCAR-study. J Invest Dermatol 2008;128:35–44.
7. Mockenhaupt M. The current understanding of Stevens-Johnson syndrome and toxic epidermal necrolysis. Expert Rev Clin Immunol 2011;7(6):803–21.
8. Dodiuk-Gad RP, Chung WH, Valeyrie-Allanore L, et al. Stevens-Johnson syndrome and toxic epidermal necrolysis: an update. Am J Clin Dermatol 2015;16:475–93.
9. Roujeau JC, Huynh TN, Bracq C, et al. Genetic susceptibility to toxic epidermal necrolysis. Arch Dermatol 1987;123:1171–3.
10. Mehta TY, Prajapati LM, Mittal B, et al. Association of HLA-B*1502 allele and carbamazepine-induced Stevens-Johnson syndrome among Indians. Indian J Dermatol Venereol Leprol 2009;75(6):579–82.
11. Chung WH, Hung SI. Recent advances in the genetics and immunology of Stevens-Johnson syndrome and toxic epidermal necrolysis. J Dermatol Sci 2012;66(3):190–6.
12. Chen P, Lin JJ, Lu CS, et al. Carbamazepine-induced toxic effects and HLA-B*1502 screening in Taiwan. New Engl J Med 2011;364:1126–33.
13. Tangamornsuksan W, Chaiyakunapruk N, Somkrua R, et al. Relationship between the HLA-B*1502 allele and carbamazepine-induced Stevens-Johnson syndrome and toxic epidermal necrolysis: a systematic review and meta-analysis. JAMA Dermatol 2013;149(90):1025–32.
14. Pichler WJ. Pharmacological interaction of drugs with antigen specific immune receptors: the p-i concept. Curr Opin Allergy Clin Immunol 2002;2(4):301–5.
15. Chung WH, Hung SI, Yang JY, et al. Granulysin is a key mediator for disseminated keratinocyte death in Stevens-Johnson syndrome and toxic epidermal necrolysis. Nat Med 2008;14(12):1343–50.
16. Viard I, Wehrli P, Bullani R, et al. Inhibition of toxic epidermal necrolysis by blockade of CD95 with

human intravenous immunoglobulin. Science 1998; 282:490–3.

17. Abe R, Shimizu T, Shibaki A, et al. Toxic epidermal necrolysis and Stevens-Johnson syndrome are induced by soluble Fas ligand. Am J Pathol 2003; 162:1515–20.

18. Arnold R, Seifert M, Asadullah K, et al. Crosstalk between keratinocytes and T lymphocytes via Fas/Fas ligand interaction: modulation by cytokines. J Immunol 1999;162:7140–70.

19. Downey A, Jackson C, Harun N, et al. Toxic epidermal necrolysis: review of pathogenesis and management. J Am Acad Dermatol 2012;66: 995–1003.

20. deProst N, Mekontso-Dessap A, Valeyrie-Allanore L, et al. Acute respiratory failure in patients with toxic epidermal necrolysis: clinical features and factors associated with mechanical ventilation. Crit Care Med 2014;42(1):118–28.

21. Powell N, Munro JM, Rowbotham D. Colonic involvement in Stevens Johnson syndrome. Postgrad Med J 2006;82(968):e10.

22. Hung CC, Liu WC, Kuo MC, et al. Acute renal failure and its risk factors in Stevens Johnson syndrome and toxic epidermal necrolysis. Am J Nephrol 2009;29(6):633–8.

23. Wolkenstein P, Roujeau JC, Revuz J. Drug-induced toxic epidermal necrolysis. Clin Dermatol 1998;16: 399–409.

24. Schulz JT, Sheridan RL, Ryan CM, et al. A 10 year experience with toxic epidermal necrolysis. J Burn Care Rehabil 2000;21:199–204.

25. McGee T, Munster A. Toxic epidermal necrolysis syndrome: mortality rate reduced with early referral to a regional burn center. Plast Reconstr Surg 1998;102:1018–22.

26. Harr T, French L. Toxic epidermal necrolysis and Stevens-Johnson syndrome. Orphanet J Rare Dis 2010;5:39–50.

27. Worswick S, Cotliar J. Stevens Johnson syndrome and toxic epidermal necrolysis: a review of treatment options. Dermatol Ther 2011;24:207–18.

28. Lebargy F, Wolkenstein P, Gisselbrecht M, et al. Pulmonary complications in toxic epidermal necrolysis: a prospective clinical study. Intensive Care Med 1997;23:1237–44.

29. Shiga S, Cartotto R. What are the fluid requirements in toxic epidermal necrolysis? J Burn Care Res 2010; 31(1):100–4.

30. Hebert PC, Wells G, Blajchman MA, et al. A multicenter, randomized, controlled clinical trial of transfusion requirements in critical care. Transfusion Requirements in Critical Care Investigators, Canadian Critical Care TrialsGroup. N Engl J Med 1999;340:409–17.

31. Mayes T, Gottschlich M, Khoury J, et al. Energy requirements of pediatric patients with Stevens Johnson syndrome and toxic epidermal necrolysis. Nutr Clin Prac 2008;23(5):547–50.

32. Heimbach DM, Engrav LH, Marvin JA, et al. Toxic epidermal necrolysis: a step forward in treatment. JAMA 1987;257:2171–5.

33. Marvin JA, Heimbach DM, Engrav LH, et al. Improved treatment of the Stevens-Johnson syndrome. Arch Surg 1984;119:601–5.

34. Davidson BL, Hunt JL. Human cadaver homograft in toxic epidermal necrolysis. J Burn Care Rehabil 1981;2:94–6.

35. Sowder LL. Biobrane® wound dressing used in the treatment of toxic epidermal necrolysis: a case report. J Burn Care Rehabil 1990;11(3):237–9.

36. Peters W, Zaidi J, Douglas L. Toxic epidermal necrolysis: a burn-centre challenge. CMAJ 1991; 144(11):1477–80.

37. Bradley T, Brown RE, Kucan JO, et al. Toxic epidermal necrolysis: a review and report of the successful use of Biobrane® for early wound coverage. Ann Plast Surg 1995;35(2):124–32.

38. Haber J, Hopman W, Gomez M, et al. Late outcomes in survivors of toxic epidermal necrolysis treated in a burn center. J Burn Care Rehabil 2005;26:33–41.

39. Mahar PD, Wasiak J, Hii B, et al. A systematic review of toxic epidermal necrolysis treated in burns centres. Burns 2014;40:1245–54.

40. Halebian PH, Madden MR, Finkelstein JL, et al. Improved burn center survival of patients with toxic epidermal necrolysis managed without corticosteroids. Ann Surg 1986;204:503–12.

41. Boorboor P, Vogt PM, Bechara FG, et al. Toxic epidermal necrolysis: use of Biobrane® or skin coverage reduces pain, improves mobilisation and decreases infection in elderly patients. Burns 2008; 34(4):487–92.

42. Rogers AD, Blackport E, Cartotto R. The use of a temporary biosynthetic skin substitute in Stevens-Johnson-Toxic Epidermal Necrolysis Syndrome [abstract]. J Burn Care Res 2016;37:S122.

43. Hsu M, Jayaram A, Verner R, et al. Indications and outcomes of amniotic membrane transplantation in the management of acute Stevens-Johnson syndrome and toxic epidermal necrolysis: a case-control study. Cornea 2012;31(12):1395–402.

44. Wolkenstein P, Iaterjet J, Roujeau JC, et al. Randomized comparison of thalidomide versus placebo in toxic epidermal necrolysis. Lancet 1998;352: 1586–9.

45. Huang YC, Li YC, Chen TJ. The efficacy of intravenous immunoglobulin for the treatment of toxic epidermal necrolysis: a systematic review and meta-analysis. Br J Dermatol 2012;167:424–32.

46. Shortt R, Gomez M, Mittman N, et al. Intravenous immunoglobulin does not improve outcome in toxic epidermal necrolysis. J Burn Care Rehabil 2004; 25:246–55.

47. Brown KM, Silver GM, Halerz M, et al. Toxic epidermal necrolysis: does immunoglobulin make a difference? J Burn Care Rehabil 2004;25:81–8.

48. Schneck J, Fagot JP, Sekula P, et al. Effects of treatments on the mortality of Stevens-Johnson syndrome and toxic epidermal necrolysis: a retrospective study of patients included in the prospective Euro-SCAR study. J Am Acad Dermatol 2008;58:33–40.

49. Yip LW, Thong BY, Tan AW, et al. High dose intravenous immunoglobulin in the treatment of toxic epidermal necrolysis: a study of ocular benefits. Eye (Lond) 2005;19(8):846–53.

50. Stella M, Clemente A, Bollero D, et al. Toxic epidermal necrolysis (TEN) and Stevens-Johnson syndrome (SJS): experience with high dose intravenous immunoglobulin and topical conservative approach. A retrospective analysis. Burns 2007;33: 452–9.

51. Gravante G, Delogu D, Marienetti M, et al. Toxic epidermal necrolysis and Stevens-Johnson syndrome: 11 years experience and outcome. Eur Rev Med Pharmacol Sci 2007;11:119–27.

52. Lee HY, Lim YL, Thirumoorthy T, et al. The role of intravenous immunoglobulin in toxic epidermal necrolysis: a retrospective analysis of 64 patients managed in a specialized centre. Br J Dermatol 2013;169:304–1309.

53. Kirchhof MG, Miliszewski MA, Sikora S, et al. Retrospective review of Stevens-Johnson syndrome and toxic epidermal necrolysis treatment comparing intravenous immunoglobulin with cyclosporine. J Am Acad Dermatol 2014;71:941–7.

54. Del Pozzo-Magana BR, Lazo-langer A, Carleton A, et al. A systematic review of drug induced Stevens Johnson syndrome and toxic epidermal necrolysis in children. J Popul Ther Clin Pharmacol 2011;18: e121–133.

55. Arévalo JM, Lorente JA, González-Herrada C, et al. Treatment of toxic epidermal necrolysis with cyclosporine A. J Trauma 2000;48:473–7.

56. Valeyrie-Allanore L, Wolkenstein P, Brochard L, et al. Open trial of ciclosporin treatment for Stevens-Johnson syndrome and toxic epidermal necrolysis. Br J Dermatol 2010;163:847–53.

57. Kelemen JJ, Cioffi WG, McManus WF, et al. Burn center care for patients with toxic epidermal necrolysis. J Am Coll Surg 1995;180:273–8.

58. Kardaun SH, Jonkman MF. Dexamethasone pulse therapy for Stevens-Johnson syndrome/toxic epidermal necrolysis. Acta Derm Venereol 2007;87: 144–8.

59. Paradisi A, Abeni D, Bergamo F, et al. Etanercept therapy for toxic epidermal necrolysis. J Am Acad Dermatol 2014;71:278–83.

60. Bastuji-Garin S, Fouchard N, Bertocchi M, et al. SCORTEN: a severity of illness score for toxic epidermal necrolysis. J Invest Dermatol 2000;115: 149–53.

61. Guegan S, Bastuji-Garin S, Poszepczynska-Guigne E. Performance of the SCORTEN during the first five days of hospitalization to predict the prognosis of epidermal necrolysis. J Investig Dermatol 2006;126:272–6.

62. Cartotto R, Mayich M, Nickerson D, et al. SCORTEN accurately predicts mortality among toxic epidermal necrolysis patients treated in a Burn Center. J Burn Care Res 2008;29:141–6.

63. Morales ME, Purdue GF, Verity SM, et al. Ophthalmic manifestations of Stevens-Johnson syndrome and toxic epidermal necrolysis and relation to SCORTEN. Am J Ophthal 2010;150(4):505–10.

Life-threatening Skin Disorders Treated in the Burn Center

Impact of Health care–associated Infections on Length of Stay, Survival, and Hospital Charges

Steven J. Hermiz, MD[a], Paul Diegidio, MD[b],
Shiara Ortiz-Pujols, MD[b], Roja Garimella, BS[c],
David J. Weber, MD, MPH[d], David van Duin, MD, PhD[d],
Charles Scott Hultman, MD, MBA[b],*

KEYWORDS

- Stevens-Johnson syndrome • Toxic epidermal necrolysis • Life-threatening skin disorders
- Hospital-acquired infections • Health care–associated infections

KEY POINTS

- Patients with life-threatening skin disorders, including those with Stevens-Johnson syndrome (SJS) and toxic epidermal necrolysis (TEN), are best treated in a burn center, because of the availability of subspecialists in surgical critical care, wound management, and rehabilitation.
- Critically ill patients with acute skin disorders have an increased need for intensive care unit care, compared with the SJS-TEN cohort, but both groups have similar length of hospital stay, survival, and incidence of hospital-acquired infections.
- Hospital-acquired infections, which are theoretically preventable, significantly increase both mortality and hospital charges, to an even greater degree, in the SJS-TEN subgroup.

INTRODUCTION

Stevens-Johnson syndrome (SJS) and toxic epidermal necrolysis (TEN) are part of a clinical syndrome that represents a medication-induced desquamation disorder. In 1922, Drs Stevens and Johnson first described SJS as an acute mucocutaneous syndrome presenting in 2 young boys.[1–3] Alan Lyell later presented 4 patients in 1956 with a cutaneous eruption and coined the term TEN.[1,2,4–7]

SJS-TEN are the 2 most common adverse drug reactions in hospitalized patients. SJS-TEN are grouped along with acute generalized exanthematous pustulosis, drug-induced hypersensitivity syndrome, and drug reaction with eosinophilia and

Funding Sources: None.
Conflicts of Interest: None.
[a] Department of Surgery, University of South Carolina School of Medicine, Columbia, SC 29209, USA; [b] Department of Surgery, University of North Carolina School of Medicine, 7038 Burnett-Womack, Campus Box 7195, Chapel Hill, NC 27599, USA; [c] Alpert Medical School, Brown University, Providence, RI 02903, USA; [d] Department of Medicine, University of North Carolina School of Medicine, Chapel Hill, NC 27599, USA
* Corresponding author.
E-mail address: cshult@med.unc.edu

Clin Plastic Surg 44 (2017) 597–602
http://dx.doi.org/10.1016/j.cps.2017.02.006

systemic symptoms (DRESS), to encompass severe cutaneous adverse reactions.[8,9] The two entities are distinguished from each other by disease severity, which is characterized by the extent of detachment of epidermis and erosions of mucous membranes.[2,4,6,8–14] The total body surface area (TBSA) involved in SJS is less than 10%, 10% to 30% in SJS-TEN overlap, and greater than 30% in TEN.[1,2,6,8–13,15,16] In more than 95% of TEN cases, the mucous membranes involved include the eyes, lips, mouth, pharynx, trachea, bronchi, vulva, glans penis, urethra, and anus.[1,8,9,11,12]

Patients admitted to a burn center with a potential diagnosis along the SJS/TEN spectrum often have high hospital morbidity and mortality. However, little is known about patients admitted to a burn center with life threatening skin disorders (LTSDs) not caused by SJS/TEN. This group includes severe rashes, nonhealing wounds, erythema multiforme, and unknown skin lesions requiring hospitalization for critical care, skin biopsy, and aggressive wound care.

This article compares and contrasts patients admitted to a single burn center and diagnosed with LTSD or SJS/TENS, focusing on intensive care unit (ICU) care, hospital charges, cost, and mortality. Furthermore, the impact of hospital-acquired infections (HAIs; also known as health care–associated infections) on these patient outcomes is assessed.

METHODS
Patient Population

Over a 10-year period from 2003 to 2013, 445 patients were admitted to the North Carolina Jaycee Burn Center with life-threatening dermatologic conditions other than thermal injury. The University of North Carolina (UNC) Health Care System is a conglomerate of health care providers and organizations that includes the School of Medicine, UNC Hospitals in Chapel Hill, and multiple hospitals and physician practices across the state of North Carolina.

Study Design

The authors conducted a retrospective, descriptive review of the 445 patients who had a diagnosis of a dermatologic condition requiring hospitalization in our burn center. Patients were identified from a prospectively managed database, and a post-hoc analysis was performed. These charts, divided into SJS-TEN and LTSD, were cross-referenced with the hospital-wide infection control database to identify patients who developed HAIs. We used the definitions developed by the Centers for Disease Control and Prevention National

Healthcare Safety Network to accurately and consistently diagnose HAIs.

Statistical Methods

Continuous discrete data (age, TBSA involved, length of stay, ventilation days, ICU days, HAI, mortality, mortality with HAI, cost, cost with HAI, catheter-associated urinary tract infection [CAUTI], blood stream infections [BSIs], and urinary tract infections [UTI]) were compared using either 2-tailed t-test or χ^2 analysis for nominal and categorical variables, respectively. Statistical significance was assigned to P values less than .05.

Study Approval

The UNC Biomedical Institutional Review Board approved this project as Institutional Review Board study number 14-1789, under the title Anticipating Changes in Bundled Payments For the Treatment of Patients with Acute, Life-threatening Dermatologic Emergencies, Through Prevention of Healthcare Associated Infections.

Data Points

The charts of 445 patients with dermatologic conditions requiring hospitalization were queried for age, gender, and TBSA involved. Main outcome measures included length of hospital stay, ventilation days, ICU days, and overall cost, generated by the facility. Complications assessed included HAIs, inpatient mortality, CAUTI, BSI, and UTI. Inpatient mortality associated with HAIs and cost associated with HAIs were also calculated.

RESULTS
Patient Demographics

Between 2003 and 2013, 445 patients were identified with dermatologic emergencies who were admitted to our burn unit. There were 316 patients in the LTSD group and 129 patients in the SJS-TEN cohort. The mean age in the LTSD group was 52.8 ± 23.3 years and 48.3 ± 22.6 years in the SJS-TEN group. Patients presenting with LTSD were more likely to be female compared with patients with SJS-TEN (78.4% vs 58.1%; P = .04). There was no difference in TBSA involvement between the two groups (19.3% vs 21.2%; P = .61).

Cause

Patients with LTSDs (n = 316) included more than 30 different diagnostic groups, with the top 11 involving drug rash (n = 43), exanthematous pustulosis (n = 22), staphylococcal scalded skin syndrome (n = 13), necrotizing fasciitis (n = 12), erythema multiforme (n = 12), pemphigoid

= 12), contact dermatitis (n = 10), exfoliative soriasis (n = 8), leukocytoclastic vasculitis ermatitis (n = 6), viral rash (n = 5), and erosive ustular dermatitis (n = 4). Although physical examination may help form a clinical diagnosis, all atients underwent skin biopsy to determine the xact dermatologic diagnosis. An additional 45 patients (23.2%) were determined to have the ollowing diagnoses: cutaneous lupus flare, cellu-is, impetigo, linear immunoglobulin A dermatosis, aumatic crush wound, DRESS syndrome, scald jury, acute spongiotic dermatitis (eczema), calci-hylaxis, suppurative hidradenitis, exfoliative xero-erma, chronic wound after burn, solar purpura, rysipelas, purpura fulminans, dermatomyositis, weet syndrome, lichen planus, soft tissue necro-s caused by Levophed, necrolytic migratory ery-ema, penile skin eruption, pressure ulcer, egloving, thrombotic skin necrosis, and fungal ash (each category with 1–3 patients).

Of the 129 patients with SJS-TEN spectrum, the citing drug was identified in 121 (93.8%). The ost common pharmacologic category was an ntimicrobial agent, which included antibacterials = 50), antivirals (n = 2), antimycobacterials = 2), and antifungals (n = 1). The next most ommon categories were anticonvulsants = 7), nonsteroidal antiinflammatory drugs = 4), and antigout agents (n = 3). Specific drugs cluded Bactrim, Lamictal, capsaicin, azithromy-n, allopurinol, ibuprofen and naproxen, acet-minophen, cephalosporins, vancomycin, ramamine, clindamycin, acyclovir, Tamiflu,

doxycycline, Dilantin, fluoroquinolone, penicillin, Macrobid, chlorphenamine, dapsone, Plaquenil, caspofungin, Lopid, and Tegretol. Bactrim, which is a combination of sulfamethoxazole and trimeth-oprim, was observed in 23 cases (17.8%).

Main Outcome Measures

The mean length of stay was 28.16 days (standard deviation [SD], 27.2 days) for the LTSD group and 22.5 days (SD, 24.5 days) for the SJS-TEN group (P = .19). Patients in the LTSD group had greater mean number of ventilator days compared with patients in the SJS-TEN group (16.39 vs 11.11 days; P<.01). The LTSD group had greater mean number of ICU days compared with the SJS-TEN group (25.35 vs 16.57 days; P<.01). The total hospital cost was higher for the LTSD group than for the SJS-TEN group ($179,316 vs $167,363; P = .01) **(Table 1)**.

Complications

The LTSD group had a 19.9% inpatient mortality compared with a 20.9% mortality for the SJS-TEN group, which was not statistically significant (P = .75). A total of 69 patients with LTSD (21.8%) and 38 patients with SJS-TEN (29.5%) had an HAI (P = .08) **(Figs. 1 and 2)**. Twelve patients (3.8%) in the LTSD group had a CAUTI, compared with 11 patients (8.5%) in the SJS-TEN group (P = .04). One patient (0.3%) in the LTSD group and 3 patients (2.3%) in the SJS-TEN group had a BSI (non–central line related)

Table 1
Patient variables

	LTSD n = 316	SJS-TEN n = 129	P Value
Age	52.8 y (23.3 y)	48.3 y (22.6 y)	.98
Female	78.4%	58.1%	.04
TBSA	19.3% (27.1%)	21.2% (27.0%)	.61
LOS	28.16 d (27.2 d)	22.5 d (24.5 d)	.19
Use of Ventilator	16.39 d (161 d)	11.11 d (24.07 d)	<.01
ICU Stay	25.35 d (197 d)	16.57 d (24.77 d)	<.01
HAIs	21.8%	29.5%	.08
Mortality	19.9%	20.9%	.75
Mortality with HAI	37%	66%	.25, .01
Cost	$179,316	$167,363	.01
Cost with HAI	$296,984	$468,542	.001, .001
CAUTI	3.8%	8.5%	.04
BSI	0.3%	2.3%	.04
UTI	3.5%	0%	.03

bbreviation: LOS, length of stay.

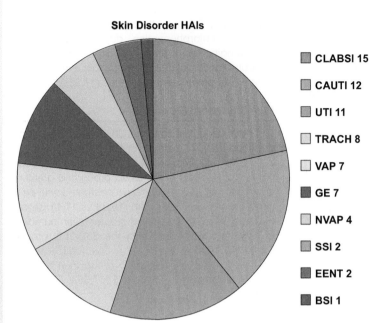

Skin Disorder HAIs

☐ CLABSI 15
☐ CAUTI 12
☐ UTI 11
☐ TRACH 8
☐ VAP 7
☐ GE 7
☐ NVAP 4
☐ SSI 2
☐ EENT 2
☐ BSI 1

Fig. 1. HAIs in the LTSD group. BS[ ] are non–central line related, an[ ] UTIs are non–catheter related CLABSI, central line–associate[ ] blood stream infection; GE, gastro enteritis (usually *Clostridium diff* *cile*); NVAP, non–ventilato[ ] associated pneumonia; SSI, surgica[ ] site infection; Trach, tracheobror chitis; VAP, ventilator-associate[ ] pneumonia.

($P = .04$). Eleven patients had a UTI (non–catheter related) in the LTSD group and no patients had a UTI (non–catheter related) in the SJS-TEN group ($P = .03$). The mortality for patients in the LTSD group with an HAI was 37% ($P = .25$), compared with 66% ($P = .01$) in the SJS-TEN group. The total hospital cost accrued for patients in the LTSD group with HAIs was

$296,984 ($P = .001$) and $468,542 ($P = .001$) for the SJS-TEN group.

The most common HAI pathogens in the LTSD group, in descending order, were *Pseudomona[ ] aeruginosa*, *Candida*, *Acinetobacter*, *Clostridiu[ ] difficile*, and methicillin-resistant *Staphylococcu[ ] aureus* (MRSA). The most common HAI pathogen in the SJS-TEN group, in descending order, wer[ ]

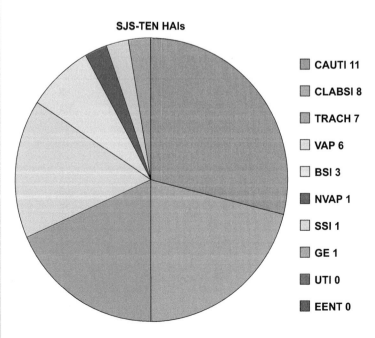

SJS-TEN HAIs

☐ CAUTI 11
☐ CLABSI 8
☐ TRACH 7
☐ VAP 6
☐ BSI 3
☐ NVAP 1
☐ SSI 1
☐ GE 1
☐ UTI 0
☐ EENT 0

Fig. 2. HAIs in the SJS-TEN group.

MRSA, *P aeruginosa*, *Candida*, *Stenotrophomonas*, and *Acinetobacter*.

SUMMARY

This article shares our experience with 445 patients presenting with dermatologic conditions requiring hospitalization in our burn center over a 10-year period. It compares patients with LTSDs and SJS-TEN, using such outcome metrics as length of stay, costs, mortality, and the incidence of HAIs. Patients with LTSD had significantly more ICU and ventilator days compared with patients with SJS-TEN. When HAIs were present, both groups had a significant increase in hospital charges, and patients with SJS-TEN had increased inpatient mortality. The two cohorts did not differ in terms of percentage TBSA, overall inpatient mortality, or incidence of HAIs. Patients with LTSD were also significantly more likely to be female, and they had a higher incidence of UTI (non–catheter related) compared with the SJS-TEN cohort. In contrast, patients with LTSD were less likely to develop a BSI (non–central line related) or CAUTI than patients with SJS-TEN.

LTSDs can be congenital, hereditary, or acquired cutaneous reactions. Acquired cutaneous reactions include meningococcal septicemia skin eruption, necrotizing fasciitis, staphylococcal scalded skin syndrome, erythema multiforme, purpura fulminans, pemphigoid, TEN, and SJS.[2,17] The incidence of SJS-TEN is approximately 1 to 2 new cases per million per year,[1,2,4,6,7,10,11,13,15,18,19] and the average mortality ranges from 25% to 40%.[5,6,9,11–13,15,16]

The average mortality for both the LTSD and SJS-TEN groups was lower than these reported figures, at 19.9% and 20.9%, respectively. Palmieri and colleagues[12] conducted a multicenter study involving 15 regional burn centers and showed that survival rate was significantly higher in patients who were transferred to a burn unit within 7 days after disease onset, compared with patients transferred after 7 days.[1,20] A delay in referral was associated with prolonged hospital stay and increased mortality.[4,6,9,11,12,15]

HAIs negatively affect morbidity, mortality, and economic cost. Infection is the main cause of mortality among patients with extensive burns and LTSDs.[21] The development of an HAI was associated with an increase in mortality from 19.9% to 37% in the LTSD group, and an increase in mortality from 20.9% to 66% in the SJS-TEN group. Similar to other published studies, BSIs that were non–central line related were more common in the SJS-TEN group, with a reported incidence in the literature of 15.5 per 1000 patient days.[15] The most common pathogens for BSI were MRSA and *P aeruginosa*, which are the most common pathogens identified in the literature.[5,11,15] Revuz and colleagues[5] reported that these 2 pathogens were the primary cause of death in 87 patients with TEN, resulting in hospital mortality of 25%.[11,15]

The economic cost of HAIs has been a significant financial burden to health care systems. For example, an episode of symptomatic UTI adds approximately $676 to hospital costs. Primary BSIs increase patient charges by $3517 per episode, and in one study yielded a mean difference of $34,508 compared with uninfected patients.[22] The annual cost of nosocomial UTIs in the United States ranges from $424 million to $451 million. The direct cost consists of the increased length of hospital stay, extra tests, and treatment required.[23,24] The Study of the Efficacy of Nosocomial Infection Control (SENIC) reported that HAIs affected approximately 6% of admitted patients in US hospitals.[23,25] The World Health Organization estimated the HAI burden to be $1.4 billion per annum.[23,25] Hospital-acquired BSIs not only cause morbidity and mortality; they add significant economic costs, ranging from $3061 to $40,000.[26]

Medicare's nonpayment policy for hospital-acquired conditions prompted a reduction in the rate of central line–associated bloodstream inflections by 11% and CAUTI by 10%.[25] Catheter-related bacteremia costs $2900 per episode. The total cost for nosocomial and community-acquired UTI is approximately $2 billion.[27] If a similar trend in Medicare nonpayment occurs for HAIs, this will pose tremendous challenges to health care systems, which have operating margins that may not be able to accommodate this decrease in reimbursement.

Despite receiving care at an American Burn Association (ABA)–verified burn center, patients in the LTSD and SJS-TEN cohorts developed HAIs at an incidence of 21.8% and 29.5%, respectively. Nonpayments for HAIs, in this setting, result in significant financial strain for all health care systems. The estimated annual cost of skin disease is $29.1 billion in direct medical costs and $10.2 billion in lost productivity costs. The economic burden on quality of life was estimated to be $56.2 billion.[28] Clearly, preventing or reducing HAIs in patients with acute LTSDs, regardless of cause, should become a primary goal of all burn centers.

Clinicians taking care of patients with SJS-TEN, as well as those with other LTSDs, should be aware of the profoundly negative impact of HAIs on number of ventilator days, length of ICU stay, length of hospitalization, and survival. With bundled payments on the horizon, and potential nonpayment of HAI complications, health care facilities may not be able to cover the cost of providing care to this group of patients, who are best managed by burn centers.

REFERENCES

1. Harr T, French LE. Toxic epidermal necrolysis and Stevens-Johnson syndrome. Orphanet J Rare Dis 2010;5(39):1–11.
2. Ugburo AO. A 12-year retrospective study of non-burn skin loss(burn-like syndromes) at a tertiary burns unit in a developing country. Burns 2008; 34(5):637–43.
3. Auquier-Durant A, Mockenhaupt M, Naldi L, et al. Correlations between clinical patterns and causes of erythema multiforme majus, Stevens-Johnson syndrome, and toxic epidermal necrolysis. Arch Dermatol 2002;138:1019–24.
4. Neff P, Meuli-Simmen C, Kempf W, et al. Lyell syndrome revisited: analysis of 18 cases of severe bullous skin disease in a burns unit. Br J Plast Surg 2005;58:73–80.
5. Revuz J, Penso D, Roujeau JC, et al. Toxic epidermal necrolysis: clinical findings and prognosis factors in 87 patients. Arch Dermatol 1987; 123:1160–5.
6. Struck MF, Hilbert P, Mockenhaupt M, et al. Severe cutaneous adverse reactions: emergency approach to non-burn epidermolytic syndromes. Intensive Care Med 2010;36(1):22–32.
7. Forman R, Koren G, Shear NH. Erythema multiforme, Stevens-Johnson syndrome and toxic epidermal necrolysis in children: a review of 10 years' experience. Drug Saf 2003;25(13):955–72.
8. Mockenhaupt M. Stevens-Johnson syndrome and toxic epidermal necrolysis: clinical patters, diagnostic considerations, etiology, and therapeutic management. Semin Cutan Med Surg 2014; 33(1):10–6.
9. Gerdts B, Vloemans AF, Kreis RW. Toxic epidermal necrolysis: 15 years' experience in a Dutch burns centre. J Eur Acad Dermatol Venereol 2007;21(6): 781–8.
10. Bastuji-Garin S, Fouchard N, Bertocchi M, et al. SCORTEN: a severity-of-illness score for toxic epidermal necrolysis. J Invest Dermatol 2000; 115(2):149–53.
11. Downey A, Jackson C, Harun N, et al. Toxic epidermal necrolysis: review of pathogenesis and management. J Am Acad Dermatol 2012;66(6):995–1003.
12. Palmieri TL, Greenhalgh DG, Saffle JR, et al. A multicenter review of toxic epidermal necrolysis treated in U.S. burn centers at the end of the twentieth century. J Burn Care Rehabil 2002;23(2):87–96.
13. Schultz JT, Sheridan RL, Ryan CM, et al. A 10-year experience with toxic epidermal necrolysis. J Burn Care Rehabil 2000;21(3):199–204.
14. Tay YK, Huff JC, Weston WL, et al. Mycoplasma pneumoniae infection is associated with Stevens-Johnson syndrome, not erythema multiforme. J Am Acad Dermatol 1996;35(5):757–60.
15. de Prost N, Ingen-Housz-Oro S, Duong TA, et al. Bacteremia in Stevens-Johnson syndrome and toxic necrolysis: epidemiology, risk factors, and predictive value of skin cultures. Medicine (Baltimore) 2010;89(1):28–36.
16. Yarborough DR. Experience with toxic epidermal necrolysis treated in a burn center. J Burn Care Rehabil 1996;17(1):30–3.
17. Atiyeh BS, Dham R, Yassin MF, et al. Treatment of toxic epidermal necrolysis with moisture-retentive ointment: a case report and review of the literature. Dermatol Surg 2003;29(2):185–8.
18. Nandha R, Gupta A, Hashmi A. Cutaneous adverse drug reactions in a tertiary care teaching hospital: a North Indian perspective. Int J Appl Basic Med Res 2011;1(1):50–3.
19. George SM, Harrison DA, Welch CA, et al. Dermatological conditions in intensive care: a secondary analysis of the Intensive Care National Audit and Research Centre (ICNARC) case mix programme database. Crit Care 2008;12(Suppl 1):S1.
20. Zajiceck R, Pintar D, Broz L, et al. Toxic epidermal necrolysis and Stevens-Johnson syndrome at the Prague Burn Centre 1998-2008. J Eur Acad Dermatol Venereol 2012;26(5):639–43.
21. Santucci SG, Gobara S, Santos CR, et al. Infections in a burn intensive care unit: experience of seven years. J Hosp Infect 2003;53:6–13.
22. DiGiovine C, Chenoweth C, Watts C, et al. The attributable mortality and costs of primary nosocomial bloodstream infections in the intensive care unit. Am J Respir Crit Care Med 1999;160:976–81.
23. Coello R, Glenister H, Fereres J, et al. The cost of infection in surgical patients: a case-control study. J Hosp Infect 1993;25(4):239–50.
24. Hassan M, Tuckman HP, Patrick RH, et al. Cost of hospital-acquired infection. Hosp Top 2010;88(3):82–9.
25. Waters TM, Daniels MJ, Bazzoli GJ, et al. Effect of Medicare's nonpayment for hospital-acquired conditions: lessons for future policy. JAMA Intern Med 2015;175(3):347–54.
26. Orsi GB, Di Stefano L, Noah N. Hospital-acquired, laboratory-confirmed bloodstream infection: increased hospital stay and direct costs. Infect Control Hosp Epidemiol 2002;23(4):190–7.
27. Foxman B. Epidemiology of urinary tract infections: incidence, morbidity, and economic costs. Dis Mon 2003;49(2):53–70.
28. Bickers DR, Lim HW, Margolis D, et al. The burden of skin diseases: 2004 a joint project of the American Academy of Dermatology Association and the Society for Investigative Dermatology. J Am Acad Dermatol 2006;55(3):490–500.

Pediatric Burn Care
Unique Considerations in Management

Amita R. Shah, MD, PhD[a,b,*], Lillian F. Liao, MD, MPH[c]

KEYWORDS

- Pediatric burn • Pediatric burn resuscitation • Pediatric burn wound care
- Pediatric burn management • Pediatric burn nutrition

KEY POINTS

- Pediatric patients with partial-thickness burns greater than 10% total body surface area (TBSA); burns of the face, head, neck, hands, feet, or genitalia; concern for intentional injury; or electrical or chemical burns should be referred to a burn center.
- Children have physiologic and psychosocial differences from adults. The Lund-Browder chart is used to estimate TBSA. The Schofield equation is used to estimate pediatric energy expenditure. Fluid requirements are estimated: 2 mL times percent of TBSA times weight in kilograms.
- Children have small airways and should be intubated immediately with a low-volume cuffed endotracheal tube if there is inhalation injury.
- Sedation and analgesia should be implemented for dressing changes to reduce pain and psychological trauma.
- Early involvement of child psychiatry, child life specialist, and therapists for the child and family is recommended.

INTRODUCTION

Burn injuries are one of the top 10 causes of unintentional deaths in children younger than 14 years old with 3892 deaths of children 0 to 14 years old reported from 2004 to 2014.[1] Most pediatric burns are minor but children with severe burns have higher mortality than nonelderly adults with similar burns.[2] Although the basic principles of burn management for pediatric patients are the same as for adults, there are key differences in the physiology and psychology of the pediatric patient. Children with severe burn injuries are best treated at a pediatric burn center that offers multidisciplinary support.

The most common types of burns experienced by young pediatric patients are thermal burns from scalding or contact with hot foods. Nonfood-related thermal burns can come from fireworks, irons, curling irons, campfires, and fire pits. Chemical burn injuries occur from topical or mucosal contact with acidic or alkaline products as seen in many common cleaning products. After enactment of the US Poison Prevention Packaging Act in the 1970s, the incidence of chemical burns decreased.[3] Electrical burns are more often seen in adolescents and occur in the setting of exposure to live electrical wires from high-voltage lines or appliances, lightning, or faulty wiring. These burns cause little visible injury because most of the injury

No commercial or financial conflicts of interests. No funding sources (A.R. Shah and L.F. Liao).
[a] Division of Plastic and Reconstructive Surgery, University of North Carolina at Chapel Hill, Chapel Hill, NC, USA; [b] Division of Plastic and Reconstructive Surgery, University of Texas Health Science Center at San Antonio, 7703 Floyd Curl Drive, San Antonio, TX 78229, USA; [c] Division of Trauma and Emergency Medicine, University of Texas Health Science Center at San Antonio, 7703 Floyd Curl Drive, San Antonio, TX 78229, USA
* Corresponding author.
E-mail address: shahar@uthscsa.edu

occurs in the deeper tissues and can also result in nerve and muscle damage and arrhythmias. Electrical burn to the commissures of the mouth can be seen when an electric cord is placed in the mouth by toddlers, leading to tissue destruction and contracture formation.[4]

INITIAL EVALUATION

Evaluation of pediatric burns occurs in different settings, ranging from an outpatient pediatrics clinic to a regional burn center. Triage involves consideration of factors, including age and medical history of the child, severity of the burn, and mechanism of injury.

Initial Triage

Children with an uncomplicated medical history and minor burns that are less than 5% total body surface area (TBSA) for partial-thickness or 2% TBSA for full-thickness thermal burns can be treated in the outpatient setting, including a pediatric or family practice clinic or urgent care clinic. If there is involvement of the face, head and neck, hands, feet, or genitalia; or if there is a concern for abuse, the child should be referred to a burn center. Children with greater than 10% TBSA burns demonstrate systemic physiologic alterations as a response to the burn and should be referred to a burn center for evaluation and treatment.[4] The American Burn Association guidelines for referral to a burn center for children states that any burned child in a hospital that does not have "qualified personnel or equipment for the care of children," including the ability for safe pediatric sedation, should be referred to a burn unit.[5]

Estimating the Severity of Burns

The Lund-Browder chart is used for estimation for TBSA of burns in children. The body surface area (BSA) varies with age; as the child ages, the BSA for the head decreases, whereas the BSA percentage for the legs increases. Superficial (first-degree) burns are not incorporated into the calculation of the TBSA. Infants and young children have thinner dermis than adults, so the extent of the burn may not be evident at first presentation and reevaluation after 48 hours is needed (**Fig. 1**).

The mechanism of burn injury should also be noted and taken into account when estimating the child's total trauma burden. Burns that occur in closed-spaces, such as house fires, may have an associated inhalation injury. Children burned in motor vehicle collisions or other blunt trauma mechanisms can have associated brain, thoracic, abdominal, and/or extremity injuries.

Emergency Department Evaluation

The initial evaluation of a child in the emergenc department with burn injuries should begin wit airway, breathing, circulation, disability, and expo sure (the ABCs). Information from the transpor team and family includes time and mechanism c injury, patient demographics and medical history the amount of prehospital fluid received, immuni zations, and medications received thus far. Bur injuries that occur in closed-spaces have a hig risk of inhalation injury. Stigmata of inhalatio injury include facial injury, singed nasal hair, soo in the airway, stridor, hoarseness, and carbona ceous sputum. The airway should be immediatel secured via a cuffed endotracheal tube if there i evidence of an inhalation injury. Depending o the development level of the child, the only sign of distress may be restlessness and irritability. A clothing and jewelry is removed to prever continued damage to the skin. The room i warmed to prevent hypothermia and the patier is covered with a clean sheet as needed.

If possible, intravenous access is obtained i intact skin or, if not, through the burned skin. Intra osseous access can be used if adequate intrave nous access cannot be obtained. A patient wit burns greater than 15% TBSA, inhalation injury intubated, or requiring multiple debridements wi likely require a central line.

Estimation of TBSA is performed using the Lund Browder chart. Burns that are circumferentia around the chest should be noted due to the ris of the burn eschar interfering with the ability t ventilate, necessitating escharotomies. Compart ment syndrome of the extremities can occur wit circumferential burns of the extremities requirin escharotomies and fasciotomies. If there are burn on or near the face, evaluation for corneal burn should be performed with fluorescein before eyeli edema prevents thorough examination.

Fluid resuscitation is started in the emergenc department using Normosol or lactated Ringer so lution. There are different formulas for determinin the amount of fluid needed for resuscitation. Th commonly used Parkland Formula is total flui over 24 hours equals 4 mL times percent c TBSA times weight in kilograms. Half of the tota fluid is given in the first 8 hours and the secon half is given over the next 24 hours. The Modifie Brooke formula is total fluid over 24 hours equal 2 mL times kg times percent of TBSA. Half of th total fluid volume is given in the first 8 hours an the other half over the next 16 hours. The amour of fluid given in transport before arrival is used i the calculation of total fluid given. Patients wit combined burn and inhalation injuries may hav

Pre-hospital fluid received:
_____

Obtain: CBC, chem 10, lactic acid, ABG or VBG
Burns>/ = 15% should have repeat labs 4 h after
arrival to aid in resuscitation

Resuscitation fluid: [normosol or LR]
Modified Brooke's: 2 **mL** x kg x %TBSA
Give half in the first 8 h after injury
Give remainder over next 16 h

Maintenance fluid: [normosol or LR]
4–2–1 rule ** add D5 to maintenance portion of fluid

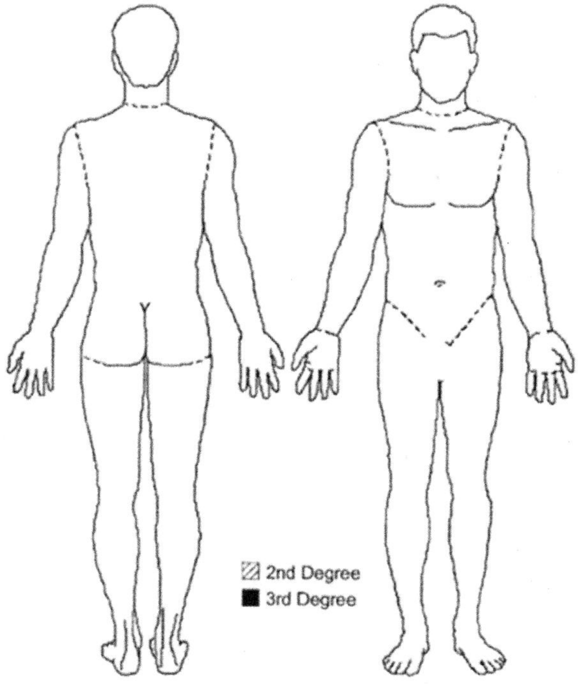

Name
_____

Age _____ Date/Time of Injury _____

CAUSE OF BURN
- ☐ Chemical ☐ Inhalation Injury
- ☐ Contact ☐ Metabolic
- ☐ Electrical ☐ Scald
- ☐ Flame ☐ Other: _____
- ☐ Questionable Circumstances

Height (cm) _____ Weight (kg) _____

Total Body Surface (m²) _____

Body Surface Area Burned (m²) _____

Preliminary Assessment Burn Diagram

☒ 2nd Degree
■ 3rd Degree

Area	Birth-1 y.	1–4 y.	5–9 y.	10–14 y.	15 y.	Adult	2°	3°	TBSA %
Head	19	17	13	11	9	7			
Neck	2	2	2	2	2	2			
Ant. Trunk	13	13	13	13	13	13			
Post. Trunk	13	13	13	13	13	13			
R. Buttock	2.5	2.5	2.5	2.5	2.5	2.5			
L. Buttock	2.5	2.5	2.5	2.5	2.5	2.5			
Genitalia	1	1	1	1	1	1			
R.U. Arm	4	4	4	4	4	4			
L.U. Arm	4	4	4	4	4	4			
R.L. Arm	3	3	3	3	3	3			
L.L. Arm	3	3	3	3	3	3			
R. Hand	2.5	2.5	2.5	2.5	2.5	2.5			
L. Hand	2.5	2.5	2.5	2.5	2.5	2.5			
R. Thigh	5.5	6.5	8	8.5	9	9.5			
L. Thigh	5.5	6.5	8	8.5	9	9.5			
R. Leg	5	5	5.5	6	6.5	7			
L. Leg	5	5	5.5	6	6.5	7			
R. Foot	3.5	3.5	3.5	3.5	3.5	3.5			
L. Foot	3.5	3.5	3.5	3.5	3.5	3.5			
						TOTAL			

Goals:
UOP: 0.5–1 mL/kg/hr
Age appropriate vital signs

Admission location:
<10% TBSA burn: floor
10–14% TBSA burn: intermediate
>/ = 15% TBSA burn, inhalational
injury, or intubated child, SJS, SSSS:
ICU

IV access:
>15% TBSA burn deep partial or full
thickness burn, inhalation injury, child
needing multiple debridement, or
intubated child → consider central
venous access for resuscitation, lab
draws, prolonged stay

Initial OR/sedation procedure for
burns >15%
nasal gastric feeding tube, foley
catheter, central venous access

Fig. 1. Emergency department pediatric burn evaluation sheet with modified Lund-Browder Chart. (*Courtesy of* The University of Texas Health Science Center at San Antonio, San Antonio, TX; with permission.)

fluid requirements that are increased by 40% to 75% and will have to be monitored closely for adequate resuscitation.[6] The key to resuscitation is to provide balanced tissue perfusion and prevent excessive tissue edema. Within the first 24 hours, volume resuscitation should be closely monitored to titrate to resuscitation parameters of urine output, lactic acid, and base deficit as indicators of end organ perfusion. After the first 24 hours, the fluid is changed to a maintenance fluid with dextrose.

Initial laboratory tests obtained include a complete blood count, electrolytes with blood urea nitrogen and creatinine, lactic acid, and arterial or venous blood gas. Laboratory tests are repeated after 4 hours to help guide resuscitation. Urinalysis is obtained to assess for myoglobin. For flame burns, a chest radiograph and blood carboxyhemoglobin levels are obtained.

Children with TBSA burns less than 10% and no other significant comorbidities can be admitted to a regular nursing floor. Patients who have greater than 15% TBSA burns, inhalation injury, and/or are intubated should be admitted to the intensive care unit.

All notes, including follow-up notes, should include the date and mechanism of the burn, the initial TBSA affected, depth and location of the burn, and the current wound care regimen. Photographs downloaded to electronic medical records or placed into a physical chart can facilitate evaluation of the wound by multiple specialties. Pictures should be taken at the time of initial evaluation, immediately after debridement, and at subsequent encounters, even after the wound is closed.

Initial Wound Management

Superficial (first-degree) burns do not need debridement and can be treated with moisturizer. Eventual peeling of the epidermis will occur with new epithelium underneath.

Superficial partial-thickness burns (second-degree) are debrided and blisters removed and covered with Mepilex Ag (Molnlycke Health Care, Gothenburg, Sweden). Mepilex Ag is a silver impregnated foam with a silicone layer that can be used over partial-thickness burns. Mepilex Ag is secured in place with Kerlex and is not taped in place. Reevaluation of the wounds is done within 7 days of the initial debridement.

Silver is an effective antimicrobial but extended use in topical ointments can result in delayed healing and cellular toxicity. Dressings such as Acticoat (Smith & Nephew, London, United Kingdom) and Mepilex Ag offer the antimicrobial effects of silver but reduce cytotoxic effects through controlled release of the silver. Additionally, because the dressing does not have to be removed from the burned surface for days, the pain of dressing changes is reduced.[7]

Deep partial-thickness burns (second-degree) are also debrided and blisters removed. If the burn is more superficial (more pink than white), Mepilex Ag is applied over the burn. Deeper burns (more white than pink) are treated with bacitracin and a nonadherent dressing, such as Telfa (Covidien, Dublin, Ireland) or Dermanet (DeRoyal, Powell, Tennessee, USA). These wounds need repeat evaluation 48 to 72 hours after the initial debridement and may be considered for excision and grafting if there is burn wound progression (**Table 1**).

Full-thickness burns (third-degree) are excised with plans for grafting within 5 days of admission. Early excision and grafting is recommended for deep burns within 1 week from injury to reduce incidence of wound infection, pain, fluid loss, and other complications from delayed wound closure, such as hypertrophic scarring.[6]

Children have a larger body surface area to body mass ratio than adults, making them more likely to become hypothermic and, with a lower total blood volume, more sensitive to blood loss. Excision and grafting is performed in a warmed operating room with warming devices over and under as much as the body as possible. Excision of the extremities is performed under tourniquet, if possible, to decrease the amount of blood loss. Hemostasis is obtained using electrocautery, epinephrine-saline–soaked laparotomy pads, and thrombin. Excision is performed down to punctate bleeding. The skin graft is harvested using a dermatome at 8-thousandths to 12-thousandths of an inch, taking into account the age of the patient and the location of the donor site because younger children have thinner skin. When taking full-thickness skin grafts from the groin, abdomen, and any other potential hair-bearing areas, the future hair growth pattern has to be taken into account because the graft will retain its ability to grow hair.

All burn patients should receive a physical therapy and occupational therapy consultation as soon as they are clinically stable. This is particularly important in patients with burns that extend over the joints. Range of motion and neutral positioning of joints needs to be stressed to prevent early contracture formation.

To prevent premature removal of the dressing by the patient, the dressing can be secured further using a 2-inch ace bandage that extends past the elbow, a splint, and/or self-adherent wrap, such as elastic bandage. When using an elastic bandage, care should be taken to not to stretch and secure it too tightly to prevent it from becoming compressive and acting as a tourniquet over the extremity.

Topical ointments, such as bacitracin, silver sulfadiazine, mafenide acetate, and silver nitrate, are commonly used. Silver sulfadiazine cannot be used on newborns or infants younger than 2 months old due to the risk of kernicterus.[8] Partial-thickness burns of 5% to 10% TBSA can

Table 1
Initial burn wound care

Depth	Debridement	Wound Care	Follow-up	Time to Healing
Superficial (1st-degree)	No	Moisturizer	As needed	2–3 d
Pink to red with minimal to no blistering, painful				
Superficial partial-thickness (2nd-degree)	Yes	Mepilex Ag		<14 d
Blistering, significant drainage, pink to red, very painful			Wound evaluation within 7 d of initial debridement	
Deep partial-thickness (2nd-degree)	Yes	Pink > white: Mepilex Ag		7–14 d
Blistering, minimal drainage, pink and white, very painful		White > pink: bacitracin + nonadherent dressing (Telfa/Dermanet)	Repeat wound evaluation 48–72 h after initial debridement	
Full-thickness (3rd-degree)	Yes	Excision and grafting		Grafting
White eschar, no pain		Within the first 5 d of admission	Admission or early follow-up if directly discharged from ED	
Facial burns	Yes	Bacitracin or cleaning q6 hours; ophthalmic bacitracin for periorbital burns	2 d	
Ear	Yes	Superficial partial-thickness: bacitracin	2 d	
		Deep partial-thickness/concern for cartilage exposure: sulfamylon		
Hands & feet	Yes	Mepilex Ag or bacitracin; wrap digits separately or use a finger separator, splint, consult OT/PT if burn crosses joints	2 d	

Courtesy of The University of Texas Health Science Center at San Antonio, San Antonio, TX; with permission.

also be biological dressings such as Biobrane (Smith & Nephew, London, United Kingdom), allograft, or xenograft. These dressing are covered with gauze until adherent and the dressing are left in place as the epithelium grows underneath. The dressing is trimmed as it becomes nonadherent, indicating epithelialization underneath.[4]

SEDATION AND ANALGESIA

The importance of appropriate and adequate sedation and analgesia has been emphasized as part of comprehensive and compassionate total burn care. Children may be willing to tolerate any dressing change the first time but once it becomes a traumatic and painful experience the child will have anxiety and fear for the subsequent treatments, decreasing the effectiveness of subsequent analgesia. The most effective way to treat pediatric burn pain is at the initial procedure.[9,10]

Procedural sedation that can be performed outside of the operating room allows for more aggressive continuous debridements to be performed, decreased incidence of anesthesia-related complications, and decreased hospital stay and cost. Methods of analgesia and sedation range from only oral medications, such as acetaminophen, nonsteroidal anti-inflammatory drugs, midazolam and oxycodone, to parenteral medications, such as morphine, midazolam, fentanyl, ketamine, and propofol. Medication choice is based on the age of the patient, depth of burn, and emotional state. Nitrous oxide alone and with oral and intravenous medications is also used.[11] Sedation for pediatric patient should be performed in a monitored setting by a provider that is experienced in pediatric anesthesia and sedation with a nearby crash cart containing flumazenil and naloxone.[10]

The psychological state is an important factor in the control of pain and anxiety. Nonpharmacological therapies, such as virtual reality, distraction, learning techniques that prepare the patient for the procedure, hypnosis, massage, and acupuncture, are also implemented.[9]

INHALATION INJURY

When the mechanism of injury involves flame burns in a closed space with exposure to smoke, inhalation injury and carbon monoxide exposure should be suspected. The child may have visible signs such as singed facial hair and soot in the airway. Hoarseness and stridor are more ominous signs of airway injury and developing obstruction, and the patient should be intubated immediately because airway edema will progress rapidly over the next 12 to 24 hours. Low-pressure cuffed endotracheal tubes should be used because c the potential for leaks compromising ventilatio and the difficulty in changing the tubes if a lea should arise.[12] Once the airway is secured, bron choscopic evaluation can be performed for bette characterization of the injury and to determine th presence of plugging. Patients with carbo monoxide exposure may be obtunded or coma tose and they should be treated with 100% oxy gen until the carboxyhemoglobin level is les than less than 10%.[13] Treatment of inhalatio injury includes chest physiotherapy, spirometry coughing, and early ambulation. Aerosolize treatments of albuterol and epinephrine trea bronchospasm, whereas aerosolized heparin N acetylcysteine and humidification help decreas plugging. If the patient is being mechanicall ventilated, care is taken to minimize barotraum and volutrauma. High-frequency percussive venti lation has also been used to decrease peak inspi ratory pressure and work of breathing.[14]

METABOLIC DEMANDS IN CHILDREN

Early and aggressive nutritional support is rec ommended. After significant burn injury, the pa tient becomes hypermetabolic with restin energy expenditure 1.6 to 2 times normal. Atten uation of the hypermetabolic state can b accomplished through non-nutritional methods such as control of the ambient temperature t 28° to 30°C, early excision and grafting of dee burns, and administration of nonselective bet blockers, such as propranolol. Nonselectiv beta-blockers are more beneficial in childre than in adults and can decrease hypermetabo lism and hypercatabolism.[15,16]

Initiation of enteral feeding either by mouth c tube feeding is recommended within 6 to 12 hour of injury. Early feeding has been associated wit decrease in the hypermetabolic response increased immunoglobulin production, reductio of stress ulceration, decreased stress hormon levels, and reduction of malnutrition and energ deficit. In children, postpyloric tube placement i easier than in adults and may occur automaticall with gastric tube placement. Parental nutrition i recommended only in cases of enteral feedin failure.[15,17]

Children have smaller reserve and greate caloric and protein requirements per kilogram c weight than an adult. Evaporative water loss i also higher in children than adults due to th higher body surface area to weight ratio. Th gold standard for measuring energy requirement after severe burn injuries is indirect calorimetry When indirect calorimetry is not available the Schofield equation is an alternative for estimating the requirements for children. The equation can underestimate requirements, so the results of the calculation should be rounded up[18] (**Table 2**).

Dextrose solutions and lipids from other infusions such as propofol should be incorporated into the total. Protein requirements are estimated to be 1.5 to 2 g/kg/d. Glutamine in doses of 0.3 g/kg/d for 5 to 10 days has been recommended.[15,19] Carbohydrates should deliver 55% to 60% of the energy requirements without exceeding 5 mg/kg/min. Glucose control targets are 6 to 8 mmol/L with caution taken with intensive insulin therapy due to the risk of hypoglycemia from frequent interruptions of feeding due to NPO requirements for anesthesia and dressing changes. Supplementation of micronutrients (trace elements and vitamins), such as copper, selenium, magnesium, and zinc, as well as vitamins B, C, E, and D, are needed. Lipids in current formulations provide 30% to 52% of total energy as fat. Nonnutritional lipid intake, such as propofol infusion for sedation, needs to be considered in the total daily lipid calculation.[15,17]

PSYCHOSOCIAL CONSIDERATIONS

Part of comprehensive acute burn care is preparing the child and family for the chronic aspects of burn care, which includes psychosocial issues. Social workers, psychologists, occupational therapists, physical therapists, and child-life specialists are integral parts of the burn team.

Pediatric psychiatry is an important part of a burn center multidisciplinary team. Evaluation of the burn patient should begin in school-aged children soon after their medical management is stabilized. The pediatric psychiatry team assists

both the patient and their parents in coping with the acute injury, as well as with chronic emotional changes associated with burn. The psychiatry team can also assist with patients' siblings who may also be affected by having a sibling injured. A review of psychosocial outcomes of burned children showed highly variable extent of psychopathology with 15% to 20% of patients experiencing significant poor psychosocial outcomes related to the burn.[20] At follow-up appointments, the child is evaluated for post-traumatic stress symptoms and referred to child psychiatry if needed. Participation at area burn camps will also help children with their psychosocial changes associated with being a burn patient. Burn camps have been shown to improve their self-image and confidence.[21]

Children who were victims of nonaccidental trauma that are age 5 years or older are evaluated by child psychiatry. If an injury prevention team or consultation service is available at the facility, they will meet with the family before discharge. All patients admitted to the hospital receive a social work consult for evaluation for prior family history of nonaccidental trauma and the determination for referral to child protective services is made.

SUMMARY

Most pediatric burn wounds are minor and can be treated in the outpatient setting with local wound care; however, in severe burns there are differences in the physiology and psychology of children at different ages, requiring that they be treated in a facility that is experienced in pediatric burn care with resources for multidisciplinary care. Because of the small size of children, there is less room for error. Equations for estimations of TBSA, fluid resuscitation, and nutrition differ from those of an adult. Adequate analgesia and sedation are also important aspects of burn care to diminish the pain and trauma of acute and chronic care. The long-term effects of the burn extend past the physical injury and cause psychological ramifications for the patient and the family. Compassionate comprehensive burn care is accomplished by a multidisciplinary team consisting of burn surgeons and nurses, therapists, pediatricians, and psychiatrists who offer healing in the acute setting and prepare the child and family for treatment and care afterward.

Table 2
Estimation of pediatric energy requirements using the Schofield equation

Age	Requirements
Girls (3–10 y old)	$(16.97 \times \text{weight in kg}) + (1618 \times \text{height in cm}) + 371.2$
Boys (3–10 y old)	$(19.6 \times \text{weight in kg}) + (1033 \times \text{height in cm}) + 414.9$
Girls (10–18 y old)	$(8365 \times \text{weight in kg}) + (4.65 \times \text{height in cm}) + 200$
Boys (10–18 y old)	$(16.25 \times \text{weight in kg}) + (1372 \times \text{height in cm}) + 515.5$

Adapted from Rousseau A, Losser M, Ichai C, et al. ESPEN endorsed recommendations: nutritional therapy in major burns. Clin Nutr 2013;32(4):499; with permission.

REFERENCES

1. Centers for Disease Control and Prevention. Injury Prevention & Control: Data & Statistics (WIS-QUARS). 2014.

2. Pereira CT, Barrow RE, Sterns AM, et al. Age-dependent differences in survival after severe burns: a unicentric review of 1,674 patients and 179 autopsies over 15 years. J Am Coll Surg 2006;202(3):536–48.

3. Walton WW. An evaluation of the poison prevention packaging act. Pediatrics 1982;69(3):363–70.

4. Jamshidi R, Sato TT, Runyan S, et al. Initial assessment and management of thermal burn injuries in children. Pediatr Rev 2013;34(9):395–404.

5. Gamelli RL. Guidelines for the operation of burn centers. J Burn Care Res 2007;28:133.

6. Klein GL, Herndon DN. Burns. Pediatr Rev 2004; 25(12):411–7.

7. Singer AJ, Dagum AB. Current management of acute cutaneous wounds. N Engl J Med 2008; 359(10):1037–46.

8. Palmieri TL, Greenhalgh DG. Topical treatment of pediatric patients with burns: a practical guide. Am J Clin Dermatol 2002;3(8):529–34.

9. Bayat A, Ramaiah R, Bhananker SM. Analgesia and sedation for children undergoing burn wound care. Expert Rev Neurother 2010;10(11):1747–59.

10. Foglia R, Moushey R, Meadows L, et al. Evolving treatment in a decade of pediatric burn care. J Pediatr Surg 2004;39(6):957–60.

11. Ebach DR, Foglia RP, Jones MB, et al. Experience with procedural sedation in a pediatric burn center. J Pediatr Surg 1999;34(6):955–8.

12. Sheridan RL. Uncuffed endotracheal tubes should not be used in seriously burned children. Pediatr Crit Care Med 2006;7(3):258–9.

13. Dries DJ, Endorf FW. Inhalation injury: epidemiology, pathology, treatment strategies. Scand J Trauma Resusc Emerg Med 2013;21:31.

14. Fidkowski CW, Fuzaylov G, Sheridan RL, et al. Inhalation burn injury in children. Paediatr Anaesth 2009; 19(Suppl 1):147–54.

15. Rousseau A, Losser M, Ichai C, et al. ESPEN endorsed recommendations: nutritional therapy in major burns. Clin Nutr 2013;32(4):497–502.

16. Finnerty CC, Herndon DN. Is propranolol of benefit in pediatric burn patients? Adv Surg 2013;47:177–97.

17. Rodriguez NA, Jeschke MG, Williams FN, et al. Nutrition in burns : Galveston contributions. JPEN J Parenter Enteral Nutr 2011;35(6):704–14.

18. Carpenter A, Pencharz P, Mouzaki M. Accurate estimation of energy requirements of young patients. J Pediatr Gastroenterol Nutr 2015;60(1):4–10.

19. De-Souza DA, Greene LJ. Intestinal permeability and systemic infections in critically ill patients: effect of glutamine. Crit Care Med 2005;33(5):1125–35.

20. Tarnowski KJ, Rasnake LK, Gavaghan-Jones MP, et al. Psychosocial sequelae of pediatric burn injuries: a review. Clin Psychol Rev 1991;11(4):371–98.

21. Maslow GR, Lobato D. Summer camps for children with burn injuries: a literature review. J Burn Care Res 2010;31(5):740–9.

Patient Safety in Burn Care

Application of Evidence-based Medicine to Improve Outcomes

Elizabeth L. Dale, MD[a],*, Charles Scott Hultman, MD, MBA[b]

KEYWORDS

- Patient safety • Quality • Value • Adverse events • Evidence-based medicine

KEY POINTS

- Patient safety is recognized as a distinct discipline that emphasizes preventing, reducing, reporting, and analyzing medical errors.
- Evidence-based medicine has evolved to not only improve patient outcomes and increase patient safety but also promote standardization of practices, reducing variability in care.
- Areas in burn care that increasingly used evidence-based medicine include resuscitation protocols, transfusion practices, vascular access, venous thromboembolic prophylaxis, and rational use of antibiotics.

PATIENT SAFETY OVERVIEW

Hippocrates may have recognized the importance of "First, do no harm" circa 400 BC, but the modern patient safety movement began in 1999, with the landmark publication of "To Err is Human" by the Institute of Medicine. In that report, the National Academy of Sciences estimated that 44,000 to 98,000 preventable deaths were due to medical errors each year. Shortly thereafter, in response to public pressure and the clear need to decrease adverse events, the Agency for Healthcare for Research and Quality defined 6 domains of health care quality that have now become the pillars for value creation: patient safety, clinical effectiveness, patient-centered care, providing timely and accessible care, improving efficiency, and correcting disparities by making health care equitable, regardless of geographic location or socioeconomic status. Today, patient safety is recognized as a distinct discipline that emphasizes preventing, reducing, reporting, and analysis of medical errors.

As we move to a value-based health care economy, replacing fee-for-service models that reward volume, quality and cost will be the key drivers that determine the value of services provided. Evidence-based medicine has evolved to not only improve patient outcomes and increase patient safety but also promote standardization of practices to reduce variability in care. Essentially, clinical practice guidelines, or "best practices," form the backbone of evidence-based medicine, which relies on the best available research to help inform physicians regarding the best treatment plans for patients. Furthermore, patient rights and preferences are brought into medical decision making, creating integrated yet personalized treatment pathways.

In the field of burn care, culture often trumps data, but times are changing. Through national registries, multicenter trials, use of benchmarks, and prevention of such "never events" as pressure ulcers, wrong-site surgery, and catheter-related

a Division of Plastic/Burn Surgery, Shriners Hospital for Children, University of Cincinnati, 231 Albert Sabin Way, Academic Health Center, Cincinnati, OH 45267-0513, USA; b Division of Plastic Surgery, Department of Surgery, University of North Carolina School of Medicine, Chapel Hill, NC, USA
* Corresponding author.
E-mail address: daleeh@ucmail.uc.edu

Clin Plastic Surg 44 (2017) 611–618
http://dx.doi.org/10.1016/j.cps.2017.02.015
0094-1298/17/© 2017 Elsevier Inc. All rights reserved.

infections, burn centers are now becoming leaders of the patient safety movement. Without doubt, the pre-existing interdisciplinary team structure of burn care has fostered the development of clinical pathways that provide internal consistency and help establish national standards. This article reviews 5 areas in burn care that increasingly use evidence-based medicine to optimize quality and safety: resuscitation protocols, transfusion practices, vascular access, venous thromboembolic prophylaxis, and rational use of antibiotics.

RESUSCITATION PROTOCOLS

A cornerstone aspect of large surface area burn injury is shock, characterized by both cellular edema and marked vascular permeability. Underhill[1] and Cope and Moore[2] provided the first clinical descriptions, with recommended therapeutic resuscitation methods. In 1968, Baxter and Shires[3] described a more precise method of estimating the fluid requirement with experiments on dogs. Baxter[4] confirmed his proposal in 1978 with a case series in human patients. As a consequence, it is now rare that patients suffer the sequelae of underresuscitation, and the concern is that overresuscitation is a more prevalent danger. Pruitt[5] described this in 2000, warning practitioners against "fluid creep," and Cancio and colleagues[6] demonstrated that clinicians are much more likely to increase fluid rates for low urine output (UOP) than to decrease it for high levels.

The current emphasis is finding ways to limit resuscitation volumes, because the consequences of excessive administered volumes can be both morbid and lethal, for example, abdominal compartment syndrome, extremity compartment syndromes, and organ failure. Chung and colleagues,[7] in a study of combat victims evacuated from the combat theater, concluded that starting with a lower calculation (2 mL/kg per% total body surface area [TBSA] vs 4 mL/kg per % TBSA) would result in lower overall volumes and may improve mortality. Their study was small and may suffer from selection bias, because only patients who survived the first days of injury and reached their center were included. Other methods to decrease resuscitation volumes are the use of colloid, and using alternative methods (than UOP) to guide resuscitation. *Cochrane Reviews* assert a 2.4 to 2.93 relative risk of death in burn patients resuscitated with colloid in addition to crystalloid.[8,9] These results have been called into question by burn providers. A recent meta-analysis found instead that use of colloid resulted in fewer gastrointestinal and central nervous

system complications and that it may reduce compartment syndrome and mortality.[10] O'Mara and colleagues[11] affirmed that intra-abdominal pressures were significantly lower in a colloid resuscitated group. Most current protocols advise use of albumin after 12 to 24 hours after burn, as a method to reduce overall volume infused.

With regards to resuscitation endpoints, UOP has long been the primary clinical indicator. Recently, noninvasive cardiac indices, for example, transpulmonary thermodilution, have been suggested as a more effective method, and one that may decrease overall infusion volumes.[12] A recent systematic review of a variety of alternative methods to determine resuscitation endpoints concluded that limited evidence exists that they resulted in improved outcomes.[13]

Unfortunately, current practice is supported only by a panoply of small studies; no large-scale multicenter trial has been performed to determine optimal methods of resuscitation. The most recent consensus guidelines by the American Burn Association recommend starting resuscitation based on formulas of 2 to 4 mL/kg body weight per % TBSA during the first 24 hours, adjusting that rate based on UOP of 0.5 to 1.0 mL/kg/h in adults and 1.0 to 1.5 mL/kg/h in children, and using colloid beginning at 12 to 24 hours after injury. Hypertonic saline is considered high risk, and there is minimal risk and possible benefit to the use of ascorbic acid (high-dose vitamin C).[14] Until large scale studies improve on this knowledge, these recommendations provide the best practice for resuscitation in the thermally injured patient.

TRANSFUSION PRACTICES

Patients with large surface area burns (>20%) nearly always require blood transfusions during their hospital stay, the number of which surpass those required by patients with other conditions. Reasons for this include acute red blood cell (RBC) destruction from thermal and inflammatory insults, suppressed marrow response to erythropoietin, substantial blood loss at each excision and graft procedure, and the repetitive phlebotomy to which all critically ill patients are subjected.[15] There is a relationship of anemia to tissue hypoxemia, and in the burn patient, the "lethal triad" of coagulopathy, acidosis, and hypothermia can happen repetitively throughout the hospital course. It is thought that maintaining adequate hemoglobin (Hgb) will avoid acidosis by replacing the oxygen-carrying capacity of the circulating blood volume. However, in recent decades, it has become clear that blood transfusion is not without its risks, with studies demonstrating increased mortality and infectious complications directly related to the number of transfusions a patient receives.[16,17] Lu and colleagues,[18] in contrast, showed no mortality or infectious detriment in the burn-injured patient directly related to number of transfusions.

In the context of burn wound excision and grafting, standard efforts made to reduce blood loss include tourniquets on extremities and the subdermal injection of epinephrine-containing tumescent solutions. Although these have decreased blood transfusion requirements, they have not omitted them. Since the TRICC Trial (Transfusion Requirements in Critical Care), there has been a trend toward adopting a lower transfusion "trigger" for RBC transfusion.[19] This multicenter trial compared using a transfusion threshold of Hgb 7 to Hgb 10. Investigators concluded that the lower threshold was at least as effective and possibly superior to the higher one, effectively changing practice. Kwan and colleagues[15] came to similar conclusions in burn patients, demonstrating lower 30-day and in-hospital mortality with a lower threshold.[1] Palmieri and colleagues[20] repeated the study in pediatric burn-injured patients in a single center and confirmed that a restricted transfusion policy was safe in that population.

Having established a lower transfusion threshold of RBC for anemia, the question of coagulopathy in the setting of acute blood loss that accompanies excision and grafting is pertinent. Pidcoke and colleagues[21] compared these procedures to the trauma patient and evaluated the direct effects of providing plasma and platelets on clotting times. Investigators demonstrated that plasma has a negligible effect in improving clot strength, and although platelets improved clot strength, it still remained below the reference range, concluding that blood product resuscitation is not hemostatic and is insufficient to address coagulopathy encountered during burn wound excision. Nonetheless, the PROPR Trial (Transfusion of Plasma, platelets and red blood cells in patients with severe trauma) provided evidence that transfusing blood products in a 1:1:1 ratio provides clinically improved rates of hemostasis at 24 hours.[22] Palmieri and colleagues[23] asked a similar question in burn-injured pediatric patients, comparing a ratio of 4:1 RBC to fresh frozen plasma to 1:1. Although the pilot study was underpowered, there was a trend toward higher hospital LOS, organ dysfunction, infection rates, and time to wound healing in the 4:1 group. The group concluded that this may be due to the detrimental effect of more units of RBC transfused. Cartotto and colleagues[24] examined whether the storage defect of RBC would increase complications and mortality in thermally injured patients. Although they found no association with the age of transfused blood, their study confirmed that the volume of blood transfused was associated directly with more bloodstream infections and trended to lengthening the time to wound healing.

Two authors have pushed the bar further in attempting to avoid the detrimental effects of blood transfusion in thermally injured patients. A very small study by Sittig and Deitch[25] used a transfusion trigger of Hgb less than 6 and found no adverse outcomes. Imai and colleagues[26] proposed autologous blood transfusion. They compared a group with preoperative phlebotomy of 800 mL of blood, and replacement with 500 mL of lactated Ringers and 6 hydroxyethylated starch during excision and graft, replacing the blood after excision and graft harvest. The control group received allogeneic RBC transfusion per their normal protocol. The blood loss was similar in both groups, and no adverse outcomes occurred. They concluded this was safer, more likely to correct coagulopathy, and less expensive.

In conclusion, it is appropriate to recognize the risk associated with blood transfusion and make every effort to limit blood loss and implement restrictive transfusion strategies in the setting of care for the burn patient. Further study is warranted in the setting of the utility of plasma and platelet transfusions during excision and grafting as well as considering an even lower Hgb as a transfusion trigger in the burn-injured patient.

CENTRAL VENOUS ACCESS

Burn intensive care units (ICUs) have higher rates of central line–associated bloodstream infections (CLABSI) than other ICUs.[27,28] The National Healthcare Safety Network reported a rate for increased numbers of line infections of 2.8/1000 line-days. CLABSIs are associated with high cost, $11,000-$56,167, which is a reflection of the increased morbidity, length of stay (LOS), and occasionally, mortality, that they cause.[29] For decades, burn surgeons have been aware of this risk, attributing it to several unique aspects of the thermally injured patient: (1) Lines are often placed on or near the burn wound; (2) Frequent transient bacteremia occurs during wound manipulation, that is, dressing changes, excision, and grafting; (3) Burn ICU LOS is prolonged.[30] In light of these unique risk factors, rigorous measures to prevent CLABSIs are essential.

Centers for Disease Control and Prevention guidelines for prevention of CLABSIs are lengthy. A few notable aspects are worth mentioning.[31]

These include the use of 2% chlorhexidine gluconate (CHG) baths to reduce infection rate and the use of antibiotic impregnated catheters if the line is expected to remain in place more than 5 days or the rate of CLABSIs is not decreasing after a comprehensive strategy to reduce rates of CLABSI. They advise against the use of routine replacement of catheters to prevent catheter-related infections as well as the routine use of guidewire exchanges for nontunneled catheters to prevent infection. Both of these practices are routine among burn practitioners.[29,32]

Burn surgeons are undecided on the ideal interval between line changes, but a number of studies have been published in support of intervals of 3 to 7 days, each demonstrating a cost/benefit analysis using binary comparison groups.[33–35] No multicenter study is available to identify the optimal interval of line change. It is clear that lines left in place more than 8 to 10 days have a markedly increased infection rate, however.[36] Two key studies demonstrate the benefit of chlorhexidine baths for reducing device-related infections. Climo and colleagues[37] did a multicenter randomized, crossover trial over several types of ICU settings that demonstrated a reduction in both multidrug-resistant organism (DRO) infections and hospital-acquired bloodstream infections with 2% CHG impregnated washcloth baths. Popp and colleagues[38] did a similar study in thermally injured patients with 0.9% chlorhexidine baths (236 mL bottle of CHG in 1 L sterile water), and eliminated CLABSI over the intervention period.

Another mode of reducing infection rates is to use antibiotic-impregnated lines. Weber and colleagues[30] demonstrated a 50% reduction in line infection rates after changes to a protocol that used antibiotic (minocycline and rifampin) -impregnated lines. Chlorhexidine and Silvadene–impregnated lines are routinely used in the authors' center. The primary concern with these lines is that they may increase rates of DRO infections. To date, there are no studies substantiating this concern in the burn population.

There is substantial evidence that using line placement and maintenance bundles and checklists consistently reduces line infection rates.[39–41] Blot and colleagues[39] demonstrated in a meta-analysis across multiple ICU types that the bundle/checklist was more effective than any other single intervention.

Finally, the role of peripherally inserted central catheters (PICC) is being investigated in the setting of burn injury. A recent review of the Trauma Registry for the American College of Surgeons in burn-injured patients demonstrated an equivalent rate of CLABSI in patients using PICC lines versus central venous catheter (CVC). Notably, the average duration of dwell was 15 days, which is much longer than most burn centers would leave a CVC.[42] A small retrospective review by Barsun and colleagues[43] demonstrated an infection rate of 12.9 per 1000 line-days in PICC lines placed through uninjured skin or healed burns/grafts. They concluded that line maintenance and rotation were warranted for PICC lines in the severely injured burn patient.

In conclusion, effective methods to decrease line infection rates in the thermally injured patient include using bundles/checklists, daily chlorhexidine baths, using antibiotic impregnated lines, and having a line change protocol of between 3 and 7 days. It is unknown what interval is ideal, and to date, there is no evidence that use of PICC lines decreases infection rates.

VENOUS THROMBOEMBOLISM PROPHYLAXIS

Venous thromboembolism (VTE), a term encompassing deep venous thrombosis (DVT) and pulmonary embolism (PE), remains a dreaded complication in the setting of burn injury. Although PE has the potential to be fatal, persistent sequelae of DVT are present in 50% of patient who suffer DVT during an acute illness. In the context of burn injury, the actual incidence of symptomatic VTE is remarkably lower than Virchow's triad of stasis, local injury, and hypercoagulability would predict. In a recent large population series and a National Burn Repository database search, the average incidence of DVT was 0.25% to 1.2%.[44–47] In smaller retrospective, single-center series where screening weekly ultrasound is used, incidence ranged from 5.92% to 23.3%.[48–50]

Although the incidence of symptomatic VTE is low, it is clear that some patients are at higher risk for DVT/PE than others and therefore should receive chemoprophylaxis. The primary questions, then, are which patients are at highest risk, and what is an effective way to provide prophylaxis?

With regard to risk assessment, the Caprini model as described in 2005 is considered a standard for surgical patients.[51] Building on the concept, Pannucci and colleagues[52] did an elegant study in 2012 in which they created and validated a risk assessment model specific to burn patients. In their model, they emphasized the importance of characterizing factors that are present at the time of admission, although they noted that other risks accumulate during the hospital stay of the burn patient. The primary risks factors are increasing TBSA burn and inhalation

jury. Interestingly, TBSA greater than 65% was
ss associated with VTE than 50% to 65%
BSA. There is speculation that the mortality at
BSA greater than 65% occurs before the occur-
ance of DVT, but does not actually represent
wer risk. Other investigators found age, obesity,
ospital LOS, and use of CVCs as predictive risk
actors.[53,54] The 2008 CHEST guidelines advocate
emoprophylaxis for patients with the following
sk factors: advanced age, morbid obesity, exten-
ve or lower-extremity trauma, use of a femoral
enous catheter, and prolonged immobility.[55] Tak-
g this group of risk assessment studies into ac-
ount, it remains to individual burn centers to
stitute protocols for mechanical and chemopro-
hylaxis. The Panucci model is the easiest to
ollow, and most centers would include morbid
obesity as an indicator to increase levels of anti-
oagulant dose.

This raises the question of adequacy of VTE pro-
hylaxis in the burn patient. Unfortunately, the ev-
ence to date is even slimmer in this area. One
tudy compared low-molecular-weight heparin
LMWH) with low-dose unfractionated heparin
LDUH) and found the incidence of heparin-
duced thrombocytopenia higher in the LDUH
roup. They advised the use of LMWH in burn pa-
ents.[56] With regards to adequacy of anticoagula-
on, efforts have been made to use antifactor Xa
vels as a benchmark. Lin and colleagues[57,58] at
e University of Utah have proposed an equation
at incorporates patient weight and TBSA to
etermine a starting dose of enoxaparin to obtain
ntifactor Xa levels of 0.2 to 0.4 U/mL.[59] Although
e group demonstrated the efficacy of the formula
or obtaining the laboratory value, they were un-
ole to demonstrate a difference in the number
f VTE events between groups. Brown and colagues[60] performed a similar study in pediatric
atients with the same disappointing outcome of
milar VTE events in each group. Each of these
udies suffered from inadequate power, because
e incidence of clinically significant events in the
urn population is already quite low. A large multi-
enter trial is necessary to demonstrate efficacy of
ne method over another. There is currently not a
roven method to demonstrate adequacy of
emoprophylaxis in the setting of burn injury.

In the trauma literature, antifactor Xa levels have
een studied more rigorously and demonstrated
 be inferior to thromboelastography (TEG) for ad-
quacy of dosing to prevent VTE.[61] TEG has not
et been studied in a burn population, but is an
ea for future research.

A recent survey of burn units in Canada
vealed that 75% of centers routinely use some
rm of chemoprophylaxis.[62] It is known that
chemoprophylaxis is more effective than mechanical prophylaxis in high-risk patients. It is reasonable to make an early risk assessment and begin
prophylactic chemoprophylaxis in patients with
known risk factors. Areas for further investigation
include type of prophylaxis and benchmarks for
adequacy of chemoprophylaxis.

RATIONAL USE OF ANTIBIOTICS

Burn-injured patients, by the nature of their injury,
are uniquely susceptible to local and systemic
infections. The implications of this are the frequent
development of DRO, necessitating a cautious
approach to antibiotic use.[63] In addition, the large
surface area burn initiates an inflammatory
response that causes systemic inflammatory
response syndrome (SIRS), making the diagnosis
of infection more difficult. In this setting, antibiotics
must be initiated appropriately, administered for
optimal bactericidal activity, and discontinued
expediently.[64,65]

In 2007, Greenhalgh and colleagues[64] led a
consensus conference to aid in the diagnosis of
acute infection. Because of the SIRS response,
burn-injured patients met criteria as defined by
the Society of Critical Care Medicine throughout
their acute illness, necessitating different measures to identify an infection.[66] The American
Burn Association group outlined 7 categories, 3
of which must be met to trigger a search for acute
infection. Practitioners should initiate broad-
spectrum antibiotics when a "change" in status indicates acute infection, proceed with a workup,
de-escalate as soon as possible, and discontinue
them as dictated by parameters specific to the
infection type, for example, 8 days for most
ventilator-associated pneumonias.[65,66]

Burn clinicians agree that topical antimicrobials
should be used as long as wounds are open; however, the use of systemic prophylactic antibiotics
and continuous versus intermittent bolus dosing
are questions recently investigated in the burn
and critical care setting. Because of the frequent
rate of ventilator-associated pneumonia in patients with inhalation injury, some physicians use
prophylactic antibiotics in this setting. Liodaki
and colleagues[67] showed no difference in the
development of pneumonia with prophylactic antibiotics. However, a multicenter database study in
Japan demonstrated a mortality benefit for burn-
injured patients requiring mechanical ventilation
to be placed on prophylactic systemic antibiotics.[68] Incidence of DRO was not specifically
sought in this population, but it was noted that
the proportion of anti-methicillin-resistant Staphylococcus aureus drug administration was not

increased. Large-scale prospective studies have not been performed to confirm this finding.

A unique aspect of the microbial flora in the burn-injured patient is the rapid development of gram-negative organisms, most frequently *Pseudomonas aeruginosa* and *Acinetobacter baumenii*. These organisms are most effectively treated with beta-lactamase antibiotics. The bactericidal activity of beta-lactamases is time dependent. Recently, studies have demonstrated improved clinical cure and decreased mortality with continuous infusion as opposed to intermittent bolus dosing.[69,70] Although these studies were done in non-burn populations, their conclusions warrant consideration. One difficulty with treating the burn-injured patient with systemic antibiotics is the increased volume of distribution caused by persistent edema and insensible fluid losses. It is, therefore, prudent to use therapeutic dose monitoring, for example, measuring trough levels, in these patients to ensure they are above the minimum inhibitory concentration for the bacterial target.[71]

Prevention and treatment of specific site infections, for example, invasive wound infection, ventilator-associated pneumonia, CLABSI, and urinary tract infection are detailed elsewhere. Many burn clinicians use routine surveillance cultures of wounds to identify colonization patterns, but abstain from systemic antimicrobials unless signs of invasive infection are present.

In conclusion, burn-injured patients present a challenge in the context of judicious use of antibiotics. Although a robust evidence-based approach is lacking, consensus guidelines and recent studies of prophylactic antibiotic use and modes of ensuring adequate dosing aid with appropriate workup and treatment regimens.

REFERENCES

1. Underhill F. The significance of anhydremia in extensive superficial burns. JAMA 1930;95:852–7.
2. Cope O, Moore FD. The redistribution of body water and the fluid therapy of the burned patient. Ann Surg 1947;126:1010–45.
3. Baxter CR, Shires T. Physiological response to crystalloid resuscitation of severe burns. Ann N Y Acad Sci 1968;150:874–94.
4. Baxter CR. Problems and complications of burn shock resuscitation. Surg Clin North Am 1978;58:1313–22.
5. Pruitt BA. Protection from excessive resuscitation: "pushing the pendulum back". J Trauma 2000;49:567–8.
6. Cancio LC, Chávez S, Alvarado-Ortega M, et al. Predicting increased fluid requirements during the resuscitation of thermally injured patients. J Traum 2004;56(2):404–13 [discussion: 413–4].
7. Chung KK, Wolf SE, Cancio LC, et al. Resuscitation of severely burned military casualties: fluid begets more fluid. J Trauma 2009;67(2):231– [discussion: 237].
8. Alderson P, Bunn F, Lefebvre C, et al, Albumin Reviewers. Human albumin solution for resuscitation and volume expansion in critically ill patients. Cochrane Database Syst Rev 2004;(4):CD001208.
9. Roberts I, Blackhall K, Alderson P, et al. Human albumin solution for resuscitation and volume expansion in critically ill patients. Cochrane Database Syst Rev 2011;(11):CD001208.
10. Navickis RJ, Greenhalgh DG, Wilkes MM. Albumin in burn shock resuscitation: a meta-analysis of controlled clinical studies. J Burn Care Res 2016 37(3):e268–78.
11. O'Mara MS, Slater H, Goldfarb IW, et al. A prospective randomized evaluation of intra-abdominal pressure with crystalloid and colloid resuscitation in burn patients. J Trauma 2005;58(5):1011–108.
12. Sánchez M, García-de-Lorenzo A, Herrero E, et al. A protocol for resuscitation of severe burn patients guided by transpulmonary thermodilution and lactate levels: a 3-year prospective cohort study. Crit Care 2013;17(4):R176.
13. Paratz JD, Stockton K, Paratz ED, et al. Burn resuscitation–hourly urine output versus alternative endpoints: a systematic review. Shock 2014;42(4) 295–306.
14. Pham TN, Cancio LC, Gibran NS, American Burn Association. American Burn Association practice guidelines burn shock resuscitation. J Burn Care Res 2008;29(1):257–66.
15. Kwan P, Gomez M, Cartotto R. Safe and successful restriction of transfusion in burn patients. J Burn Care Res 2006;27(6):826–34.
16. Corwin HL. The CRIT Study: anemia and blood transfusion in the critically ill—current clinical practice in the United States. Crit Care Med 2004 32(1):39–52.
17. Palmieri TL, Caruso DM, Foster KN, et al. American Burn Association Burn Multicenter Trials Group: effect of blood transfusion on outcome after major burn injury: a multicenter study. Crit Care Med 2006;34(6):1602–7.
18. Lu RP, Lin FC, Ortiz-Pujols SM, et al. Blood utilization in patients with burn injury and association with clinical outcomes (CME). Transfusion 2013;53(10) 2212–21 [quiz: 2211].
19. Hebert PC, Wells G, Blajchman MA, et al. A multicenter, randomized, controlled clinical trial of transfusion requirements in critical care. Transfusion Requirements in Critical Care Investigators, Canadian Critical Care Trials Group. N Engl J Med 1999;340(6):409–17.

20. Palmieri TL, Lee T, O'Mara MS, et al. Effects of a restrictive blood transfusion policy on outcomes in children with burn injury. J Burn Care Res 2007; 28(1):65–70.

21. Pidcoke HF, Isbell CL, Herzig MC, et al. Acute blood loss during burn and soft tissue excisions: an observational study of blood product resuscitation practices and focused review. J Trauma Acute Care Surg 2015;78(6 Suppl 1):S39–47.

22. Holcomb JB, Tilley BC, Baraniuk S, et al, PROPPR Study Group. Transfusion of plasma, platelets, and red blood cells in a 1:1:1 vs a 1:1:2 ratio and mortality in patients with severe trauma: the PROPPR randomized clinical trial. JAMA 2015;313(5):471–82.

23. Palmieri TL, Greenhalgh DG, Sen S. Prospective comparison of packed red blood cell-to-fresh frozen plasma transfusion ratio of 4: 1 versus 1: 1 during acute massive burn excision. J Trauma Acute Care Surg 2013;74(1):76–83.

24. Cartotto R, Yeo C, Camacho F, et al. Does the storage age of transfused blood affect outcome in burn patients? J Burn Care Res 2014;35(2): 186–97.

25. Sittig KM, Deitch EA. Blood transfusions: for the thermally injured or for the doctor? J Trauma 1994;36: 369–72.

26. Imai R, Matsumura H, Uchida R, et al. Perioperative hemodilutional autologous blood transfusion in burn surgery. Injury 2008;39(1):57–60.

27. CDC NNIS System. National nosocomial infection surveillance (NNIS) system report, data summary from January 1992 through June 2004, issued October 2004. Am J Infect Control 2004;32:470.

28. Dudeck MA, Horan TC, Peterson KD, et al. National Healthcare Safety Network (NHSN) report, data summary for 2010, device-associated module. Am J Infect Control 2011;39:798–816.

29. Sood G, Heath D, Adams K, et al. Survey of central line-associated bloodstream infection prevention practices across american burn association-certified adult burn units. Infect Control Hosp Epidemiol 2013;34(4):439–40.

30. Weber JM, Sheridan RL, Fagan S, et al. Incidence of catheter-associated bloodstream infection after introduction of minocycline and rifampin antimicrobial-coated catheters in a pediatric burn population. J Burn Care Res 2012;33(4):539–43.

31. O'Grady NP, Alexander M, Burns LA, et al. Guidelines for the prevention of intravascular catheter-related infections. Atlanta (GA): CDC; 2011. Available at: http://www.cdc.gov/hicpac/pdf/guidelines/bsiguidelines-2011.pdf. Accessed June 21, 2016.

32. Sheridan RL, Neely AN, Castillo MA, et al. A survey of invasive catheter practices in U.S. burn centers. J Burn Care Res 2012;33:741–6.

33. O'Mara MS, Reed NL, Palmieri TL, et al. Central venous catheter infections in burn patients with scheduled catheter exchange and replacement. J Surg Res 2007;142(2):341–50.

34. King B, Schulman CI, Pepe A, et al. Timing of central venous catheter exchange and frequency of bacteremia in burn patients. J Burn Care Res 2007;28(6): 859–60.

35. Kagan RJ, Neely AN, Rieman MT, et al. A performance improvement initiative to determine the impact of increasing the time interval between changing centrally placed intravascular catheters. J Burn Care Res 2014;35(2):143–7.

36. Sheridan RL, Weber JM. Mechanical and infectious complications of central venous cannulation in children: lessons learned from a 10-year experience placing more than 1000 catheters. J Burn Care Res 2006;27:713–8.

37. Climo MW, Yokoe DS, Warren DK, et al. Effect of daily cholorhexidine bathing on hospital-acquired infection. N Engl J Med 2013;368:533–42.

38. Popp JA, Layon AJ, Nappo R, et al. Hospital-acquired infections and thermally injured patients: chlorhexidine gluconate baths work. Am J Infect Control 2014;42(2):129–32.

39. Blot K, Bergs J, Vogelaers D, et al. Prevention of central line-associated bloodstream infections through quality improvement interventions: a systematic review and meta-analysis. Clin Infect Dis 2014;59(1):96–105.

40. Remington L, Faraklas I, Gauthier K, et al. Assessment of a central line-associated bloodstream infection prevention program in a burn-trauma intensive care unit. JAMA Surg 2016; 151(5):485–6.

41. van Duin D, Jones SW, Dibiase L, et al. Reduction in central line-associated bloodstream infections in patients with burns. Infect Control Hosp Epidemiol 2014;35(8):1066–8.

42. Austin RE, Shahrokhi S, Bolourani S, et al. Peripherally inserted central venous catheter safety in burn care: a single-center retrospective cohort review. J Burn Care Res 2015;36(1):111–7.

43. Barsun A, Sen S, Palmieri TL, et al. Peripherally inserted central line catheter infections in burn patients. J Burn Care Res 2014;35(6):514–7.

44. Fecher AM, O'Mara MS, Goldfarb IW, et al. Analysis of deep vein thrombosis in burn patients. Burns 2004;30(6):591–3.

45. Barret JP, Dziewulski PG. Complications of the hypercoagulable status in burn injury. Burns 2006; 32(8):1005–8.

46. Pannucci CJ, Osborne NH, Wahl WL. Venous thromboembolism in thermally injured patients: analysis of the National Burn Repository. J Burn Care Res 2011; 32(1):6–12.

47. Rue LW III, Cioffi WG, Rush R, et al. Thromboembolic complications in thermally injured patients. World J Surg 1992;16:1151–5.

48. Mullins F, Mian MA, Jenkins D, et al. Thromboembolic complications in burn patients and associated risk factors. J Burn Care Res 2013;34(3):355–60.

49. Wibbenmeyer LA, Hoballah JJ, Amelon MJ, et al. The prevalence of venous thromboembolism of the lower extremity among thermally injured patients determined by duplex sonography. J Trauma 2003; 55:1162–7.

50. Wahl WL, Brandt MM, Ahrns KS, et al. Venous thrombosis incidence in burn patients: preliminary results of a prospective study. J Burn Care Rehabil 2002; 23(2):97–102.

51. Caprini JA. Thrombosis risk assessment as a guide to quality patient care. Dis Mon 2005;51(2–3):70–8.

52. Pannucci CJ, Osborne NH, Wahl WL. Creation and validation of a simple venous thromboembolism risk scoring tool for thermally injured patients: analysis of the National Burn Repository. J Burn Care Res 2012;33(1):20–5.

53. Harrington DT, Mozingo DW, Cancio L, et al. Thermally injured patients are at significant risk for thromboembolic complications. J Trauma 2001;50(3):495–9.

54. Wahl WL, Brandt MM. Potential risk factors for deep venous thrombosis in burn patients. J Burn Care Rehabil 2001;22(2):128–31.

55. Geerts WH, Bergqvist D, Pineo GF, et al, American College of Chest Physicians. Prevention of venous thromboembolism: American College of Chest Physicians Evidence-Based Clinical Practice Guidelines (8th edition). Chest 2008;133(6 Suppl):381S–453S.

56. Hejl CG, Leclerc T, Bargues L, et al. Incidence and features of heparin-induced thrombocytopenia (HIT) in burn patients: a retrospective study. Thromb Haemost 2008;99:974–6.

57. Lin H, Faraklas I, Saffle J, et al. Enoxaparin dose adjustment is associated with low incidence of venous thromboembolic events in acute burn patients. J Trauma 2011;71(6):1557–61.

58. Lin H, Faraklas I, Cochran A, et al. Enoxaparin and antifactor Xa levels in acute burn patients. J Burn Care Res 2011;32(1):1–5.

59. Faraklas I, Ghanem M, Brown A, et al. Evaluation of an enoxaparin dosing calculator using burn size and weight. J Burn Care Res 2013;34(6):621–7.

60. Brown A, Faraklas I, Ghanem M, et al. Enoxaparin and antifactor Xa levels in pediatric acute burn patients. J Burn Care Res 2013;34(6):628–32.

61. Van PY, Cho SD, Underwood SJ, et al. Thrombelastography versus AntiFactor Xa levels in the assessment of prophylactic-dose enoxaparin in critically ill patients. J Trauma 2009;66:1509–15 [discussion: 1515–7].

62. Abedi N, Papp A. A survey of current practice patterns in prophylaxis against venous thromboembolism (VTE) and gastrointestinal (GI) ulceration among Canadian burn centers. Burns 2011;37(7): 1182–6.

63. Weber DJ, van Duin D, DiBiase LM, et al. Healthcare-associated infections among patients in a large burn intensive care unit: incidence and pathogens, 2008-2012. Infect Control Hosp Epidemiol 2014; 35(10):1304–6.

64. Greenhalgh DG, Saffle JR, Holmes JH 4th, et al. American Burn Association consensus conference to define sepsis and infection in burns. J Burn Care Res 2007;28:776–90.

65. Mosier MJ, Pham TN. American Burn Association Practice guidelines for prevention, diagnosis, and treatment of ventilator-associated pneumonia (VAP) in burn patients. J Burn Care Res 2009;30(6): 910–28.

66. Bone RC, Balk RA, Cerra FB, et al. Definitions for sepsis and organ failure and guidelines for the use of innovative therapies in sepsis. The ACCP/SCCM consensus conference Committee. American College of Chest Physicians/Society of Critical Care Medicine. Chest 1992;101:1644–55.

67. Liodaki E, Kalousis K, Schopp BE, et al. Prophylactic antibiotic therapy after inhalation injury. Burns 2014; 40(8):1476–80.

68. Tagami T, Matsui H, Fushimi K, et al. Prophylactic antibiotics may improve outcome in patients with severe burns requiring mechanical ventilation: propensity score analysis of a Japanese Nationwide Database. Clin Infect Dis 2016;62(1):60–6.

69. Abdul-Aziz MH, Sulaiman H, Mat-Nor MB, et al. Beta-Lactam Infusion in Severe Sepsis (BLISS): a prospective, two-centre, open-labelled randomised controlled trial of continuous versus intermittent beta-lactam infusion in critically ill patients with severe sepsis. Intensive Care Med 2016;42(10): 1535–45.

70. Roberts JA, Abdul-Aziz MH, Davis JS, et al. Continuous versus intermittent beta-lactam infusion in severe sepsis: a meta-analysis of individual patient data from randomized trials. Am J Respir Crit Care Med 2016;194(6):681–91.

71. Cotta MO, Roberts JA, Lipman J. Antibiotic dose optimization in critically ill patients. Med Intensiva 2015;39(9):563–72.

Resurfacing

Surgical Excision of Burn Wounds

Best Practices Using Evidence-Based Medicine

Timothy H.F. Daugherty, MD, MS[a], Amanda Ross, MD[a],
Michael W. Neumeister, MD, FRCSC[b],*

KEYWORDS

- Burns • Excision • Immune function • Wound healing • Scar minimization

KEY POINTS

- The ability to evaluate burn depth is critical to planning surgical excision.
- Assessment of tissue viability is key to proper burn excision and can be achieved by evaluating for punctate bleeding, patent vessels, pearly white appearance of the dermis, absence of ecchymosis, and bright yellow fat.
- Early excision has improved outcomes by decreasing overall mortality, incidence of wound sepsis, and length of hospital stay.

INTRODUCTION

The management of burns is a multidisciplinary cooperation of all specialties from surgeons and nurses to therapists and nutritionists, and all who have patient contact. Unfortunately, burn wounds can lead to scarring, wound sepsis, and even death, mandating early, safe, and efficient treatment. The decisions to remove the burn tissue are critical to survival in many patients. The most important decision making in burns then, is deciding when to perform surgery and at what depth to debride for the most optimum healing and patient recovery.

EVALUATION AND DEPTH OF BURN WOUNDS

The surgical management of burn injury is influenced by the depth of injury. Superficial (first-degree) burns involve only epidermis and are treated entirely nonsurgically. Partial-thickness (second-degree) burns penetrate into the dermis with a variable depth. Superficial partial-thickness burns penetrate to the papillary dermis, whereas deep partial-thickness burns penetrate deeper into the reticular dermis. Partial-thickness burns have the ability to re-epithelialize naturally from stem cells surrounding the dermal appendages (hair follicles, sebaceous glands, sweat glands, and apocrine glands). Often times, superficial partial-thickness injury can be treated without excision and grafting, with expected healing within 10 to 14 days. Deep partial-thickness burns, however, often take longer to heal, with an increased incidence of hypertrophic scarring. Finally, full-thickness burns cause a level of injury down to subcutaneous fat, eradicating the dermal appendages and eliminating a source for cutaneous regeneration, therefore requiring surgical debridement and grafting.

[a] Institute for Plastic Surgery, Southern Illinois University School of Medicine, Springfield, IL 62702, USA;
[b] Department of Surgery, Institute for Plastic Surgery, Southern Illinois University School of Medicine, Baylis Medical Building, 747 North Rutledge Street, 3rd Floor, Suite 357, Springfield, IL 62702, USA
* Corresponding author.
E-mail address: mneumeister@siumed.edu

Clin Plastic Surg 44 (2017) 619–625
http://dx.doi.org/10.1016/j.cps.2017.02.018

When evaluating depth of burn injury, one must take into consideration the thickness of the skin layers in the area of injury, which can offer varying degrees of protection from thermal exposure. The epidermal thickness can vary from less than 1 mm in the genitalia and eyelids to greater than 10 mm on the back. The dermis also varies in thickness depending on the age of the patient, with thinner dermis present in children and elderly patients. Therefore, surgical management may vary based on the patient's age and the location of the burn.

Burn wounds have been described as 3 concentric zones with varying tissue injury including a central zone of coagulation, a surrounding zone of stasis, and an outer zone of hyperemia.[1] The zone of stasis is an ischemic, yet initially viable portion of skin that surrounds the nonviable zone of coagulation. This zone is particularly susceptible to insults that can induce conversion to nonviable tissue including improper resuscitation or delayed excision of burn eschar, causing inflammation or bacterial infection.[2-4]

HISTORY OF SURGICAL MANAGEMENT OF BURN WOUNDS

Prior to the mid 1900s, the management of burn injuries was primarily medical, where wounds were treated with topical medications only. When full-thickness burns were treated nonsurgically, the natural progression was separation of the eschar from the underlying wound bed weeks to months after the initial insult. This left a granulating wound that was still in need of grafting or was allowed to scar in, leading to prolonged hospital stay, hypertrophic scarring, contractures, wound sepsis, multisystem organ failure, and at times death.[5]

The paradigm shift toward early burn excision occurred in 1970 when Janzekovic showed improved patient outcomes with tangential excision and complete removal of necrotic tissue with autografting on the preserved well-vascularized deep tissue.[6] This ground-breaking study showed a reduction in pain, total number of procedures for wound closure, and length of hospital stay. The study was followed by multiple others in support of early excision due to additional benefits including quicker healing, less incidence of hypertrophic scarring, decreased incidence of wound sepsis and need for antibiotics, and a greater than 3-fold decrease in mortality rate.[7-11] Early excision had already become the standard of care when the relationship between burn eschar, inflammation, and systemic inflammatory response syndrome was discovered. Systemic instability was shown to be induced by inflammatory mediators from burn eschar, and this response can be attenuated with early excision.[2,12] As the burn size approaches 15% to 20% total body surface area (TBSA), the inflammatory mediators are prevalent enough to cause a systemic inflammatory response, therefore justifying the need for massive fluid resuscitation to prevent conversion of burn and early excision to abort the inflammatory cascade.

Recent work on animal models has given further insight into the benefits of early burn wound excision. Although animals exhibit a much quicker capacity to heal burn wounds, they have contributed to the basic understanding of certain phases of the healing process in respect to people. Singer and colleagues[13] have shown that tangential excision and grafting of full-thickness burns in a porcine model can decrease timing to heal as well as produce significantly thinner scars when performed early at day 2 versus later at day 14. Additional porcine studies have shown delayed excision and grafting to correlate with significantly worse Vancouver scar scale scores and increased fibrosis and alpha-smooth muscle, suggesting that delays in excision can increase incidence of hypertrophic scarring.[14] Wang and colleagues[15] used a rabbit model to show that tissue edema, wound contracture, and graft loss was significantly greatest when excision and grafting occurred at 18 to 24 hours, suggesting that it may be beneficial to perform excision and grafting either ultra-early or after 48 hours.

Burn injury has been shown to have suppressive effects on both the innate and adaptive immune response, leaving patients at risk for viral and bacterial infections. The effect of timing of excision on the immune system has therefore also been the target of animal models. Early complete excision of burn wounds in mice has been shown to restore cytotoxic lymphocyte function and viral-specific T lymphocyte cytotoxicity for the innate immune system.[16,17] Immediate excision and grafting have also been shown to improve the adaptive immune system with restoration of antibody synthesis to bacterial antigens, suggesting that earlier excision may decrease risk of bacterial infections in burn patients.[18] Fear and colleagues[19] reported that early excision is less disruptive to the immune response by looking at markers for the innate and adaptive immune system. This study suggests that early excision during the phase of immune down-regulation initiated by the burn trauma maintains the innate and adaptive immune cell responses compared with delayed excision, which causes these to be down-regulated.

To this day, no exact recommendation for timing of early excision or safe percentage of burn to excise has been elucidated (**Table 1**). Common

Table 1
Timing of burn excision depends on different factors including the stability of the patient and the size of the wounds

Ultra early	<24 h
Early	24–96 h
Delayed	>96 h

ming depends on different factors including the stability of the patient and the size of the wounds. This table ustrates some of the timepoints surgeons use to describe ie timing of burn excision relative to burn injury.

ractice is toward excision on postinjury day 3 to 5 ue to the older recommendations by Janzekovic. ewer surveys suggest approximately 56% of urn surgeons will perform excision on postinjury ay 1, and 57% will excise up to 20% TBSA at 1 me.[20] Recent meta-analysis of randomized conol trials looking at timing of excision show that xcision between day 1 and day 6 is beneficial or mortality reduction in patients without inhalaon injury and length of stay but increases the equirement for blood transfusion.[5] Excision can e performed in a staged or complete fashion. tudies report safe total excision of all burn as arly as the first 24 hours.[21] Herndon and colagues[22] showed both staged and complete excion of large burns with immediate use of autograft nd allograft to be safe and effective within 2 hours of injury.

URN WOUND EXCISION
reoperative Considerations

lanning for the surgical care of burn patients reuires much thought. One must first consider tact skin for harvesting as well as recipient sites or the skin grafts. If there is little intact skin for haresting, if possible, priority should be given to xcision and grafting areas critical for central enous and arterial lines, tracheostomy sites, nd gastrostomy sites, as patients with larger urns are expected to have a prolonged critical ourse with need for monitoring and long-term rway and nutritional supplementation. Larger reas not at high risk of contamination or shear lay be considered next as engraftment is more kely. Getting early stable coverage may be critical survival depending on the TBSA involved and ie overall patient condition. Occasionally, priority given to major joints or hands, since delays can ad to increased scar tissue formation and elayed range of motion during therapy, therefore ausing an increased incidence of joint contracres. The exact order of burn excision is surgeon

dependent but should be well planned and communicated to all parties involved to optimize outcomes.

Harvesting skin is performed with a dermatome and involves shaving of the epidermis and the superficial portion of the dermis. This leaves behind the remainder of the dermis to regenerate the epidermis through epidermal appendages; however, the dermis does not regenerate. Therefore, the thickness of the dermis at the harvest site should be taken into consideration, as it may limit the number of skin graft harvests one can take from a single site. If donor skin is limited, one may need to consider the need for skin harvest for growth of cultured epithelial autografts.

Patients with greater than 20% burns have an impaired ability for thermoregulation and therefore require close monitoring of body temperature. This loss of surface area able to contribute to thermoregulation, in addition to massive excision and blood loss, can contribute to temporary hypothermia intraoperatively. This can be countered by maintaining the ambient operative room temperature at 37° Celsius and keeping the patient covered with warm blankets, Bair huggers (3M, St Paul, MN), and the use of warmed intravenous fluids. Should the patient's temperature drop below 35° C, coagulopathies may develop contributing to perioperative blood loss.

Types of Excision

The most important concept with excision of burn eschar is that debridement should be carried down to a level where only viable tissue remains. Burn wound excision can be performed as either tangential or fascial excision. Tangential excision is performed using a hand-held knife or dermatome that excises the burn eschar in a serial fashion to a depth of viable tissue capable of accepting a skin graft. This allows for preservation of as much viable tissue as possible with better contour and cosmesis than the fascial excision.

Fascial excision involves a full-thickness excision of skin and subcutaneous tissue down to the level of muscle fascia. Fascial excision is usually reserved for large, life-threatening burns where there is a need for rapid excision, or extremely deep full-thickness burns where only minimal fat is remaining. Advantages of this over tangential excision include its ease of dissection, limited blood loss, and a well-vascularized fascial layer for skin graft placement. Disadvantages include obvious contour deformities, permanent loss of all cutaneous sensation, and removal of viable subcutaneous elements including lymphatics, which can lead to bothersome lymphedema distal to the excision, precluding its use in the routine patient.

Tools Used for Excision

Prior to formal excisional debridement, mechanical debridement can be performed using a Norsen blade to remove pseudoeschar or eschar overlying burn wounds.

Tangential excision is mainly performed using hand-held knives: Weck, Watson, Goulian, Braitwaithe, or Humby blades. These are placed at the edge of the burn eschar with light pressure on the blade and used with a quick back-and-forth motion to pass across the length of the wound (**Fig. 1**). Appropriate tension on the skin will assist with ease of uniformity of excision. Sequential passes can be made until a viable level of tissue is reached. Bovi electrocautery is used for fascial excision as well as to maintain hemostasis in tangential excision for larger punctate bleeding vessels.

Recently, newer tools such as hydrodissectors (Versajet; Smith & Nephew, London, UK) have become popular for excision of smaller, more superficial burns. These are passed over the area of eschar, debriding portions of the eschar off with each subsequent pass, working in a similar manner as tangential excision. These newer tools, however, are more expensive and have not been shown to have an advantage over traditional hand-held knives.[23]

Assessment of Tissue Viability During Excision

The ability to accurately assess the underlying tissue following excision is the key to a successful

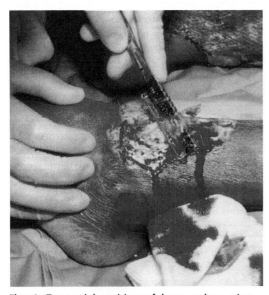

Fig. 1. Tangential excision of burn eschar using a Weck blade down to punctate bleeding.

debridement and to assure survival of a split thickness skin graft on the recipient site. The viability of the tissue is mainly determined by patient blood flow in the depth of excision. Often punctate bleeding is used as an indicator of tissue viability, but one must take caution, as the appearance of bleeding can vary depending on the depth of the dermis. The distribution of the capillaries in the papillary dermis is close together, in contrast to the arterioles, which are farther apart in the reticular dermis. Therefore, tangential excision of a superficial partial-thickness burn will cause close punctate bleeding from capillaries, whereas deeper excision in a deep partial-thickness burn will cause more widely spaced punctate bleeding from arterioles. Other indicators of tissue viability in the dermal layer are the appearance of a pearly white dermis and absence of ecchymosis.

If nonviable tissue necessitates that tangential excision be carried down through the subcutaneous fat, one must judge viability by looking for both patent blood vessels and bright yellow greasy-appearing fat. Careful attention must be paid to remove all coagulated vessels, ecchymotic tissue, and gray/brown fat. If fascial excision is performed, one must look for patent vessels within the fascia.

When to Abort Excision

As mentioned previously, massive excision of burn wounds can be performed safely in a single-stage operation; however, the surgeon must hold criteria to abort the procedure if the patient becomes unstable. This requires close communication with anesthesiologists. The surgeon should consider aborting the procedure and temporizing the wounds if a patient becomes hemodynamically unstable or hypothermic (less than 35° C).

HEMOSTASIS

Excision of burn wounds can induce massive blood loss if meticulous hemostasis is not maintained. This is due to inflammatory cytokines, coagulopathies, and large surface area excision of burn eschar. Hemostasis should be maintained during the excision in order to limit complications, sustain hemodynamic stability, and limit the number of blood transfusions necessary. Several methods have been used in order to maintain hemostasis, including tourniquets on extremities, tumescence with epinephrine solutions, or topically applied epinephrine.

The use of tourniquets and tumescence can alter the surgeon's ability to assess the viability of the remaining tissue after excision. When using these methods, one must pay even closer attention to the appearance of the dermis or fat, patency of vessels, and absence of ecchymosis as indicators of tissue viability rather than punctate bleeding alone.

Epinephrine-soaked Telfas (Medtronic, Minneapolis, MN) and compression are useful in the attenuation of bleeding following excision down to an acceptable level. The epinephrine-soaked Telfas can be combined with hydrogen peroxide or thrombin to assist in hemostasis. Bovi electrocautery can then be used to control any larger vessels. Finally, tissue factor in skin autograft or allograft is beneficial in stopping the punctate bleeding.

SPECIALIZED AREAS

Hands

Hands are susceptible to deeper burns on account of exposure during the burn injury. Partial-thickness burns to the hand can be treated with mechanical debridement with a Norsen blade (Belmed Inc, Bellingham, WA) followed by xeno-grafting for pain control. This can allow for quicker return to therapy.

For deep partial- and full-thickness burns to the hand, early excision and grafting are beneficial in order to prevent joint contracture and expedite therapy. Deep partial-thickness and full-thickness burns usually require tangential excision and auto-grafting if the patient has shown no healing within 10 to 14 days. Debridement should be carried down to the subcutaneous tissue in order to prevent retention of epidermal appendages and subsequent inclusion cysts.

Sheet grafts should be used whenever possible in order to minimize secondary contracture of the graft and lessen the chance of joint contractures. The thickness of the graft has not been shown to affect appearance, and 15/1000 of an inch is sufficient and has less donor site morbidity.[24] If there is peritenon present following excision, in order to allow for tendon glide, coverage should be attempted with a dermal-regenerative template (Integra LifeSciences Corporation, Plainsboro, NJ). Application of Integra to the hand has been shown to be beneficial in burn patients with good cosmetic and functional results.[25] The thick glaberous skin on the palmar surface of the hand rarely requires grafting. This is best treated with mechanical debridement and dressing changes.

Face

Because of the rich blood supply to the face, most facial burns are partial-thickness burns and therefore will heal without surgical intervention. Partial-thickness burns should initially be treated

nonsurgically to allow healing. Mechanical debridement at the bedside with a Norsen blade can be used to assist with removal of eschar to facilitate re-epithelialization.

Approximately 5% to 10% of facial burns will not heal within 10 to 14 days and therefore may require excision and grafting.[26,27] Deep partial-thickness facial burns that take more than 18 days have been found to carry increased risk for hypertrophic scarring and therefore should be grafted prior to this time if the patient is showing no signs of healing.[28] If the burn is frankly full thickness, excision and grafting should be performed as soon as edema has subsided to obtain the best cosmetic result. Excision is best performed tangential in order to maintain facial contour.

As mentioned previously, the skin around the eyelids represents some of the thinnest dermis and epidermis in the body and therefore is more susceptible to full-thickness burn. If this is present, excision and grafting should be performed early in order to prevent cicatricial ectropion, xerophthalmia, bacterial infection, and eye injury affecting vision.[29]

Coverage to the face should always be performed with sheet grafts in order to limit secondary contraction of the skin graft. Whenever possible, the donor site should be obtained from skin of similar color. The scalp provides a good possible source for similar skin.

Genitals and Perianal Burns

Burns in the genital and perianal area can present challenges due to potential contamination from the nearby anus. To prevent contamination, it is best to establish an effective bowel regimen with placement of a rectal tube, especially prior to operative care if indicated. Genital burns are typically superficial or partial-thickness burns that can be treated without excisional debridement but rather with topical antimicrobials.

The thin skin of the genitalia can, however, leave them susceptible to full-thickness burns. This is more common in males on account of external anatomy. If full-thickness burns are present, these should be promptly treated with excision and grafting. Delayed treatment leads to increased incidence of infection, longer recovery, increased length of hospital stay, and scar contracture.[30] The scrotum can be treated by grafting or reconstruction with thigh pouch creation. For circumferential penile shaft injury affecting only a portion of the shaft, severe lymphedema and lymphatic obstruction can occur, and therefore all viable skin distal to the burn injury should also be excised up to the subcorona.[30] The glans has a robust blood supply and therefore rarely requires excisional debridement unless it is grossly necrotic. Urethral catheters should be avoided in males with full-thickness burns on the ventral glans or shaft of the penis. These patients are better suited with a suprapubic tube as urethral catheters, can cause pressure necrosis leading to severe hypospadias.[30]

SUMMARY

Early excision of burn eschar has improved outcomes in burn care including decreasing length of hospital stay, wound sepsis, and overall mortality. Adequate assessment of the tissue following excision is essential to skin graft viability and can be determined by patent vessels, punctate bleeding, pearly white dermis, absence of ecchymosis, and yellow fat.

REFERENCES

1. Jackson D. The diagnosis of the depth of burning. Br J Surg 1953;40:588–96.
2. Drost A, Burleson D, Cioffi W, et al. Plasma cytokines following thermal injury and their relationship with patient mortality, burn size, and time postburn. J Trauma 1993;35:335–9.
3. Nguyen T, Cox C, Traber D, et al. Free radical activity and loss of plasma antioxidants, vitamin E, and sulfhydryl groups in patients with burns. J Burn Care Rehabil 1993;14:602–9.
4. Nguyen T, Gilpin D, Meyer N, et al. Current treatment of severely burned patients. Ann Surg 1996;223:14–25.
5. Ong Y, Samuel M, Song C. Meta-analysis of early excision of burns. Burns 2006;32(2):145–50.
6. Janzekovic Z. A new concept in the early excision and immediate grafting of burns. J Trauma 1970; 10:1103–8.
7. Burke J, Bondoc C, Quinby W. Primary burn excision and immediate grafting: a method for shortening illness. J Trauma 1974;14:389–95.
8. Burke J, Quinby W, Bondoc C, et al. Primary excision and prompt grafting as routine therapy for the treatment of thermal burns in children. Surg Clin North Am 1976;56:447–94.
9. Gray D, Pine R, Harner T, et al. Early surgical excision versus conventional therapy in patients with 20 to 40 percent burns: a comparative study. Am J Surg 1982;144:76–80.
10. Tompkins RG, Burke J, Schoenfeld DA, et al. Prompt eschar excision: a treatment system contributing to reduced burn mortality. Ann Surg 1986;204(3):272–81.
11. Engrav L, Heimbach D, Reus J, et al. Early excision and grafting versus nonoperative treatment of burns of indeterminant depth: a randomized prospective study. J Trauma 1983;23:1001–4.
12. Demling R, Lalonde C. Early burn excision attenuates the postburn lung and systemic response to edotoxin. Surgery 1990;108:28–35.
13. Singer AJ, Toussaint J, Chung WT, et al. Early versus delayed excision and grafting of full-thickness burns in a porcine model: a randomized study. Plast Reconstr Surg 2016;137:972e–9e.
14. Chan QE, Harvey JG, Graf NS, et al. The correlation between timing to skin grafting and hypertrophic scarring following an acute contact burn in a porcine model. J Burn Care Res 2012;33:e43–8.
15. Wang YB, Ogawa Y, Kakudo N, et al. Survival and wound contracture of full-thickness skin grafts are associated with the degree of tissue edema of the graft bed in immediate excision and early wound excision and grafting in a rabbit model. J Burn Care Res 2007;28:182–6.
16. Hultman CS, Cairns BA, deSerres S, et al. Early, complete burn wound excision partially restores cytotoxic T lymphocyte function. Surgery 1995; 118(2):421–9.
17. Hultman CS, Yamamoto H, deSerres S, et al. Early but not late burn wound excision partially restores viral-specific T lymphocyte cytotoxicity. J Trauma 1997;43(3):441–7.
18. Yamamoto H, Siltharm S, deSerres S, et al. Immediate burn wound excision restores antibody synthesis to bacterial antigen. J Surg Res 1996;62(1):157–62.
19. Fear VS, Poh W, Valvis S, et al. Timing of excision after a non-severe burn has a significant impact on the subsequent immune response in a murine model. Burns 2016;42:815–24.
20. Israel J, Greenhalgh D, Gibson A. Variations in burn excision and grafting: a survey of the American Burn Association. J Burn Care Res 2017;38:e125–32.
21. Sorensen B, Fisker N, Steensen J, et al. Acute excision or exposure treatment: final results of a three-year-old randomized control clinical trial. Scand J Plast Reconstr Surg 1984;18:87–93.
22. Herndon D, Parks D. Comparison of serial debridement and autografting and early massive excision with cadaver skin overlay in treatment of large burns in children. J Trauma 1986;26:149–52.
23. Klein M, Hunter S, Heimbach D, et al. The versajet water dissector: a new tool for tangential excision. J Burn Care Rehabil 2005;26:483–7.
24. Mann R, Gibran NS, Engrav LH, et al. Prospective trial of thick vs standard split thickness skin grafts in burns of the hand. J Burn Care Rehabil 2001; 22(6):390–2.
25. Dantzer E, Queruel P, Salinier L, et al. Dermal regeneration template for deep hand burns: clinical utility for both early grafting and reconstructive surgery. Br J Plast Surg 2003;56(8):764–74.
26. Engrav LH, Heimbach DM. Early reconstruction of facial burns. West J Med 1991;154(2):203–4.

27. Engrav LH, Heimbach DM, Walkinshaw MD, et al. Excision of burns of the face. Plast Reconstr Surg 1986;77(5):744–51.

28. Fraulin FO, Illmayer SJ, Tredget EE. Assessment of cosmetic and functional results of conservative versus surgical management of facial burns. J Burn Care Rehabil 1996;17(1):19–29.

29. Barrow RE, Jeschke MG, Hendon DN, et al. Early release of third-degree eyelid burns prevents eye injury. Plast Reconstr Surg 2000;105(3): 860–3.

30. Chang AJ, Brandes S. Advances in diagnosis and management of genital injuries. Urol Clin North Am 2013;40:427–38.

Skin Substitutes and Bioscaffolds
Temporary and Permanent Coverage

Anthony G. Haddad, MD[a], Giorgio Giatsidis, MD[b],
Dennis P. Orgill, MD, PhD[b], Eric G. Halvorson, MD[c],*

KEYWORDS

- Skin substitutes • Bioscaffolds • Allografts • Xenografts • Dermal templates

KEY POINTS

- The goals of skin substitutes are prevention of wound infection, maintenance of moist wound healing environment, and replacement of normal skin to restore function and aesthetics.
- Allografts have always been the temporary coverage of choice when donor autografts are limited, but factors such as availability and cost are of concern.
- Xenografts can provide temporary coverage, but because of their inability to revascularize fully they should be viewed more as a dressing than as a skin substitute.
- Despite constant evolution in the development of skin substitutes, no single product stands out as the gold standard.
- When choosing a skin substitute, several practical issues, including wound indication, ease of application, storage time, and cost, factor into the choices made by clinicians.

INTRODUCTION

Skin serves as a protective layer from microorganisms and external forces, in addition to having sensory and immune functions, controlling fluid loss, and serving important aesthetic functions. The 2 layers (dermis and epidermis) are linked by epidermal derivatives or appendages, such as sebaceous glands and hair follicles, that invaginate into the dermis. The dermis hosts a rich vascular network that helps regulate temperature. For most minor injuries, such as a paper cut, the skin is able to self-repair without scarring.[1] Deeper skin injuries caused by burns or degloving injuries can cause significant physiologic derangement, expose the body to a risk of systemic infection,

and become a life-threatening problem. Large skin losses have pushed researchers to develop technologies to improve wound coverage and attempt to restore skin. Although much has been accomplished in burn research, developments in the areas of acute and chronic surgical wound treatment have propelled advances in the burn field even further.

Injuries and burns that extend into the deep dermis or through the entire dermis heal only after a prolonged time or may become chronic wounds. A reliable coverage option includes autologous skin grafts, which can be divided into full-thickness skin grafts (FTSGs) or split-thickness skin grafts (STSGs). FTSGs consist of the entire epidermis and dermis, whereas STSGs consist of the

Disclosure: D.P. Orgill is a consultant for Integra LifeSciences Corporation and has previously received research funding from Integra LifeSciences Corporation. The other authors have nothing to disclose.
[a] Department of Surgery, Brigham and Women's Hospital, 75 Francis Street, Boston, MA 02115, USA; [b] Division of Plastic Surgery, Brigham and Women's Hospital, 75 Francis Street, Boston, MA 02115, USA; [c] Plastic Surgery Center of Asheville, 5 Livingston Street, Asheville, NC 28801, USA
* Corresponding author.
E-mail address: eric.halvorson@gmail.com

Clin Plastic Surg 44 (2017) 627–634
http://dx.doi.org/10.1016/j.cps.2017.02.019

epidermis and only part of the dermis. Scarring, donor site pain, graft loss, and limited supply of donor sites have pushed clinicians and researchers to consider alternative methods for wound coverage, such as skin substitutes and bioscaffolds.

The most important functions of skin substitutes are prevention of wound infection, maintenance of a moist wound healing environment, and replacement of normal skin to restore function and aesthetics. Despite constant evolution in the development of skin substitutes, no single product stands out as the gold standard. Allografts, xenografts, bovine/porcine collagen sheets, and dermal matrices are commonly used in burned patients to support wound closure. When choosing a skin substitute, several practical issues, including ease of application, storage time, and cost, factor into the choices made by clinicians.

This article explores skin substitutes and bioscaffolds currently available to treat patients with burns.

BURN WOUND COVERAGE

Burn wound closure or coverage should ideally be done as soon as possible to avoid the serious consequences that result from burn injury. These consequences typically include dehydration, shock, and sepsis, in addition to a variety of other physiologic derangements that are mainly driven by the profound catabolic state and systemic inflammation resulting from the burn insult. Most burns should ideally be covered using autografts, which remain the current standard of care. The lack of sufficient donor sites or the need for a temporary dressing are challenges met by the current array of available temporary dressings and skin substitutes.

TEMPORARY DRESSINGS
Allografts

Cadaveric allograft skin has always been the temporary coverage of choice. Despite the potential infection risks that come with its use and its high cost, it has gained popularity given its ability to take as an allograft and provide durable coverage for an extended period of time (compared with other temporary dressings), providing wound coverage for 3 to 4 weeks.[2] Refrigerated allograft remains viable for up to 14 days when preserved in adequate nutrient media (RPMI [Roswell Park Memorial Institute]-1640).[3] Cryopreserved allograft can be stored for a longer period of time and retain good viability. It has an indefinite shelf life and can be accumulated for future use. It is usually prepared by controlled-rate freezing in cryopreservation solution. Despite the conditions of storage,

cryopreservation itself does not eliminate the risk of viral or bacterial transmission. However, most cryopreserved allografts are processed and stored on an elective basis, which gives time for cautious and adequate donor screening for potential pathogens. Human immunodeficiency virus and hepatitis C were cited as causes in the past, but tighter US Food and Drug Administration (FDA) regulations and extensive tissue donor screening have limited such occurrences.

Another limiting factor is the availability of allografts. Fresh allografts usually need to be used within a few days to a week at most or otherwise have to be cryopreserved. The careful selection of donors further compromises availability because patients with systemic malignancy, sepsis, and viral illnesses need to be excluded. Cost should also be taken into consideration because fresh allografts cost up to $2.65/cm^2 whereas the price for cryopreserved allograft is $2.15/cm^2 (quote from Allosource, Centennial, CO). The development of tissue banks providing high-quality, safe, and viable allografts has contributed to the increased cost of this coverage option.

Xenografts

Over the years, skin from multiple animal species has been used as temporary coverage. In the late nineteenth century, the first xenograft to be used in the United States was harvested from sheep.[4] Frog skin has also been used in some instances, but the only commercially available products to date are taken from pigs.[5] However, given the high potential for antigenicity, there needs to be a careful preparation process. Several methods have been used, including silver impregnation, irradiation, and freezing and thawing.[6] Xenografts can provide temporary coverage when allografts are unavailable or cost-prohibitive. Because of its inability to revascularize fully, they should be viewed more as a dressing than as a true skin substitute. Xenografts have been shown to retard evaporative water loss, reduce infection, and encourage autologous epidermal growth.[4] Most clinicians have used xenografts as dressings for covering partial-thickness burns, donor sites, and wounds in toxic epidermal necrolysis.[7] Advantages of xenografts include lower cost, prolonged shelf life, and availability. Disadvantages include the potential for transmission of infectious agents in addition to some cultural and religious considerations.

Amnion

Temporary wound coverage with inner amnion and outer chorion has been described for many ears. Outer chorion carries the disadvantage of a igher antigenic potential; hence amnion has ained more popularity. The main use of amnion for ophthalmologic (corneal) burns.[8] Multiple ommercial products have been made available the past few years (eg, AmnioGraft, Bio-issue, Doral, FL; AmnioGuard, Bio-Tissue, Doral, L; Acelagraft; Celgene Cellular Therapeutics, Ce-ar Knolls, NJ) and have been used as overlay af-er autografting or as a dressing in superficial and iid-dermal burns.[9,10] Amnion has also been used small areas, such as the diabetic foot. Advan-iges of amnion include that it is available, readily dherent, transparent (thus allowing wound moni-oring), has the potential to reduce the risk of ound infection, and may have an analgesic ef-ect. Disadvantages include difficulty in handling nd fast degradation, in addition to the lack of dherence in full-thickness burns, making it a tem-orary dressing for such wounds.[11]

ther Temporary Dressings

cticoat (Smith & Nephew Inc, Andover, MA) is a lver antimicrobial dressing containing nanocrys-lline silver that offers a slow release of silver ns over time. It is indicated in both full-ickness and partial-thickness wounds. It has road antimicrobial coverage, but it has to be nanged every 2 to 4 days. Silver-impregnated mporary dressings have been shown to reduce ealing time and pain.[12]

Aquacel Ag (ConvaTec, Princeton, NJ) is a ydrofiber dressing with silver. It has been useful treating second-degree burns, chronic wounds, nd donor sites. Aquacel maintains a moist wound nvironment by controlling exudate and hence re-uces the likelihood of infection. It has also shown improve wound healing time and to be superior silver sulfadiazine.[12]

Biobrane (Smith & Nephew Inc, Andover, MA) is nother temporary burn wound coverage alterna-ve consisting of a woven nylon membrane ated with silicone to which collagen is chemi-ally bound.[13] Like Acticoat and Aquacel, it has een shown to be as effective as topical silver ılfadiazine in reducing pain and decreasing ound healing time.[12] The main advantage of obrane remains in its cost-effectiveness ecause it has the potential to remain in place r a prolonged period of time if the wound is ean. It can adhere firmly in superficial partial-ickness burns until healing occurs,[14] and this how most clinicians have used this dressing. owever, it is susceptible to infection and epi-des of life-threatening toxic shock syndrome ave been reported.[15]

Although no longer produced, TransCyte (Advanced BioHealing, Westport, CT, USA) is similar to Biobrane and composed of a nylon mesh covered with fibroblasts from neonatal hu-man foreskin. It was previously suggested as a temporary coverage for wounds waiting to be covered with autografts. One postulated mecha-nism is that the harvested fibroblasts secrete extracellular matrix components and growth fac-tors that contribute to the healing process.[16]

Apligraf (Orthogenesis Inc, Canton, MA) is made from neonatal foreskin fibroblasts and keratino-cytes (dermal components from cultured fibro-blasts with bovine type I collagen and cultured keratinocytes eventually added to form a stratum corneum). Apligraf is currently FDA approved for use in treating diabetic foot and venous ulcers although it is also used in burn treatment. Cost is a significant concern and has prevented its use for larger wounds.

Like TransCyte, OrCel (OrCel International Inc, New York, NY) is no longer available. OrCel is an allogeneic, bilayered substitute composed of cultured human fibroblasts and keratinocytes. However, the fibroblasts in OrCel are seeded onto a preformed matrix instead of being cocultured with collagen in solution. Also, OrCel lacks Apli-graf's stratum corneum. OrCel is FDA approved for use on split-thickness skin graft donor sites in patients with burns and in reconstructive hand sur-gery in patients with epidermolysis bullosa. A study performed by Still and colleagues[17] found OrCel to be more effective than Biobrane with regard to wound closure time and scar appearance.

PERMANENT SKIN SUBSTITUTES

In an article from 1999 published in *Burns*, Sheri-dan and Tompkins[5] described the characteristics of an ideal skin substitute. The ultimate substitute should be inexpensive; be available off the shelf; have a long shelf life; be nonantigenic, durable, and flexible; prevent water loss; provide a barrier to bacteria; conform to irregular surfaces; be easy to secure; grow with children; be applied in 1 operation; and not have the ability to become hypertrophic.[5]

Although burn dressings and the products previ-ously described may provide a temporary solution for wound coverage, some wounds require a more permanent form of coverage, but patients may not be candidates for a standard autograft. Skin sub-stitutes can be thought of as replacing either or both layers of the skin and have dermal and/or epidermal components.

Given how debilitating the extent of burn injuries can be, the availability of alternatives with good coverage may eventually provide faster recovery and better quality of life. Many severe burn injuries are now survivable thanks to progress in intensive care management, hence research in skin substitutes and permanent coverage is expanding to catch up with the current state of burn care.[18]

Cultured Epidermal Autografts

Cultured epidermal autografts (CEAs) are an available approach for wound coverage. These skin grafts are grown in a laboratory after obtaining a biopsy from the patient's own skin and several weeks later the grafts are applied to the wound bed. Most clinicians reserve the use of CEA for extensive burn injuries when there is very little donor site remaining. This approach is extremely costly, and there are disadvantages to CEAs, chiefly related to the thin and fragile nature of these grafts. Graft take is highly susceptible to shear forces, and once the grafts have taken they remain fragile and prone to injury for a prolonged period of time compared with standard STSGs.

Epicel (Genzyme Biosurgery, Cambridge, MA) is the best known commercially available CEA system on the market. The grafts are produced by obtaining a patient's own keratinocytes from a full-thickness skin biopsy, treating them with trypsin, and expanding them ex vivo in coculture with murine 3T3 fibroblast feeder cells. The medium also contains fetal calf serum, insulin, transferrin, hydrocortisone, epidermal growth factor, and cholera toxin.[5] As a result, a neoepidermis made of keratinocyte layers of variable thickness is arranged into sheets. Its use has been reserved for patients with large surface area burns (>30%), especially when donor availability is severely diminished or absent. Various studies have shown different rates of graft take for Epicel. Williamson and colleagues[19] studied 28 patients with a mean total body surface area burned of 52.2% and a mean total full-thickness injury of 42.4% treated with Epicel over a mean period of 5 years. Mean take rate was 26.9% of the grafted area. Despite the hope for durable wound coverage, many complications of CEA have been reported. Blistering and shearing caused by the thin layer of graft in addition to contractures and pruritus remain an issue.[20] Long in-vitro expansion times, high cost, susceptibility to infection, and prolonged hospital stays have all rendered it a last-resort option when other alternatives are not applicable.[21,22]

DOUBLE-LAYER DERMAL SUBSTITUTES
Dermal Substitutes

A breakthrough in burn wound coverage was achieved with the development of Integra (Integra LifeSciences Corporation, Plainsboro, NJ) by Yannas and Burke.[23] This product was derived from bovine collagen and contains glycosaminoglycans. Subsequently, additional coverage alternatives have been developed using collagen and other scaffolds with or without a silicone layer (single layer or double layer).

Integra

Integra remains one of the most popular bilaminate dermal substitutes. In addition to its use in patients with burns, it can also be used in trauma, skin excisions for cancerous conditions, and other clinical scenarios. Since its development as a collaborative project between the Massachusetts General Hospital and the Massachusetts Institute of Technology it has received FDA approval for use in burns. It is composed of a dermal layer of bovine collagen and chondroitin-6-sulfate glycosaminoglycan (GAG) in addition to an epidermal layer of synthetic silicone.[24] The 2-mm-thick inner layer has pores allowing vascular invasion and eventual degradation of the matrix. The outer silicone layer (0.23 mm thick) acts like an epidermis and is functionally close to normal epithelium.[2] Integra is designed to be used on freshly excised full-thickness burn wounds. The outer silicone layer is left in place for 2 to 3 weeks and then removed and replaced by an STSG. The STSG should ideally be thin, and it is thought that Integra with a thinner STSG gives the same result as an open wound treated with a thicker STSG alone.[2] The use of negative pressure wound therapy to the silicone layer has been described and has been shown in some instances to decrease the time needed for revascularization down to 10 days. Advantages of using Integra include adequate long-term wound coverage in addition to some decrease hypertrophic scars and pruritus.[24] Disadvantages include high cost and some reported infectious complications. Contributing to the high cost is the need for staged procedures and extended hospital stays, which have been barriers to adopting Integra as a universal and popular skin substitute.

Renoskin

Renoskin (Symatese, Ivry-le-Temple, France) is a 2-mm-thick bilaminar skin substitute that used to be available in Europe. It is composed of bovine type 1 collagen and a silicone film. It has been suggested for use in acute burns.[26] The same manufacturer now produces NEVELIA, a bilayer matrix consisting of a collagen layer to promote dermal regeneration and a reinforced silicone layer acting as a pseudoepidermis.

Hyalomatrix

Hyalomatrix (Anika, Boston, MA) is a dermal substitute made of HYAFF, an extended derivative of hyaluronic acid. It is a bioresorbable dermal substitute that has been described to be used for coverage in acute burns. The product allows rapid granulation tissue formation and requires a secondary skin graft.[27]

SINGLE-LAYER DERMAL SUBSTITUTES
Alloderm

Alloderm (LifeCell Corporation, Branchburg, NJ) provides additional alternatives for dermal replacement. Alloderm is a cryopreserved allogenic dermis that is prepared from cadaveric allograft skin. After a thorough infection screening process all epidermal and dermal cells are removed chemically and using freeze drying. Basement membrane proteins and collagen fibers are unharmed by the process (laminin and type IV and VII collagen). Alloderm is available in different thicknesses; however, for burn surgery, the thin material is preferred. It can be used in acute, freshly excised burn wounds. It has successfully been described in full-thickness burn wounds. To provide an alternative for the lost epidermal layer, a split-thickness autograft can be applied simultaneously.[28] In a large, multicenter, prospective clinical trial evaluating Alloderm as a coverage alternative in a 1-stage procedure, superior graft take was obtained with meshed Alloderm and thin STSGs. Good aesthetic and functional results have also been obtained.[29] Alloderm is revascularized by superficial wound beds, as well as fascial structures.[30] Despite its availability as an alternative, the high cost of the product has been a barrier to its wide application as an option in patients with burns. Despite multiple available case series, the small sample size of most of them makes it challenging to draw conclusions about the role of Alloderm in burn care. A more rigorous evaluation is needed to establish it as a reliable means for burn wound coverage.

Integra (Single Layer)

Integra Life Science has also developed a single-layer version of their traditional product. Integra single layer is an acellular permanently cross-linked collagen and glycosaminoglycan-based matrix. It measures 1.3 mm in thickness and only consists of a dermal replacing component. The main goal of the product was to spare a 2-stage procedure and transition to a single-step procedure with simultaneous application of an STSG.[31,32] Given its recent emergence on the market, the product is currently under investigation; however, there have been reports of its successful use as a 1-step procedure with an STSG to reconstruct defects.[33]

Matriderm

Although not available in the United States, Matriderm (MedSkin Solutions DR. Suwelack AG, Billerbeck, Germany) is another available dermal regeneration construct, consisting of a matrix based on 1-mm-thick (also available in thicknesses of 0.5 and 2 mm) acellular lyophilized collagen (type I, III, IV) and elastin. Matriderm (1 mm thickness) has been described for use in combination with an STSG as a 1-step procedure for wound coverage.[34] In a comparative study with single-layer Integra in rats, there was no difference in rate of take, vascularization, and inflammatory response between the two and both were judged suitable for a 1-stage coverage procedure with an STSG.[35] Further studies are needed to establish the role of Matriderm in burn care.

ReCell

Autologous noncultured cell therapy is an alternative for burn wound treatment. The ReCell system (Avita Medical, Cambridge, United Kingdom) is a technique that relies on harvesting cells from the dermal-epidermal junction of the skin through a biopsy in order to deliver them to the wound as a cellular suspension. The processing typically produces a complete cell population, including keratinocytes, melanocytes, Langerhans cells, and fibroblasts. Wood and colleagues[36] showed that a cell suspension obtained with this technology consists of 1.7×10^6 cells/cm^2 of harvested skin consisting of approximately 65% keratinocytes, 30% fibroblasts, and 3.5% melanocytes, in contrast with standard CEAs, which consist almost entirely of keratinocytes (reepithelialization depends on the ability of keratinocytes to form holoclones).

In a recent randomized controlled trial, ReCell was compared with STSG for epidermal replacement in patients with deep dermal partial-thickness burn wounds. Both techniques seemed to provide adequate epidermal replacement but the reepithelialization rate was faster with STSG. However, ReCell had less postoperative pain compared with STSG. Despite the overall results, ReCell remains an interesting alternative given that there is no need to harvest large areas.[37] Its main advantages are that application is quick and no scaffold is needed. High cost remains a disadvantage in addition to loss of cells caused by mechanical pressure while spraying.[38]

SKIN SUBSTITUTES UNDER INVESTIGATION

StrataGraft (Stratatech Corporation, Madison, WI) is a full-thickness skin substitute consisting of a dermal component that contains human dermal fibroblasts and a fully stratified epidermis. StrataGraft has been granted an orphan product designation by the FDA for use in the treatment of partial-thickness and full-thickness burns.[39]

The Tissue Biology Research Unit of the Department of Surgery of the University Children's Hospital at the University of Zurich has developed 2 new skin substitutes. DenovoDerm is a dermal substitute and DenovoSkin is a full-thickness skin substitute. Both are currently under investigation.

Novosorb (Polynovo, Melbourne, Australia), a biodegradable temporizing matrix (BTM), is a fully synthetic dermal regeneration template that is currently under investigation. Preliminary data compared with Integra show a more extensive vascular network for Novosorb BTM but also a greater inflammatory response, requiring further investigation.[40]

FURTHER STRATEGIES
Composite Bilayered Skin Structures with Adnexal Structures

Complete regeneration of functional skin must include all the skin appendages (hair follicles, sweat glands, and sensory organs) and layers (epidermis, dermis, and subcutaneous fat), and a preformed functional vascular and neuronal network. Few products currently provide a bilayered skin substitute. Apligraf consists of a cultured system with fibroblasts seeded on a collagen gel covered by cultured epithelial cells.[41–43] Collagen-GAG scaffolds have also been cocultured with autologous fibroblasts and keratinocytes or used directly with uncultured keratinocytes or stem cells obtained at the point of care in the operating room.[44] Both these approaches have shown potential in addressing the current limits of skin substitute but more research is needed.

Despite the advances in epidermal and dermal repair, regeneration of skin adnexal structures remains elusive. Some, but not all, of the functions can be restored with existing skin substitutes. Bioengineered skin substitutes currently contain only 2 cell types: fibroblasts and keratinocytes. Ongoing studies are addressing the possibility of bioengineering fully functional skin grafts containing all structures of native skin, including vasculature, hair, pigmentation, sweat and sebaceous glands, resident immune-regulatory cells, and nerve endings. Recently, a bioengineered human dermoepidermal bilayered skin substitute has been developed containing functional dermal blood and lymphatic vessels.[44]

Skin Three-Dimensional Printing

Three-dimensional cell printing technology has been explored to develop trilayered skin substitutes with the potential to introduce other elements into the system in the future and the capacity to integrate a vascular network.[45–47] Commercially available skin substitutes are mostly produced with fixed dimensions either in a cellular or acellular form to provide off-the-shelf availability. Collagen-based bio-ink and various other biomaterials have been used for bioprinting and skin engineering.[45–47]

At present, no bioprinted skin can fully replicate native skin in terms of its morphologic, biochemical, and physiologic properties. However, despite being at the very early developmental stages, three-dimensional skin printing offers fascinating scenarios for the future of skin regeneration. The feasibility of in-situ printing (directly on a wound) has also been explored with some success in animal models.[48] Bioprinting enables the deposition of a thin layer of melanocytes, can construct hollow channels to replicate the skin vascular network, and can recreate the hair-inducing microenvironment found in dermal papilla cells.[45–47] In the future, skin bioprinting could lead to the on-demand fabrication of skin substitutes that are customized to a patient's characteristics or bioprinted in situ for direct wound treatment.

LIMITS OF CURRENTLY AVAILABLE SKIN SUBSTITUTES

Commercially available skin substitutes mostly replace a single layer or function of the skin. Almost all products are single layered and do not provide both the epidermal and dermal skin layers.[49,50] Epidermal skin substitutes are effective in providing rapid and temporary external coverage of wounds but lack the underlying connective tissue (dermal and subcutaneous) that provides the elasticity and mechanical stability of regenerated skin.[49] Furthermore, the dermal layer not only restores the mechanical strength of skin but also provides the blood supply that nourishes epidermal layers.[51] In contrast, dermal substitutes are limited by the need for gradual revascularization after in-vivo implantation. Revascularization of skin substitutes occurs by ingrowth of bed vessels (angiogenesis) into the graft. This process can take up to 3 weeks and significantly limits the apacity to obtain wound closure in a short period f time.[50] Some available skin substitutes allow ngiogenesis but usually this is insufficient and ould benefit from further improvements. Advances in research have suggested the possibility f scaffolds with adequate mechanical properties o mimic native skin elasticity and resistance, but ot all scaffolds provide acceptable outcomes.[50] eripheral scarring is another significant limit unctional, mechanical, and aesthetic) of skin subtitutes that has not found a proper solution. uture skin substitutes should address this problem. Significant efforts have been undertaken to ddress these issues by including cellular components in skin substitutes. The use of laboratoryultured cells seeded into scaffolds has been hown to be time/resource intensive because xtensive cell culture procedures are involved for he different cell types used.[52] Cells usually require to 3 weeks of cell culture before they are ready or grafting. This time lag constrains regular use f cell-seeded skin substitutes in clinical scenarios, in particular in traumatic causes.

EFERENCES

1. Dunkin CSJ, Pleat JM, Gillespie PH. REF scarring occurs at a critical depth of skin injury: precise measurement in a graduated dermal scratch in human volunteers. Plast Reconstr Surg 2007;119:1722–34.
2. Saffle JR. Closure of the excised burn wound: temporary skin substitutes. Clin Plast Surg 2009;36(4):627–41.
3. Robb EC, Bechmann N, Plessinger RT, et al. Storage media and temperature maintain normal anatomy of cadaveric human skin for transplantation to full-thickness skin wounds. J Burn Care Rehabil 2001;22:393–6.
4. Song IC, Bromberg BE, Mohn MP, et al. Heterografts as biological dressings for large skin wounds. Surgery 1966;59:576–83.
5. Sheridan RL, Tompkins RG. Skin substitutes in burns. Burns 1999;25(2):97–103.
6. Ersek RA, Denton DR. Silver-impregnated porcine xenografts for treatment of meshed autografts. Ann Plast Surg 1984;13:482–7.
7. Heimbach DM, Engrav LH, Marvin JA, et al. Toxic epidermal necrolysis. A step forward in treatment. JAMA 1987;257:2171–5.
8. Lineen E, Namias N. Biologic dressing in burns. J Craniofac Surg 2008;19:923–8.
9. Lin SD, Lai CS, Hou MF, et al. Amnion overlay meshed autograft. Burns Incl Therm Inj 1985;11:374–8.
0. Sawhney CP. Amniotic membrane as a biological dressing in the management of burns. Burns 1989;15:339–42.
11. Fairbairn NG, Randolph MA, Redmond RW. The clinical applications of human amnion in plastic surgery. J Plast Reconstr Aesthet Surg 2014;67(5):662–75.
12. Wasiak J, Cleland H, Campbell F. Dressings for superficial and partial thickness burns. Cochrane Database Syst Rev 2008;(4):CD002106.
13. Whitaker IS, Prowse S, Potokar TS. A critical evaluation of the use of Biobrane as a biologic skin substitute: a versatile tool for the plastic and reconstructive surgeon. Ann Plast Surg 2008;60:333–7.
14. Lal S, Barrow RE, Wolf SE, et al. Biobrane improves wound healing in burned children without increased risk of infection. Shock 2000;14:314–8.
15. Bacha EA, Sheridan RL, Donohue GA, et al. Staphylococcal toxic shock syndrome in a paediatric burn unit. Burns 1994;20:499–502.
16. Noordenbos J, Dore C, Hansbrough JF. Safety and efficacy of TransCyte for the treatment of partial-thickness burns. J Burn Care Rehabil 1999;20:275–81.
17. Still J, Glat P, Silverstein P, et al. The use of a collagen sponge/living cell composite material to treat donor sites in burn patients. Burns 2003;29(8):837–41.
18. Sheridan R. Closure of the excised burn wound: autografts, semipermanent skin substitutes, and permanent skin substitutes. Clin Plast Surg 2009;36(4):643–51.
19. Williamson JS, Snelling CF, Clugston P, et al. Cultured epithelial autograft: five years of clinical experience with twenty-eight patients. J Trauma 1995;39:309–19.
20. Sood R, Roggy D, Zieger M, et al. Cultured epithelial autografts for coverage of large burn wounds in eighty-eight patients: the Indiana University experience. J Burn Care Res 2010;31:559–68.
21. Paddle-Ledinek JE, Cruickshank DG, Masterton JP. Skin replacement by cultured keratinocyte grafts: an Australian experience. Burns 1997;23:204–11.
22. Barret JP, Wolf SE, Desai MH, et al. Cost-efficacy of cultured epidermal autografts in massive pediatric burns. Ann Surg 2000;231:869–76.
23. Yannas IV, Burke JF. Design of an articial skin. I. Basic design principles. J Biomed Mater Res 1980;14(1):65–81.
24. Heimbach DM, Warden GD, Luterman A, et al. Multicenter postapproval clinical trial of Integra dermal regeneration template for burn treatment. J Burn Care Rehabil 2003;24:42–8.
25. Yannas IV, Burke JF, Orgill DP, et al. Wound tissue can utilize a polymeric template to synthesize a functional extension of skin. Science 1982;215:174–6.
26. Druecke D, Lamme E, Hermann S, et al. Modulation of scar tissue formation using different dermal regeneration templates in the treatment of

experimental full-thickness wounds. Wound Repair Regen 2004;12(5):518–27.

27. Erbatur S, Coban YK, Aydin EN. Comparision of clinical and histopathological results of Hyalomatrix usage in adult patients. Int J Burns Trauma 2012;2(2):118–25.

28. Metcalfe AD, Ferguson MW. Tissue engineering of replacement skin: the crossroads of biomaterials, wound healing, embryonic development, stem cells and regeneration. J R Soc Interface 2007;4:413–37.

29. Wainwright D, Madden M, Luterman A, et al. Clinical evaluation of an acellular allograft dermal matrix in full-thickness burns. J Burn Care Rehabil 1996;17:124–36.

30. Menon NG, Rodriguez ED, Byrnes CK, et al. Revascularization of human acellular dermis in full-thickness abdominal wall reconstruction in the rabbit model. Ann Plast Surg 2003;50:523–7.

31. Stiefel D, Schiestl C, Meuli M. Integra artificial skin for burn scar revision in adolescents and children. Burns 2010;36(1):114–20.

32. Branski LK, Herndon DN, Pereira C, et al. Longitudinal assessment of Integra in primary burn management: a randomized pediatric clinical trial. Crit Care Med 2007;35(11):2615–23.

33. Koenen W, Felcht M, Vockenroth K, et al. One-stage reconstruction of deep facial defects with a single layer dermal regeneration template. J Eur Acad Dermatol Venereol 2011;25(7):788–93.

34. Atherton DD, Tang R, Jones I, et al. Early excision and application of Matriderm with simultaneous autologous skin grafting in facial burns. Plast Reconstr Surg 2010;125(2):60e–1e.

35. Bottcher-Haberzeth S, Biedermann T, Schiestl C, et al. Matriderm® 1 mm versus Integra® Single Layer 1.3 mm for one-step closure of full thickness skin defects: a comparative experimental study in rats. Pediatr Surg Int 2012;28:171–7.

36. Wood FM, Giles N, Stevenson A, et al. Characterisation of the cell suspension harvested from the dermal epidermal junction using a ReCell kit. Burns 2012;38:44–51.

37. Gravante G, Di Fede MC, Araco A, et al. A randomized trial comparing ReCell system of epidermal cells delivery versus classic skin grafts for the treatment of deep partial thickness burns. Burns 2007;33:966–72.

38. Singh M, Nuutila K, Kruse C, et al. Challenging the conventional therapy: emerging skin graft techniques for wound healing. Plast Reconstr Surg 2015;136(4):524e–30e.

39. Varkey M, Ding J, Tredget EE. Advances in skin substitutes—potential of tissue engineered skin for facilitating anti-fibrotic healing. J Funct Biomate 2015;6:547–63.

40. Cheshire PA, Herson MR, Cleland H, et al. Artificia dermal templates: a comparative study o NovoSorb™ Biodegradable Temporising Matri: (BTM) and Integra® Dermal Regeneration Template Burns 2016;42(5):1088–96.

41. Veves A, Falanga V, Armstrong DG, et al, Apligra Diabetic Foot Ulcer Study. Graft skin, a human ski equivalent, is effective in the management of nonin fected neuropathic diabetic foot ulcers: a prospec tive randomized multicenter clinical trial. Diabetes Care 2001;24(2):290–5.

42. Falanga V, Margolis D, Alvarez O, et al. Rapid heal ing of venous ulcers and lack of clinical rejectio with an allogeneic cultured human skin equivalen Human Skin Equivalent Investigators Group. Arcl Dermatol 1998;134(3):293–300.

43. Sabolinski ML, Alvarez O, Auletta M, et al. Cultured ski as a 'smart material' for healing wounds: experience i venous ulcers. Biomaterials 1996;17(3):311–20.

44. Rossi A, Gabbrielli E, Villano M, et al. Human micro vascular lymphatic and blood endothelial cells pro duce fibrillin: deposition patterns and quantitative analysis. J Anat 2010;17(6):705–14.

45. Patra S, Young V. A review of 3D printing technique and the future in biofabrication of bioprinted tissue Cell Biochem Biophys 2016;74(2):93–8.

46. Bauermeister AJ, Zuriarrain A, Newman MI. Three dimensional printing in plastic and reconstructive surgery: a systematic review. Ann Plast Surg 2015 [Epub ahead of print].

47. Algzlan H, Varada S. Three-dimensional printing o the skin. JAMA Dermatol 2015;151(2):207.

48. Michael S, Sorg H, Peck CT, et al. Tissue engineered skin substitutes created by laser-assisted bio printing form skin-like structures in the dorsal ski fold chamber in mice. PLoS One 2013;8(3):e57741

49. Golas AR, Hernandez KA, Spector JA. Tissue engi neering for plastic surgeons: a primer. Aestheti Plast Surg 2014;38(1):207–21.

50. Nyame TT, Chiang HA, Leavitt T, et al. Tissue-eng neered skin substitutes. Plast Reconstr Surg 2015 136(6):1379–88.

51. Yannas IV, Orgill DP, Burke JF. Template for ski regeneration. Plast Reconstr Surg 2011;127(Supp 1):60S–70S.

52. Cherubino M, Valdatta L, Balzaretti R, et al. Huma adipose-derived stem cells promote vascularizatio of collagen-based scaffolds transplanted into nud mice. Regen Med 2016;11(3):261–71.

Stem Cells and Tissue Engineering
Regeneration of the Skin and Its Contents

Amy L. Strong, MD, PhD, MPH[a],
Michael W. Neumeister, MD, FRCSC[b], Benjamin Levi, MD[c,d],*

KEYWORDS

- Epithelial stem cells • Interfollicular epidermal stem cells • Hair follicle stem cells
- Mesenchymal stem cells • Bone marrow-derived mesenchymal stem cells
- Adipose-derived stem cells • Umbilical cord mesenchymal stem cells

KEY POINTS

- The current gold standard of care for full-thickness burn injuries is to debride and use skin grafts to cover the wounds.
- These approaches are limited by the amount of skin available for grafting, particularly when the burns cover a large total body surface area.
- Stem cells are a unique cell population characterized by self-renewal and differentiation capabilities, which may allow for regeneration of the skin and its contents.
- Advances in tissue engineering have increased the interest in applying stem cells onto tissue engineered scaffolds to further reconstitute the damaged tissue and develop skin regenerative therapies.

INTRODUCTION

Skin functions to preserve processes such as hydration, to protect against the external environment, and to regulate temperature. Severe damage to the skin as in burn injuries may interfere with these processes and, in severe cases, may be life threatening. Although the current gold standard of care for full-thickness burn injuries is to debride and use skin grafts to cover the wounds, these approaches are limited by the amount of skin available for grafting, particularly when the burns cover a large total body surface area. Recently, there has been significant interest in the use of stem cells for skin regeneration. Stem cells are a unique cell population characterized by self-renewal and differentiation capabilities. Several populations of stem cells have been identified that have shown to assist in wound healing through immunomodulation, reepithelialization, revascularization, and collagen deposition. Furthermore, the advances in tissue engineering have increased the interest in applying stem cells

Disclosure Statement: Dr B. Levi was supported by funding from National Institutes of Health/National Institute of General Medical Sciences grant K08GM109105, American Association of Plastic Surgery Academic Scholarship, International FOP Association, Plastic Surgery Foundation Pilot Award and American College of Surgeons Clowes Award. Dr B. Levi collaborates on a project unrelated to this article with Boehringer Ingelheim on a project not examined in this study.

[a] Division of Plastic Surgery, Department of Surgery, University of Michigan, 1500 East Medical Center Drive, Ann Arbor, MI 48109, USA; [b] Department of Surgery, Institute for Plastic Surgery, Southern Illinois University School of Medicine, 747 North Rutledge Street, Springfield, IL 62702, USA; [c] Division of Plastic Surgery, Department of Surgery, University of Michigan, 1500 East Medical Center Drive, Ann Arbor, MI 48109, USA; [d] Burn Wound and Regenerative Medicine Laboratory, University of Michigan, 1150 West Medical Center Drive, Ann Arbor, MI 48109, USA
* Corresponding author. Division of Plastic Surgery, Department of Surgery, University of Michigan, 1500 East Medical Center Drive, Ann Arbor, MI 48109.
E-mail address: blevi@med.umich.edu

onto tissue engineered scaffolds to further reconstitute the damaged tissue. Although these applications of stem cells in wound regenerative therapies have provided encouraging results, long-term clinical studies are necessary to determine whether the observed effects are clinically significant and whether regeneration can be achieved. In this review, we discuss the stages of skin wound healing, the role of stem cells in accelerating skin wound healing, and the mechanism by which these stem cells may reconstitute the skin in the context of tissue engineering.

BACKGROUND

Skin is a soft tissue that forms roughly 8% of the total body mass and covers the entire surface area of the body. It is a self-repairing, self-renewing organ that forms an important barrier that separates the outer environment from the internal organs. The skin is composed of the epidermis, dermis, and hypodermis (**Fig. 1**). The epidermis is the outermost layer of the skin and is characterized by a stratified structure and acts as a protective barrier. The layers of the epidermis include the stratum corneum, stratum granulosum, stratum lucidum, stratum spinosum, and stratum basale (see **Fig. 1**). Underneath the epidermis is the dermis, which is enriched for dermal fibroblasts that produce collagens and elastin fibers and provides the skin with structural support and elasticity. The dermis is divided into 2 layers—the more superficial papillary layer and deeper reticular layer. Within the dermis are also epidermal appendages that give rise to hair follicles, sebaceous glands, and sweat glands that provide sensation and support to the skin. Important differences exist between the papillary and reticular layers of the dermis that play a role in scarring depending on the depth of burn injury.[1] The dermal fibroblasts located in the papillary dermis are heterogeneous in terms of morphology and proliferation kinetics, whereas dermal fibroblasts located in the reticular dermis have myofibroblast-like characteristics.[2] Thus, with progressively deeper wounds, the fibroblasts in the reticular dermis are activated producing more alpha-smooth muscle protein and higher collagen lattice contraction, leading to scarring. In contrast, burns affecting the papillary dermis are less likely to result in hypertrophic scar formation.

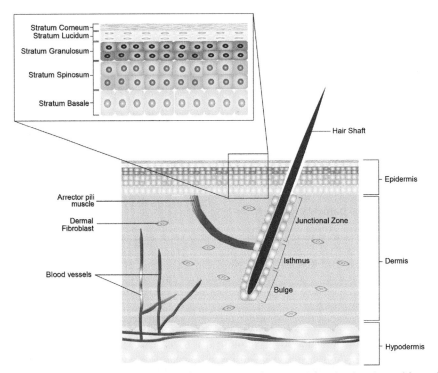

Fig. 1. Human skin and its cell populations. The skin contains 3 layers: epidermis, dermis, and hypodermis. The epidermis is a stratified epithelium composed of 4 to 5 layers: stratum corneum, stratum lucidium, stratum granulosum, stratum spinosum, and stratum basale. Other structures in the skin include the hair follicles, arrector pili muscle, and blood vessels. The hair follicle is further divided into the junction zone, the isthmus, and the bulge. Epithelial stem cells, located in the stratum basale and the isthmus and bulge of the hair follicle, have the ability to self-renew and differentiate into epithelial cells.

below the dermis lies the hypodermis, which consists mainly of adipose tissue and blood vessels. The hypodermis not only insulate the skin and provide an energy reservoir, but it also ensures the life-saving mechanical and thermoregulatory characteristics of the skin. Deep to the hypodermis is fascia, muscle, and bone, which provide mechanical and structural support for all the layers more superficial to it. Together, these components form a highly organized and complex environment for which different cell types must communicate to continuously repair and regenerate the skin during normal homeostasis and during injury.

Any disruption in the normal anatomic structure and functional integrity of the skin ultimately leads to a wound. Wound healing relies on a complex dynamic process that involves the interaction of many cell types, growth factors, cytokines, and chemokines.[3,4] Dysfunction of this mechanism can result in chronic, nonhealing wounds that lead to infection, sepsis, insensible fluid loss, impaired temperature regulation, and, in severe cases, death. Disruption in the wound-healing process can also lead to the formation of excess granulation tissue, which can ultimately lead to hypertrophic scar formation.[5,6]

Particularly challenging wounds are large burn wounds. In addition to the acute systemic responses that occur immediately after the injury, these large burn wounds are also more likely to enter a prolonged period of hypermetabolism, chronic inflammation, and lean body mass wasting, all of which may impair wound healing.[7] Furthermore, an increased susceptibility to infection owing to altered immune status may lead to sepsis, which can be lethal if not treated appropriately.[8] With respect to sustained hypermetabolism and inflammation, these processes impair wound healing through delayed reepithelialization.[9] Furthermore, limited availability of donor skin grafts becomes a significant challenge in large burn wounds. Split thickness skin grafts, often meshed to maximize the harvested skin, can cause secondary contracture during the healing process owing to variable thickness of the dermis. In addition to the thickness of the skin graft, the depth of the underlying wound bed also affects the extent and type of scarring.[10] Autologous keratinocytes cultured in vitro have been used as an alternative to treat serious burns; however, this approach requires weeks to generate enough material to cover large burn wounds.[11,12] Current treatment strategies require 2 biopsies followed by shipping of the samples, expansion, and return of the cultured tissue. These cultured tissues represent the only option for large burn injury patients; however, when used alone, they have increased risk of infection and take longer to incorporate. Epicel (Genzyme

Biosurgery, Cambridge, MA) is the most commonly used cultured epithelial autograft. To help mitigate the high risk of infection and graft failure, special antimicrobial soaks such as sulfamylon and silver nitrate can be used. Additionally, the cultured epithelial autograft can be used on top of a widely meshed autograft (4:1, 6:1, or MEEK) to help autograft incorporation. A cultured epithelial autograft is not without risks as squamous cell carcinoma has been reported in grafted regions.

Others have focused their efforts on regenerating the dermal component of the skin with tissue engineered skin substitutes or acellular dermal substitutes, and although these efforts have been promising, disadvantages of these substitutes include slow vascularization, poor integration, and rejection.[13,14] Acellular dermal substitutes are also often applied in a 2-step procedure that still requires skin grafting.[14] Thus, there is an increased interest to identify an alternative treatment plan to augment the wound healing process to accelerate wound closure, minimize scar formation, and minimize additional operations.

Interest in the use of stem cells to regenerate different aspects of the skin has increased in the last decade. The skin harbors several distinct populations of stem cells and a rich array of cell types that have the potential to repair the skin. Studies have focused recently on characterizing the capacity of these cells for wound healing and tissue engineering purposes. In this review, we discuss the various stem cell populations found within the different layers of the skin and their potential application for skin regeneration. Enriching these stem cell populations and cultivating a microenvironment that facilitates the survival of these stem cells may assist in the regeneration of the skin and its contents.

SKIN REGENERATION AND HAIR FOLLICLE DEVELOPMENT

Wound healing is a complex and dynamic process that begins immediately after injury. Normal wound healing is divided into overlapping phases: hemostasis, inflammation, proliferation, and remodeling. Hemostasis is the first phase and starts immediately after the initial injury to prevent exsanguination and initiate clot formation. In the second phase, inflammatory cells are recruited to the site of injury to remove cellular debris and initiate cellular signaling cascades for further wound healing. During the proliferative phase, keratinocytes proliferate to close the wound while the myofibroblasts contract to decrease the wound size. Endothelial cells are simultaneously proliferating throughout all phases of wound healing to revascularize the damaged tissue. Last, over weeks to years, the extracellular matrix (ECM) remodels and forms a scar with a tensile strength close to 80% compared with normal uninjured skin.

Most wounds to the skin cause leakage of blood from damaged blood vessels and a clot forms to serve as a temporary shield to protect the denuded wound tissue and provide a provisional matrix through which cells can migrate during the reparative process.[15] The clot consists of platelets embedded in a mesh of cross-linked fibrin fibers together with small amounts of plasma fibronectin, vitronectin, and thrombospondin.[15] It also serves as a reservoir of cytokines and growth factors, such as platelet-derived growth factor, transforming growth factor-β (TGF-β), epidermal growth factor, and insulin-like growth factor-1, which are released by degranulating platelets.[16] Owing to the high concentration of cytokines and growth factors, the clot also provides chemotactic cues to recruit circulating inflammatory cells to the wound site and initiates and stimulates angiogenesis. After hemostasis is achieved (within minutes), chemotactic signals released by degranulating platelets as well as byproducts of proteolysis of fibrin and other matrix components recruit neutrophils and monocytes to the wound site.[17] Neutrophils arrive within minutes of injury at the wound site and serve to clear the initial rush of contaminating bacteria as well as provide a source of proinflammatory cytokines that serve as the earliest signals to activate local fibroblast and keratinocytes.[17] In contrast, macrophages accumulate at the wound site several days after the initial injury and are essential for effective wound healing.[18] The macrophages phagocytose any remaining pathogenic organisms and cellular debris.[18,19] Once activated, macrophages also release a battery of growth factors and cytokines at the wound site, thus amplifying the earlier wound signals released by degranulating platelets and neutrophils.[20] Therefore, these crucial M2 macrophages secrete growth factors and antiinflammatory cytokines to mediate the reparative process.[21]

When ongoing injury has ceased, hemostasis has been achieved, and an immune response successfully set in place, the acute wound shifts toward tissue repair. The proliferative phase starts on the third day after wounding and lasts for approximately 2 weeks thereafter. This phase is characterized by fibroblast migration and deposition of newly synthesized ECM to replace the provisional fibrin network. Fibroblasts and myofibroblasts in the surrounding tissue are stimulated to proliferate for the first 3 days, after which these cells migrate into the wound.[22] Once in the wound,

these cells proliferate profusely and produce the matrix proteins fibronectin, hyaluronan, and proteoglycans.[22,23] By the end of the first week, abundant ECM accumulates, which provides support for the wound and further supports cell migration. The fibroblasts then convert into myofibroblasts, which initiates wound contraction in the reparative process that helps to approximate the wound edges.[24]

In the proliferative phase, reepithelialization through migration of keratinocytes also occurs and starts from the wound edges within a few hours of wounding. In the unwounded skin, the basal keratinocyte layer attaches to the basement membrane. These keratinocytes are anchored primarily to hemidesmosomes, which bind to laminin in the basement membrane by way of integrins and have intracellular links to the keratin–cytoskeletal network. During wound healing, the hemidesmosomes dissolve and the leading edge keratinocytes express new integrins that allow for the cells to migrate over the provisional wound matrix.[25,26] In addition, the leading-edge keratinocytes also have the ability to dissolve the fibrin barrier ahead of them to allow for the migration.[26] The chief fibrinolytic enzyme is plasmin, which is derived from plasminogen within the clot itself and can be activated by either tissue-type plasminogen activator or urokinase-type plasminogen activator (uPA).[26] Both of these activators and the receptor for uPA are upregulated in the migrating keratinocyte. Furthermore, various members of the matrix metalloproteinase (MMP) family are also upregulated by the wound edge keratinocytes. More specifically, MMP-9 can cut collagen type IV and VII and is thought to be responsible for releasing keratinocytes from the basement membrane.[27] Additional MMPs have been identified in the wound that degrades native collagens and presumably aids keratinocyte crawling by cutting collagen type I and III at the sites of focal adhesion attachment to the dermis.[28] Once the denuded wound surface has been covered by a monolayer of keratinocytes, epithelial migration ceases and a new stratified epidermis with underlying basal lamina is reestablished from the margins of the wound inward.[29]

In the final phase of wound healing, the remodeling phase is responsible for the development of new epithelium and scar tissue formation, which can last for up to 1 to 2 years. In this phase, the ECM begins to mature. The collagen bundles increase in diameter and the tensile strength of the wound increases progressively to approximately 80% of the original strength compared with unwounded tissue. In addition to collagen deposition, the collagen fibers become more organized which leads to increased contraction that initially began in the inflammatory phase.[30,31] As the wound matures, the density of fibroblasts and macrophages is reduced by apoptosis. With time, the growth of the capillaries stops, blood flow to the area declines, and metabolic activity at the wound site decreases.[32] The end result is a fully mature scar with a reduced number of cells, decreased blood vessels, and high tensile strength.

EPITHELIAL STEM CELLS: INTERFOLLICULAR EPIDERMAL STEM CELLS AND HAIR FOLLICLE STEM CELLS

Epithelial stem cells, in general, fit a broader definition of adult tissue resident stem cells. Scores of epithelial stem cell populations have been identified based on both in vitro and in vivo methods and are believed to interact to accelerate skin repair and regeneration during injury. Epithelial stem cells are divided into 2 broad categories: interfollicular epidermal stem cells and hair follicle stem cells, each of which have their own distinct characteristics.

Interfollicular epidermal stem cells are located in the basal layer of the epidermis and are believed to have self-renewal capacity. Because epidermal renewal is continuous throughout life, it has been postulated that at least a portion of the epidermal basal cells behave like stem cells.[33] After injury, these epidermal stem cells undergo a limited number of replications before undergoing differentiation. Thus, these cells are unipotent and differentiate to form the mature epidermis in adult skin.[34]

In contrast, hair follicle stem cells isolated from the bulge region have been shown to have the potential to regenerate hair follicles as well as contribute to epidermal regeneration in response to wounding. These bulge stem cells are located in the deepest portion of the permanent hair follicle and represent a promising source of multipotent stem cells.[35,36] Human stem cells extracted from the bulge region of the hair follicle have been induced to form epidermal and sebaceous cells and have the potential to differentiate toward other hair follicle components in vitro.[37,38] In response to injury, these bulge stem cells can be rapidly mobilized and migrate to repair damaged epidermis in vivo.[38,39] Studies have also shown that defects in the hair follicle bulge lead to an acute delay in reepithelialization of cutaneous wounds.[40]

Additional epidermal stem cells have been identified in the isthmus of the hair follicle, which is the region between the bulge and the sebaceous gland.[41] These isthmus stem cells have been shown to have the potential to differentiate into all epidermal cell lineages after transplantation.[41] Recently, an additional population of hair follicle stem cells has been isolated from the isthmus that expressed Lgr6.[42] These Lgr6-expressing stem cells have been shown to give rise to all epidermal lineages after transplantation and contribute to the homeostasis of the isthmus region and sebaceous gland.[43]

Clinically, transplantation of cultured epithelial cells containing epidermal stem cells and keratinocytes, either in cell suspension or as cell sheets, has been well-established for the treatment of extensive and deep wounds, particularly when using fibrin matrices as vehicles to facilitate the transplantation of epidermal stem cells.[44,45] The use of cultured epithelial allografts to treat chronic skin ulcers or deep dermal burns has also been reported.[45] Meanwhile, there is increasing evidence to suggest immune privilege of skin–dermal stem cells. For instance, it was reported that hair follicles were produced surprisingly without inducing immunogenic rejection after transplantation of allogenic follicle dermal sheath cells.[46] Considering their capacity to regenerate the epidermis in a relatively simple manner, the epidermal stem cells may become an important source for novel therapeutic approaches in the management of wounds. In the future, clinical trials will be necessary to determine the safety and efficacy of these cells for skin regeneration and repair.

MESENCHYMAL STEM CELLS

In addition to epidermal stem cells, our current understanding and development of stem cell therapy for the treatment of wounds has been through the study of mesenchymal stem cells (MSCs). MSCs have been isolated not only from bone marrow aspirates but also from adipose tissue and umbilical cord blood.[47] Their role in wound closure has been well-documented through the years and their potential use in tissue engineering and skin regeneration has gained significant interest in recent years. MSCs have been shown to traffic to areas of injury and secrete cytokines, chemokines, and growth factors to stimulate repair in a paracrine fashion (**Fig. 2**). These factors have been shown to immunomodulate the inflammatory process, recruit various cell types for neovascularization, and stimulate proliferation during this regenerative process (see **Fig. 2**). Furthermore, studies have demonstrated that MSCs are capable of self-renewal and differentiation into various lineages, including osteogenic, adipogenic, and chrondrogenic lineages, to replace the damaged tissue.[47]

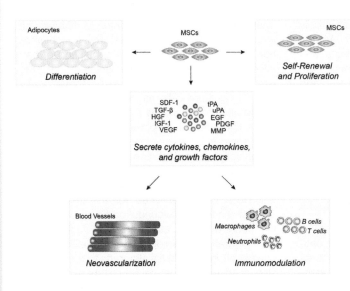

Fig. 2. Mechanism of mesenchymal stem cells (MSCs). MSCs have both direct and indirect effects of wound healing. Direct effects of MSCs are associated with the differentiate into dermal fibroblast, endothelial cells, and keratinocytes. Paracrine effects of MSCs include the secretion of antiinflammation cytokines and chemokines to modulate the inflammatory process and promote neovascularization through endothelial cells. EGF, epidermal growth factor; HGF, hepatocyte growth factor; IGF-1, insulin-like growth factor-1; MMP, matrix metalloproteinase; PDGF, platelet-derived growth factor; SDF-1, stromal cell-derived factor-1; TGF-β, transforming growth factor-β; tPA, tissue-type plasminogen activator; uPA, urokinase-type plasminogen activator; VEGF, vascular endothelial growth factor.

Bone Marrow

Bone marrow-derived MSCs (BMSCs) are isolated from bone marrow aspirates and are an attractive source of stem cells owing to their easy accessibility, expandable capacity in vitro, and low immunogenic potential.[48] Little to no rejection has been observed after transplantation, when allogenic MSCs were administered systematically.[49,50] Therefore, the application of BMSCs to facilitate wound repair has been of particular interest. Studies have shown that distant BMSCs contribute to the reconstruction of the dermal fibroblast population in cutaneous wounds in a chimeric mouse model.[51] Moreover, BMSCs have been shown to express higher amounts of collagen, basic fibroblast growth factor (bFGF), and vascular endothelial growth factor (VEGF), compared with native dermal fibroblasts, indicating their potential use in accelerating the healing process. Furthermore, BMSCs were found to improve cutaneous healing by accelerating reepithelialization, increasing angiogenesis, as well as directly differentiating into epithelial cells expressing keratinocyte specific marker.[52,53] These findings support the use of BMSCs to assist in the reparative process.

Emerging preclinical evidence also supports the therapeutic application of BMSCs. Injection of human BMSCs into the incisional wound led to improved wound closure with better tensile strength and significant reduction in scar formation in rabbits.[54] Murine BMSCs applied to full-thickness excisional wounds exhibited an equivalent ability as control fibroblast to migrate

through the tissue and to attenuate the local inflammatory response, thereby facilitating cutaneous healing in mice.[55] Application of a fibrin polymer spray with cultured autologous BMSCs aided in the healing of acute and nonhealing wounds in both human and mice.[56] This approach might represent a practical method to introduce cells to the wound and might eventually facilitate the clinical use of MSC-based therapies.

The application of BMSCs in cutaneous healing has been explored in the management of various clinical conditions as well. Studies have shown that the application of BMSCs impregnated in collagen matrices onto chronic leg ulcers that resisted conventional treatment for more than 1 year responded to BMSC treatment with reduced wound size, increased vascularity of the dermis, and increased dermal thickness of the wound bed.[57] Moreover, application of autologous BMSCs together with skin fibroblast on biodegradable collagen on the wound edges of patients with diabetic foot ulcers improved healing.[58] Promising results were reported in a case series that demonstrated the efficacy of transplanting BMSCs into lower extremity wounds.[59] Together, the data demonstrated that topical application and peripheral injection of BMSCs into the wound were both safe and efficacious in healing wounds.

Adipose Tissue

Adipose tissue has been identified as another source for multipotent stem cells, with characteristics resembling those of BMSCs. The adipose-derived stem cells (ASCs) are capable of differentiating into cells of adipogenic, chondrogenic, myogenic, and osteogenic lineages in response to specific stimuli.[60,61] ASCs can be isolated from liposuction aspirates or excised fat, which are obtained more easily in adequate quanties with minimal patient discomfort and negligible donor site morbidity as compared with bone marrow procurement. The application of ASCs in wound repair and tissue regeneration has been shown in a number of experimental models both in vitro and in vivo.[62] Application of ASCs significantly accelerated the reepithelialization of cutaneous wounds by promoting human dermal fibroblast proliferation through direct cell–cell contact or through paracrine secretion of a variety of growth factors, including bFGF and TGF-.[63,64] Furthermore, these ASCs differentiate into adipocytes to provide a supportive architecture for dermal regeneration and reepithelialization.[65]

In addition to the direct effects of administering ASCs directly into the wounds, the application of ASCs in tissue engineered constructs for the production of a new skin substitute has also been proposed. The application of autologous ASCs onto an atelocollagen matrix accelerated wound healing of diabetic ulcers in impaired diabetic mice.[66] Topical application of human ASCs seeded on a silk fibrin–chitosan scaffold also showed improvement in wound repair, and these cells were shown to differentiate and contribute to fibrovascular, endothelial, and epithelial components of the reconstituted tissue.[67] In addition to the promising results obtained in preclinical studies, ASCs were reported to improve tissue hydration and new vessel formation during the treatment of radiation-induced tissue damage in clinical studies.[68] Although the mechanism of healing has not been understood completely, ASCs have been speculated to contribute to wound repair and tissue regeneration by actively secreting growth factors, such as VEGF and hepatocyte growth factor, and thus promote subsequent angiogenesis and proliferation of keratinocytes or dermal fibroblasts.[69] These results together also suggest that ASCs are a viable option for wound repair and tissue engineering.

Umbilical Cord Derived

Umbilical cord blood has been proposed to be the largest untouched source of stem cells with naïve immune status. Stem cells isolated from umbilical cord blood have been shown to differentiate into epithelial cells in vitro.[70,71] A recent in vivo study further confirmed that umbilical cord blood could improve obstinate skin wound healing by accelerating wound closure.[72] The authors showed that these MSCs derived from umbilical cord blood were able to differentiate into keratinocytes in the wound bed. Thus, these stem cells isolated from umbilical cord blood could be used as a starting material for the expansion of cells needed for the treatment of large skin defects. However, although the studies have been promising, it should be noted that transplantation or transfusion of umbilical cord blood–derived stem cells may lead to immunologic rejection owing to their allogenic nature and thus their immunogenicity must be evaluated carefully before their use in clinical applications.

In addition to umbilical cord blood being used as a source of stem cells, different layers of the umbilical cord tissue could serve as a source of stem cells.[73] The stem cells isolated from the umbilical cord have been termed umbilical cord MSCs (UC-MSCs). In general, UC-MSCs exhibited similar immunophenotypic and functional characteristics of BMSCs.[74,75] Therefore, UC-MSCs are considered as a promising alternative to BMSCs in tissue repair and regeneration. Both in vitro and in vivo studies have demonstrated their potential to differentiate into epidermal tissue, and these studies suggest the potential clinical application of UC-MSCs for epithelial reconstitution in wound healing. Several ongoing clinical trials are underway currently to evaluate the application of these cells in the treatment of partial and full thickness burns, and chronic diabetic wounds. Immunologic rejection has not been observed in these trials and confirms the safety of amniotic stem cells and attenuates the concerns regarding their neoplastic potential in clinical applications.[76] However, there remain questions regarding the effect of donor selection and culture condition on clinical outcomes, long-term therapeutic effect, and product consistency that require additional investigation before their use in the clinic.

Muscle Satellite Cells

Severe burns have the ability to damage structures that extend deep to the adipose tissue into the skeletal muscle. Interestingly, the damaged skeletal muscles have been shown to have the capacity to regenerate. Adult skeletal muscle is a stable tissue under normal circumstances, and has remarkable ability to repair itself after injury. Skeletal muscle regeneration is a highly orchestrated process involving the activation of various cellular and molecular responses. As a skeletal muscle stem cell, muscle satellite cells play an indispensable role in in the regeneration of skeletal muscle through the activation of various cellular and molecular responses.[77] These satellite stem cells not only maintain the stem cell population through self-renewal, but also provide numerous myogenic cells that reconstitute a functional contractile apparatus. Studies demonstrate that these satellite cells express high levels of Pax3 and Pax7, and mutations in the Pax3 and Pax7 genes impair muscle regeneration.[78] Animal studies have supported the importance of Pax7 in normal muscle development, as a mutation in Pax7 results in the loss of satellite cells in the postnatal period.[79]

Interestingly, studies have revealed recently that satellite cells exhibit heterogeneity with respect to their cell fate potential and have the intrinsic potential to differentiate into multiple mesenchymal lineages.[80] When cultured on solubilized basement membrane matrix (Matrigel), satellite cells from single myofibers spontaneously differentiated into myocytes, adipocytes, and osteocytes.[80] These findings indicate that satellite cells may functionally resemble BMSCs. This notion is substantiated by other studies wherein satellite cells cultured in oxygen-rich culture conditions were found to assume mesenchymal lineage cells.[81] Clonal analysis revealed that myogenic and adipogenic satellite cells have 2 separate populations in the satellite cell compartment. Both populations express the myogenic marker Pax7 and adipogenic markers, including peroxisome proliferator-activated receptors gamma and CCAAT/enhancer binding proteins.[82] These results indicate that muscle satellite cells may represent a heterogeneous population of stem cells that have the potential to not only regenerate damaged skeletal muscle, but it highlights the possibility of these cells to develop into other mesenchymal lineage cells. Future advances in systems biology and bioengineering will be necessary to develop therapeutic approaches to regenerate loss skeletal muscle and other deeper structures.

PARACRINE EFFECTS OF STEM CELLS
Neovascularization

Neovascularization is important in providing nutrients to the regenerating wound bed and removing waste products. Although various stem cells contribute to the development of new blood vessels, MSCs have been studied widely in the last decade. MSCs have been shown to secrete and release many factors, such as epidermal growth factor, bFGF, platelet-derived growth factor, TGF-β, VEGF, hepatocyte growth factor, and insulinlike growth factor-1, as well as enzymes, such as tissue-type plasminogen activator, uPA, and MMPs, that contribute to angiogenesis. Transplantation of BMSCs into the skin has also been shown to enhance angiogenesis through the

specific secretion of epidermal growth factor.[83,8] Human MSCs express VEGF as well as nitric oxide, which promote endothelial cell proliferation and vascular permeability.[85,86] Despite similar multipotency and phenotypes, MSCs from different tissue promote angiogenesis through distinct mechanisms. ASCs mediate vessel morphogenesis through the plasmin system and minimally with MMPs, whereas BMSC stimulate capillary formation solely using membrane-type MMPs.[87,88] In addition, the expression patterns of angiogenic factors, such as uPA and hepatocyte growth factor, differ in ASCs and BMSCs during angiogenesis.[87,88] Nevertheless, these findings suggest that, regardless of the mechanism of action, MSCs enhance neovascularization.

Proliferation

The effects of stem cells on proliferation that allows for rapid regeneration of cells and lost ECM has been shown to be multifold. Interfollicular epidermal stem cells undergo rapid self renewal and proliferation to regenerate the most superficial layer of the skin. Fibroblasts, located in the dermis, are a major stromal cell population in the skin and their main function is to maintain the structural integrity of connective tissue by continuously secreting precursors of the ECM. MSCs have been shown to regulate dermal fibroblast proliferation, migration, and gene expression to accelerate wound healing and also play a role in the orderly transition of the matrix product and organization to minimize scar formation MMPs.[89,90] Conditioned medium generated from MSCs expresses high concentrations of cytokines and chemokines, including interleukin (IL) 6, IL-8, TGF-β, tumor necrosis factor-α and VEGF, all of which are important in increasing proliferation for normal wound healing.[89] In vitro studies have shown that dermal fibroblasts increase the expression of integrin alpha 7 and downregulate the expression of intracellular adhesion molecule-1, vascular cell adhesion molecule-1, and MMP-11, when exposed to BMSCs.[91] Increased abundance of these factors in the wound bed likely accelerates the closure of the wound. ASCs have also been shown to stimulate the migration of fibroblasts and upregulate collagen types I and III and fibronectin, which contribute to wound closure and increased tensile strength of the healed wound.[92] Furthermore muscle satellite cells have been shown to undergo proliferation and differentiation to regenerate any skeletal muscle that has been lost. Various stem cells undergo proliferation to assist in the reconstitution of the damaged tissue.

Migration

Stem cells have also been shown to contribute to the migration of immune cells and endothelial cells during would repair, particularly MSCs. Cultured MSCs secrete a variety of chemoattractant molecules, which include CCL2 (MCP-1), CCL5 (RANTES), CCL7 (MCP-3), CCL20 (MIP-3alpha), CCL26 (eotaxin-3), CX3CL1 (fractalkine), CXCL5 (ENA-78) CXCL11 (i-TAC), CXCL1 (GROalpha), CXCL12 (stromal derived factor-1; SDF-1), CXCL8 (IL-8), CXCL2 (GRObeta), and CXCL10 (IP-10).[93–96] Target cells for these molecules are predominantly inflammatory cells, including monocytes, eosinophils, neutrophils, basophils, memory and naïve T cells, B cells, natural killer cells, dendritic cells, and hematopoietic and endothelial cells. As such, the recruitment of these vital cells to the wound bed assist in recruiting cells for the inflammatory phase of wound healing. Furthermore, MSC-conditioned medium has been shown to promote proliferation and migration of endothelial cells in a dose-dependent manner with VEGF and bFGF, which promotes angiogenesis and enhances collateral flow recovery and remodeling of the wound and the contents deep to the wound.[97,98]

Osteogenic Differentiation (Bone Morphogenetic Protein)

In severe cases where bone has been compromised owing to burns that extend deep to the hypodermis, the skeletal architecture may be compromised. In these cases, preliminary results using stem and progenitor cells have been promising and have been shown to regenerate the damaged tissue. A number of studies on enhanced bone repair with stem cells and genetically modified cells have been conducted. Studies have demonstrated that genetically modified BMSCs, ASCs, UC-MSC, and muscle satellite cells overexpressing a number of bone morphogenetic proteins (BMPs), including BMP-2, BMP-4, BMP-7, BMP-9, and insulinlike growth factor-1 have proven successful in the use of these cells to repair bone defects.[99] Others have shown that overexpression of BMP-4 alone resulted in enhanced recruitment of stem cells, cell survival, and endochondral cartilage formation compared with unmodified cells. Transduction of BMSCs with BMP-2 not only accelerated bone formation and regeneration, but also increased angiogenesis in the injured tissue.[100] Additional studies have shown the addition of BMSCs or ASCs seeded onto biodegradable scaffolds enhanced osteogenic differentiation of the stem cells.[101–103] In a study by Sándor and colleagues,[103] defects were reconstructed with either bioactive glass or beta-tricalcium phosphate scaffolds seeded with ASCs, and in some cases, with the addition of recombinant human BMP-2. This study demonstrated successful integration of the construct to the surrounding skeleton and good long-term outcomes. Together, these results indicate that BMSCs, ASCs, UC-MSCs, and muscle satellite cells may provide a viable cell source capable of modulating bone regeneration when implanted with biocompatible scaffolds along with the addition of growth factors.

IMMUNOMODULATORY PROPERTIES OF STEM CELLS

MSCs express intermediate levels of major histocompatibility complex class I but do not expression major histocompatibility complex class II or the costimulatory molecules CD80, CD86, or CD40, which are involved in controlling humoral or cell-mediated immune responses. A large body of studies has indicated that MSCs have low inherent immunogenicity and possess an immunomodulation and immunosuppression function, which makes these cells attractive candidates for autologous and allogenic transplantation to treat diseases involving immune dysfunction.[104–106]

In response to injury, proinflammatory cytokines are secreted into the wound that induces the migration of MSCs into the wound to immunomodulate the microenvironment. Proinflammatory cytokines, including tumor necrosis factor-α and IL-1, secreted by activated lymphocytes and monocytes leads to the upregulation of SDF-1 in the inflamed tissue.[107,108] The high concentration of SDF-1 in the damaged tissue induces appreciable migration of MSCs to mediate the inflammatory response. Although the immunosuppressive effect of MSCs is not intrinsic, the exposure to inflammatory cytokines or chemokines induces MSCs to secrete abundant antiinflammatory cytokines and chemokines.[109] Thus, in injured states, the recruited MSCs can be activated by the supernatant of activated lymphocytes and monocytes.[110] Activated MSCs have potent immunosuppressive effects on inflammatory responses and any type of immune cells.[111] MSCs also secrete soluble mediators, such as nitric oxide, prostaglandin E2, indoleamine 2,3-dioxygenase, and IL-6, which inhibit T-cell proliferation and B-cell differentiation into plasma cells, prevent the development of cytotoxic T cells, and interfere with dendritic cell differentiation, maturation, and function.[112–114] Additionally, studies have shown that MSCs have the ability to modulate the inflammatory response by exposing macrophages to microRNA (miRNA) through exosomes.[115] These RNA incorporate into immune cells and quench the secretion of proinflammatory cytokines. The effect is then propagated through the exchange of these miRNA among immune cells, further modulating the immune system.[115]

SYNERGIST EFFECT OF STEM CELLS AND BIOMATERIALS DURING REPAIR AND REGENERATION

Traditionally, the ECM has been considered to be an inert, space-filling material providing mechanical support and tissue integrity. However, in recent years, it has become clear that the matrix also provides a bioactive structure that controls cell behavior through chemical and mechanical signals.[116] Several ECM-based therapeutic systems for skin repair and regeneration have reached the clinics or are in clinical trials.[117–119] In recent years, dermal substitutes have gained significant attention owing to their ability to repair full-thickness skin defects both in acute and chronic wounds.[120] There is also evidence to suggest that these dermal substitutes have the ability to control pain and improve scar quality.[121]

Dermal substitutes are designed to mimic the basic properties of the ECM and share the same functions as normal dermis. These dermal products are categorized currently based on the source of the dermal substitutes as biological or synthetic material. Natural biological dermal substitutes, which include Alloderm, Integra, Glyaderm, Matriderm, Permacol, Strattice, Xenoderm, and Primatrix, are generated from human, porcine, or bovine tissue. The cells within the matrix are eliminated to decrease the risk of immune response, leaving behind a porous, structurally enact ECM. The major advantage of these matrices is in their high similarity to native dermis, rich in collagen and elastin. Furthermore, preparation of these scaffolds results in partial conservation of the basement membrane, which favors keratinocyte adherence.[122] Synthetic materials, such as Dermagraft and Transcyte, are generated with biocompatible material and are advantageous owing to their resistance to tearing, ease of handling, and lack of rejection.[123] These dermal substitutes are often used as temporary coverage for excised burns before autografting to assist in the generation of a neodermis. With the loss of the dermis in extensive full-thickness wounds, the application of dermal substitutes followed by split thickness skin grafting in a 2-stage surgical approach assist in closing the wound and minimize contracture and scar formation.[124]

Although dermal matrices have the potential to form a neodermis, others have proposed the use of scaffolds to deliver stem cells to assist in wound healing. The transplantation of Lgr6+ epithelial stem cell-enriched scaffold has been shown to repair full thickness soft tissue defects and induce hair regeneration.[125] BMSCs and ASCs have also been seeded on acellular dermal matrices and have been shown to enhance proliferation of the epithelial cells, increase angiogenesis, enhance collagen deposition, and minimize scar formation.[126–132] Full-thickness skin wounds treated with BMSCs seeded on acellular dermal matrix demonstrated an increased number of cells colonizing the dermal substitute, suggesting either the recruitment of cells into the wound or the proliferation of seeded cells, as well as increased vascular density, compared with acellular dermal matrix without BMSCs.[133] A comparative analysis of acellular dermal matrix with and without the addition of ASCs demonstrated superior volume retention, vascular density, and collagen content with the application of ASCs on the acellular dermal matrix.[127,129,134] Future studies are needed to provide the functionality of these complex synthetic material for encouraging new tissue growth in vivo under physiologic and pathologic wound conditions. Nevertheless, engineering synthetic biomaterials opens up avenues for investigating the systematic and independent variation of biomolecular and mechanical features of wound healing. In this regard, biomaterials research could provide a better understanding of how the ECM and its mechanical forces affect cell invasion, growth, and differentiation.[135,136] Thus, although synthetic biomaterials are currently simplified mimics of natural ECM, the capacity to manipulate and direct fundamental cell functions and to apply this knowledge to tissue growth and repair will be a cornerstone for the future of regenerative medicine.

STEM CELLS IN CLINICAL TRIALS AND FUTURE PERSPECTIVE

Food and Drug Administration–approved cellular products for regenerative therapies in the clinic have been focused on primary human cells. Over the years, epidermal stem cells, hair follicle stem cells, BMSCs, ASCs, UC-MSC, and muscle satellite cells have been investigated in numerous preclinical studies and a few pilot clinical studies. Cultured epidermal autografts were explored initially to regenerate sheets of epidermal cells; however, the use of epidermal stem cells or hair follicle stem cells, which would reconstitute similar differentiated cells, have not been approved for linical use. Clinical studies have shown that MSCs and ASCs can augment the repair process when applied locally to chronic wounds.[137,138] However, although these studies have been promising, there is no Food and Dug Administration–approved stem cell product on the market for the treatment of wounds. Several steps need to be taken in the future to develop stem cell–based therapies. Identification of the optimal cell populations for the wounds, the most favorable route of delivery, and the time point of cell delivery will be necessary before use of these cells for clinical purposes.[139] Additional biological analyses investigating the mechanism of action, survival, and integration of transplanted cells, and whether cells can establish and maintain their identity in a new microenvironment will also be necessary.[139] Additional large-scale clinical trials are necessary to investigate the safety of these stem cells, both immediately after transplantation and years after transplantation.[140,141] Nevertheless, with the versatility of adult stem cells and the increased interest in coupling bioengineering products with stem cells for regenerative purposes, stem cell therapy may be more promising than just a hypothetical option.

SUMMARY

Over the past decade, considerable insights into the molecular pathways driving skin repair and regeneration have suggested new therapeutic targets and provided scientific rationale for future clinical trials. Recognition of the complexity of the wound healing process and its associated diseases as well as acceptance of the seriousness and mortality related to repair pathologies is critical in these future efforts. Stem cells have gained significant interest, both owing to their self-renewal and differentiation capabilities. In addition, tissue engineering has pioneered biomaterials that allow for the delivery of the stem cells to a specific wound. Further understanding of the interaction with the different stem cells along with their interaction with the biomaterials and the wound bed will lead to the development of novel therapeutic options. Through the use of clinical trials, we can then test the efficacy of these treatments for patients to reduce the burden of large wounds.

REFERENCES

1. Tredget EE, Nedelec B, Scott PG, et al. Hypertrophic scars, keloids, and contractures. The cellular and molecular basis for therapy. Surg Clin North Am 1997;77:701–30.

2. Tredget EE, Levi B, Donelan MB. Biology and principles of scar management and burn reconstruction. Surg Clin North Am 2014;94:793–815.

3. Bielefeld KA, Amini-Nik S, Alman BA. Cutaneous wound healing: recruiting developmental pathways for regeneration. Cell Mol Life Sci 2013;70:2059–81.

4. Singer AJ, Clark RA. Cutaneous wound healing. N Engl J Med 1999;341:738–46.

5. Gauglitz GG, Korting HC, Pavicic T, et al. Hypertrophic scarring and keloids: pathomechanisms and current and emerging treatment strategies. Mol Med 2011;17:113–25.

6. Yang L, Scott PG, Dodd C, et al. Identification of fibrocytes in postburn hypertrophic scar. Wound Repair Regen 2005;13:398–404.

7. Porter C, Hurren NM, Herndon DN, et al. Whole body and skeletal muscle protein turnover in recovery from burns. Int J Burns Trauma 2013;3:9–17.

8. Sommer K, Sander AL, Albig M, et al. Delayed wound repair in sepsis is associated with reduced local pro-inflammatory cytokine expression. PLoS One 2013;8:e73992.

9. Farina JA Jr, Rosique MJ, Rosique RG. Curbing inflammation in burn patients. Int J Inflam 2013;2013:715645.

10. Rose LF, Wu JC, Carlsson AH, et al. Recipient wound bed characteristics affect scarring and skin graft contraction. Wound Repair Regen 2015;23:287–96.

11. Compton CC, Hickerson W, Nadire K, et al. Acceleration of skin regeneration from cultured epithelial autografts by transplantation to homograft dermis. J Burn Care Res 1993;14:653–62.

12. Munster AM. Cultured skin for massive burns. A prospective, controlled trial. Ann Surg 1996;224:372–7.

13. Wainwright DJ. Use of an acellular allograft dermal matrix (AlloDerm) in the management of full-thickness burns. Burns 1995;21:243–8.

14. Debels H, Hamdi M, Abberton K, et al. Dermal matrices and bioengineered skin substitutes: a critical review of current options. Plast Reconstr Surg Glob Open 2015;3:e284.

15. Gurtner GC, Werner S, Barrandon Y, et al. Wound repair and regeneration. Nature 2008;453:314–21.

16. Barrientos S, Stojadinovic O, Golinko MS, et al. Growth factors and cytokines in wound healing. Wound Repair Regen 2008;16:585–601.

17. Knighton DR, Silver IA, Hunt TK. Regulation of wound-healing angiogenesis-effect of oxygen gradients and inspired oxygen concentration. Surgery 1981;90:262–70.

18. Brancato SK, Albina JE. Wound macrophages as key regulators of repair: origin, phenotype, and function. Am J Pathol 2011;178:19–25.

19. Rodero MP, Khosrotehrani K. Skin wound healing modulation by macrophages. Int J Clin Exp Pathol 2010;3:643–53.

20. Koh TJ, DiPietro LA. Inflammation and wound healing: the role of the macrophage. Expert Rev Mol Med 2011;13:e23.

21. Ferrante CJ, Leibovich SJ. Regulation of macrophage polarization and wound healing. Adv Wound Care 2012;1:10–6.

22. Darby IA, Laverdet B, Bonté F, et al. Fibroblasts and myofibroblasts in wound healing. Clin Cosmet Investig Dermatol 2014;7:301–11.

23. Gabbiani G. The myofibroblast in wound healing and fibrocontractive diseases. J Pathol 2003;200:500–3.

24. Abe R, Donnelly SC, Peng T, et al. Peripheral blood fibrocytes: differentiation pathway and migration to wound sites. J Immunol 2001;166:7556–62.

25. Hart J. Inflammation. 1: Its role in the healing of acute wounds. J Wound Care 2002;11:205–9.

26. Skover GR. Cellular and biochemical dynamics of wound repair. Wound environment in collagen regeneration. Clin Podiatr Med Surg 1991;8:723–56.

27. Salo T, Mäkelä M, Kylmäniemi M, et al. Expression of matrix metalloproteinase-2 and -9 during early human wound healing. Lab Invest 1994;70:176–82.

28. Gill SE, Parks WC. Metalloproteinases and their inhibitors: regulators of wound healing. Int J Biochem Cell Biol 2008;40:1334–47.

29. Natarajan S, Williamson D, Stiltz AJ, et al. Advances in wound care and healing technology. Am J Clin Dermatol 2000;1:269–75.

30. Berry DP, Harding KG, Stanton MR, et al. Human wound contraction: collagen organization, fibroblasts, and myofibroblasts. Plast Reconstr Surg 1998;102:124–31.

31. Marks MG, Doillon C, Silvert FH. Effects of fibroblasts and basic fibroblast growth factor on facilitation of dermal wound healing by type I collagen matrices. J Biomed Mater Res 1991;25:683–96.

32. Greenhalgh DG. The role of apoptosis in wound healing. Int J Biochem Cell Biol 1998;30:1019–30.

33. Mascre G, Dekoninck S, Drogat B, et al. Distinct contribution of stem and progenitor cells to epidermal maintenance. Nature 2012;489:257–62.

34. Morasso MI, Tomic-Canic M. Epidermal stem cells: the cradle of epidermal determination, differentiation and wound healing. Biol Cell 2005;97:173–83.

35. Blanpain C, Lowry WE, Geoghegan A, et al. Self-renewal, multipotency, and the existence of two cell populations within an epithelial stem cell niche. Cell 2004;118:635–48.

36. Christiano AM. Epithelial stem cells: stepping out of their niche. Cell 2004;118:530–2.

37. Ohyama M. Hair follicle bulge: a fascinating reservoir of epithelial stem cells. J Dermatol Sci 2007;46:81–9.

38. Ito M, Liu Y, Yang Z, et al. Stem cells in the hair follicle bulge contribute to wound repair but not to homeostasis of the epidermis. Nat Med 2005;11:1351–4.

39. Blanpain C, Fuchs E. Epidermal homeostasis: a balancing act of stem cells in the skin. Nat Rev Mol Cell Biol 2009;10:207–17.

40. Nowak JA, Polak L, Pasolli HA, et al. Hair follicle stem cells are specified and function in early skin morphogenesis. Cell Stem cell 2008;3:33–43.

41. Jensen UB, Yan X, Triel C, et al. A distinct population of clonogenic and multipotent murine follicular keratinocytes residing in the upper isthmus. J Cell Sci 2008;121:609–17.

42. Jensen KB, Collins CA, Nascimento E, et al. Lrig1 expression defines a distinct multipotent stem cell population in mammalian epidermis. Cell Stem cell 2009;4:427–39.

43. Lough DM, Yang M, Blum A, et al. Transplantation of the LGR6+ epithelial stem cell into full thickness cutaneous wounds results in enhanced healing, nascent hair follicle development, and augmentation of angiogenic analytes. Plast Reconstr Surg 2014;133:579–90.

44. Pellegrini G, Ranno R, Stracuzzi G, et al. The control of epidermal stem cells (holoclones) in the treatment of massive full-thickness burns with autologous keratinocytes cultured on fibrin. Transplantation 1999;68:868–79.

45. Ronfard V, Rives JM, Neveux Y, et al. Long-term regeneration of human epidermis on third degree burns transplanted with autologous cultured epithelium grown on a fibrin matrix. Transplantation 2000;70:1588–98.

46. Meyer KC, Klatte JE, Dinh HV, et al. Evidence that the bulge region is a site of relative immune privilege in human hair follicles. Br J Dermatol 2008;159:1077–85.

47. Laverdet B, Micallef L, Lebreton C, et al. Use of mesenchymal stem cells for cutaneous repair and skin substitute elaboration. Pathol Biol (Paris) 2014;62:108–17.

48. Bianco P, Robey PG, Simmons PJ. Mesenchymal stem cells: revisiting history, concepts, and assays. Cell Stem cell 2008;2:313–9.

49. Cizkova D, Rosocha J, Vanicky I, et al. Transplant of human mesenchymal stem cells improve functional recovery after spinal cord injury in the rat. Cell Mol Neurobiol 2006;26:1167–80.

50. Liu H, Kemeny DM, Heng BC, et al. The immunogenicity and immunomodulatory function of osteogenic cells differentiated from mesenchymal stem cells. J Immunol 2006;176:2864–71.

51. Fathke C, Wilson L, Hutter J, et al. Contribution of bone marrow-derived cells to skin: collagen deposition and wound repair. Stem Cells 2004;22:812–22.

52. Sasaki M, Abe R, Fujita Y, et al. Mesenchymal stem cells are recruited into wounded skin and contribute to wound repair by transdifferentiation into multiple skin cell type. J Immunol 2008;180: 2581–7.

53. Wu Y, Chen L, Scott PG, et al. Mesenchymal stem cells enhance wound healing through differentiation and angiogenesis. Stem Cells 2007;25:2648–59.

54. Stoff A, Rivera AA, Sanjib Banerjee N, et al. Promotion of incisional wound repair by human mesenchymal stem cell transplantation. Exp Dermatol 2009;18:362–9.

55. Chen L, Tredget EE, Liu C, et al. Analysis of allogenicity of mesenchymal stem cells in engraftment and wound healing in mice. PLoS One 2009;4: e7119.

56. Falanga V, Iwamoto S, Chartier M, et al. Autologous bone marrow-derived cultured mesenchymal stem cells delivered in a fibrin spray accelerate healing in murine and human cutaneous wounds. Tissue Eng 2007;13:1299–312.

57. Badiavas EV, Falanga V. Treatment of chronic wounds with bone marrow-derived cells. Arch Dermatol 2003;139:510–6.

58. Kwon DS, Gao X, Liu YB, et al. Treatment with bone marrow-derived stromal cells accelerates wound healing in diabetic rats. Int Wound J 2008;5(3): 453–63.

59. Rogers LC, Bevilacqua NJ, Armstrong DG. The use of marrow-derived stem cells to accelerate healing in chronic wounds. Int Wound J 2008;5:20–5.

60. Mizuno H, Tobita M, Uysal AC. Concise review: adipose-derived stem cells as a novel tool for future regenerative medicine. Stem cells 2012;30: 804–10.

61. Gimble JM, Katz AJ, Bunnell BA. Adipose-derived stem cells for regenerative medicine. Circ Res 2007;100:1249–60.

62. Sheng L, Yang M, Liang Y, et al. Adipose tissue-derived stem cells (ADSCs) transplantation promotes regeneration of expanded skin using a tissue expansion model. Wound Repair Regen 2013;21:746–54.

63. Kim WS, Park BS, Sung JH, et al. Wound healing effect of adipose-derived stem cells: a critical role of secretory factors on human dermal fibroblasts. J Dermatol Sci 2007;48:15–24.

64. Strong AL, Bowles AC, MacCrimmon CP, et al. Adipose stromal cells repair pressure ulcers in both young and elderly mice: potential role of adipogenesis in skin repair. Stem Cells Transl Med 2015;4: 632–42.

65. Koellensperger E, Lampe K, Beierfuss A, et al. Intracutaneously injected human adipose tissue-derived stem cells in a mouse model stay at the site of injection. J Plast Reconstr Aesthet Surg 2014;67:844–50.

66. Nambu M, Ishihara M, Kishimoto S, et al. Stimulatory effect of autologous adipose tissue-derived stromal cells in an atelocollagen matrix on wound healing in diabetic db/db mice. J Tissue Eng 2011;2011:158105.

67. Altman AM, Gupta V, Rios CN, et al. Adhesion, migration and mechanics of human adipose-tissue-derived stem cells on silk fibroin-chitosan matrix. Acta Biomater 2010;6:1388–97.

68. Akita S, Akino K, Hirano A, et al. Mesenchymal stem cell therapy for cutaneous radiation syndrome. Health Phys 2010;98:858–62.

69. Kilroy GE, Foster SJ, Wu X, et al. Cytokine profile of human adipose-derived stem cells: expression of angiogenic, hematopoietic, and pro-inflammatory factors. J Cell Physiol 2007;212:702–9.

70. Kamolz LP, Kolbus A, Wick N, et al. Cultured human epithelium: human umbilical cord blood stem cells differentiate into keratinocytes under in vitro conditions. Burns 2006;32:16–9.

71. Mortier L, Delesalle F, Formstecher P, et al. Human umbilical cord blood cells form epidermis in the skin equivalent model. Exp Dermatol 2010;19: 929–30.

72. Luo G, Cheng W, He W, et al. Promotion of cutaneous wound healing by local application of mesenchymal stem cells derived from human umbilical cord blood. Wound Repair Regen 2010;18: 506–13.

73. Huang L, Wong YP, Gu H, et al. Stem cell-like properties of human umbilical cord lining epithelial cells and the potential for epidermal reconstitution. Cytotherapy 2011;13:145–55.

74. Musina RA, Bekchanova ES, Belyavskii AV, et al. Differentiation potential of mesenchymal stem cells of different origin. Bull Exp Biol Med 2006; 141:147–51.

75. Suzdal'tseva YG, Burunova VV, Vakhrushev IV, et al. Capability of human mesenchymal cells isolated from different sources to differentiation into tissues of mesodermal origin. Bull Exp Biol Med 2007;143:114–21.

76. Miki T, Lehmann T, Cai H, et al. Stem cell characteristics of amniotic epithelial cells. Stem cells 2005; 23:1549–59.

77. Allen RE, Boxhorn LK. Regulation of skeletal muscle satellite cell proliferation and differentiation by transforming growth factor-beta, insulin-like growth factor I, and fibroblast growth factor. J Cell Physiol 1989;138:311–5.

78. Montarras D, Morgan J, Collins C, et al. Direct isolation of satellite cells for skeletal muscle regeneration. Science 2005;309:2064–7.

79. Relaix F, Montarras D, Zaffran S, et al. Pax3 and Pax7 have distinct and overlapping functions in adult muscle progenitor cells. J Cell Biol 2006; 172:91–102.

80. Asakura A, Komaki M, Rudnicki M. Muscle satellite cells are multipotential stem cells that exhibit myogenic, osteogenic, and adipogenic differentiation. Differentiation 2001;68:245–53.

81. Csete M, Walikonis J, Slawny N, et al. Oxygen-mediated regulation of skeletal muscle satellite cell proliferation and adipogenesis in culture. J Cell Physiol 2001;189:189–96.

82. Shefer G, Wleklinski-Lee M, Yablonka-Reuveni Z. Skeletal muscle satellite cells can spontaneously enter an alternative mesenchymal pathway. J Cell Sci 2004;117:5393–404.

83. Zhou SB, Chiang CA, Liu K, et al. Intravenous transplantation of bone marrow mesenchymal stem cells could effectively promote vascularization and skin regeneration in mechanically stretched skin. Br J Dermatol 2015;172:1278–85.

84. Yang M, Li Q, Sheng L, et al. Bone marrow-derived mesenchymal stem cells transplantation accelerates tissue expansion by promoting skin regeneration during expansion. Ann Surg 2011; 253:202–9.

85. Bassaneze V, Barauna VG, Lavini-Ramos C, et al. Shear stress induces nitric oxide-mediated vascular endothelial growth factor production in human adipose tissue mesenchymal stem cells. Stem Cells Dev 2010;19:371–8.

86. Colazzo F, Alrashed F, Saratchandra P, et al. Shear stress and VEGF enhance endothelial differentiation of human adipose-derived stem cells. Growth Factors 2014;32:139–49.

87. Ghajar CM, Kachgal S, Kniazeva E, et al. Mesenchymal cells stimulate capillary morphogenesis via distinct proteolytic mechanisms. Exp Cell Res 2010;316:813–25.

88. Kachgal S, Putnam AJ. Mesenchymal stem cells from adipose and bone marrow promote angiogenesis via distinct cytokine and protease expression mechanisms. Angiogenesis 2011;14:47–59.

89. Yoon BS, Moon JH, Jun EK, et al. Secretory profiles and wound healing effects of human amniotic fluid-derived mesenchymal stem cells. Stem Cells Dev 2010;19:887–902.

90. Chen L, Tredget EE, Wu PY, et al. Paracrine factors of mesenchymal stem cells recruit macrophages and endothelial lineage cells and enhance wound healing. PLoS One 2008;3:e1886.

91. Smith AN, Willis E, Chan VT, et al. Mesenchymal stem cells induce dermal fibroblast responses to injury. Exp Cell Res 2010;316:48–54.

92. Kim WS, Park BS, Park SH, et al. Antiwrinkle effect of adipose-derived stem cell: activation of dermal fibroblast by secretory factors. J Dermatol Sci 2009;53:96–102.

93. Boomsma RA, Geenen DL. Mesenchymal Stem cells secrete multiple cytokines that promote angiogenesis and have contrasting effects on chemotaxis and apoptosis. PLoS One 2012;7: e35685.

94. Burlacu A, Grigorescu G, Rosca AM, et al. Factors secreted by mesenchymal stem cells and endothelial progenitor cells have complementary effects on angiogenesis in vitro. Stem Cells Dev 2013;22: 643–53.

95. Lavoie JR, Rosu-Myles M. Uncovering the secretes of mesenchymal stem cells. Biochimie 2013;95: 2212–21.

96. Kapur SK, Katz AJ. Review of the adipose derived stem cell secretome. Biochimie 2013;95:2222–8.

97. Kinnaird T, Stabile E, Burnett MS, et al. Marrow-derived stromal cells express genes encoding a broad spectrum of arteriogenic cytokines and promote in vitro and in vivo arteriogenesis through paracrine mechanisms. Circ Res 2004; 94:678–85.

98. Kinnaird T, Stabile E, Burnett MS, et al. Local delivery of marrow-derived stromal cells augments collateral perfusion through paracrine mechanisms. Circulation 2004;109:1543–9.

99. Waese EY, Kandel RA, Stanford WL. Application of stem cells in bone repair. Skeletal Radiol 2008;37: 601–8.

100. Gamradt SC, Lieberman JR. Genetic modification of stem cells to enhance bone repair. Ann Biomed Eng 2004;32:136–47.

101. Schantz JT, Teoh SH, Lim TC, et al. Repair of calvarial defects with customized tissue-engineered bone grafts I. Evaluation of osteogenesis in a three-dimensional culture system. Tissue Eng 2003;9(Suppl 1):S113–26.

102. Romagnoli C, Brandi ML. Adipose mesenchymal stem cells in the field of bone tissue engineering. World J Stem Cells 2014;6:144–52.

103. Sándor GK, Numminen J, Wolff J, et al. Adipose stem cells used to reconstruct 13 cases with cranio-maxillofacial hard-tissue defects. Stem Cells Transl Med 2014;3:530–40.

104. Bartholomew A, Sturgeon C, Siatskas M, et al. Mesenchymal stem cells suppress lymphocyte proliferation in vitro and prolong skin graft survival in vivo. Exp Hematol 2002;30:42–8.

105. Krampera M, Glennie S, Dyson J, et al. Bone marrow mesenchymal stem cells inhibit the response of naive and memory antigen-specific T cells to their cognate peptide. Blood 2003;101: 3722–9.

106. Rasmusson I, Ringden O, Sundberg B, et al. Mesenchymal stem cells inhibit lymphocyte proliferation by mitogens and alloantigens by different mechanisms. Exp Cell Res 2005;305:33–41.

107. Avniel S, Arik Z, Maly A, et al. Involvement of the CXCL12/CXCR4 pathway in the recovery of skin following burns. J Invest Dermatol 2006;126: 468–76.

08. Toksoy A, Muller V, Gillitzer R, et al. Biphasic expression of stromal cell-derived factor-1 during human wound healing. Br J Dermatol 2007;157: 1148–54.

09. Yoo KH, Jang IK, Lee MW, et al. Comparison of immunomodulatory properties of mesenchymal stem cells derived from adult human tissues. Cell Immunol 2009;259:150–6.

10. Ren G, Su J, Zhang L, et al. Species variation in the mechanisms of mesenchymal stem cell-mediated immunosuppression. Stem Cells 2009; 27:1954–62.

11. Shi Y, Hu G, Su J, et al. Mesenchymal stem cells: a new strategy for immunosuppression and tissue repair. Cell Res 2010;20:510–8.

12. DelaRosa O, Lombardo E, Beraza A, et al. Requirement of IFN-gamma-mediated indoleamine 2,3-dioxygenase expression in the modulation of lymphocyte proliferation by human adipose-derived stem cells. Tissue Eng Part A 2009;15: 2795–806.

13. Xu G, Zhang L, Ren G, et al. Immunosuppressive properties of cloned bone marrow mesenchymal stem cells. Cell Res 2007;17:240–8.

14. Spaggiari GM, Capobianco A, Abdelrazik H, et al. Mesenchymal stem cells inhibit natural killer-cell proliferation, cytotoxicity, and cytokine production: role of indoleamine 2,3-dioxygenase and prostaglandin E2. Blood 2008;111:1327–33.

15. Alexander M, Hu R, Runtsch MC, et al. Exosome-delivered microRNAs modulate the inflammatory response to endotoxin. Nat Commun 2015;6:7321.

16. Eming SA, Martin P, Tomic-Canic M. Wound repair and regeneration: mechanisms, signaling, and translation. Sci Transl Med 2014;6:265sr266.

17. Badylak SF, Weiss DJ, Caplan A, et al. Engineered whole organs and complex tissues. Lancet 2012; 379:943–52.

18. Berthiaume F, Maguire TJ, Yarmush ML. Tissue engineering and regenerative medicine: history, progress, and challenges. Annu Rev Chem Biomol Eng 2011;2:403–30.

19. Orlando G, Wood KJ, Stratta RJ, et al. Regenerative medicine and organ transplantation: past, present, and future. Transplantation 2011;91:1310–7.

20. Shahrokhi S, Arno A, Jeschke MG. The use of dermal substitutes in burn surgery: acute phase. Wound Repair Regen 2014;22:14–22.

21. Hodgkinson T, Bayat A. Dermal substitute-assisted healing: enhancing stem cell therapy with novel biomaterial design. Arch Dermatol Res 2011;303: 301–15.

22. Wilshaw SP, Kearney J, Fisher J, et al. Biocompatibility and potential of acellular human amniotic membrane to support the attachment and proliferation of allogeneic cells. Tissue Eng Part A 2008; 14:463–72.

123. Harding K, Sumner M, Cardinal M. A prospective, multicentre, randomised controlled study of human fibroblast-derived dermal substitute (Dermagraft) in patients with venous leg ulcers. Int Wound J 2013;10:132–7.

124. Pham C, Greenwood J, Cleland H, et al. Bioengineered skin substitutes for the management of burns: a systematic review. Burns 2007;33: 946–57.

125. Lough DM, Wetter N, Madsen C, et al. Transplantation of an LGR6+ epithelial stem cell-enriched scaffold for repair of full-thickness soft-tissue defects: the in vitro development of polarized hair-bearing skin. Plast Reconstr Surg 2016;137: 495–507.

126. Nie C, Yang D, Morris SF. Local delivery of adipose-derived stem cells via acellular dermal matrix as a scaffold: a new promising strategy to accelerate wound healing. Med Hypotheses 2009;72:679–82.

127. Orbay H, Takami Y, Hyakusoku H, et al. Acellular dermal matrix seeded with adipose-derived stem cells as a subcutaneous implant. Aesthetic Plast Surg 2011;35:756–63.

128. Iyyanki TS, Dunne LW, Zhang Q, et al. Adipose-derived stem-cell-seeded non-cross-linked porcine acellular dermal matrix increases cellular infiltration, vascular infiltration, and mechanical strength of ventral hernia repairs. Tissue Eng Part A 2015; 21:475–85.

129. Huang SP, Hsu CC, Chang SC, et al. Adipose-derived stem cells seeded on acellular dermal matrix grafts enhance wound healing in a murine model of a full-thickness defect. Ann Plast Surg 2012;69:656–62.

130. Meruane MA, Rojas M, Marcelain K. The use of adipose tissue-derived stem cells within a dermal substitute improves skin regeneration by increasing neoangiogenesis and collagen synthesis. Plast Reconstr Surg 2012;130:53–63.

131. Lafosse A, Desmet C, Aouassar N, et al. Autologous adipose stromal cells seeded onto a human collagen matrix for dermal regeneration in chronic wounds: clinical proof of concept. Plast Reconstr Surg 2015;136:279–95.

132. Chawla R, Tan A, Ahmed M, et al. A polyhedral oligomeric silsesquioxane-based bilayered dermal scaffold seeded with adipose tissue-derived stem cells: in vitro assessment of biomechanical properties. J Surg Res 2014;188:361–72.

133. Leonardi D, Oberdoerfer D, Fernandes MC, et al. Mesenchymal stem cells combined with an artificial dermal substitute improve repair in full-thickness skin wounds. Burns 2012;38: 1143–50.

134. Lequeux C, Oni G, Wong C, et al. Subcutaneous fat tissue engineering using autologous

adipose-derived stem cells seeded onto a collagen scaffold. Plast Reconstr Surg 2012;130:1208–17.

135. Discher DE, Mooney DJ, Zandstra PW. Growth factors, matrices, and forces combine and control stem cells. Science 2009;324:1673–7.

136. Conway A, Schaffer DV. Biophysical regulation of stem cell behavior within the niche. Stem Cell Res Ther 2012;3:50.

137. Mulder GD, Lee DK, Jeppesen NS. Comprehensive review of the clinical application of autologous mesenchymal stem cells in the treatment of chronic wounds and diabetic bone healing. Int Wound J 2012;9:595–600.

138. Ojeh N, Pastar I, Tomic-Canic M, et al. Stem cells in skin regeneration, wound healing, and their clinical applications. Int J Mol Sci 2015;16:25476–501.

139. Doulatov S, Daley GQ. Development. A stem cell perspective on cellular engineering. Science 2013;342:700–2.

140. Schneider CK, Salmikangas P, Jilma B, et al. Challenges with advanced therapy medicinal products and how to meet them. Nat Rev Drug Discov 2010;9:195–201.

141. von Tigerstrom BJ. The challenges of regulating stem cell-based products. Trends Biotechnol 2008;26:653–8.

Even Better Than the Real Thing? Xenografting in Pediatric Patients with Scald Injury

Paul Diegidio, MD[a], Steven J. Hermiz, MD[b],
Shiara Ortiz-Pujols, MD[a], Samuel W. Jones, MD[a],
David van Duin, MD, PhD[c], David J. Weber, MD, MPH[c],
Bruce A. Cairns, MD[a], Charles Scott Hultman, MD, MBA[a],*

KEYWORDS

• Scald injury • Pediatric burn • Xenograft • Infections

KEY POINTS

- Xenografting seems a reasonable option for patients with partial-thickness scald injuries.
- Although nonoperative management may be appropriate for small/superficial burns, and autografting may be required for large/deep burns, xenografting provides rapid wound closure.
- Xenografting also permits earlier hospital discharge, reduces need for reconstruction, and should strongly be considered as first-line therapy for intermediate-depth pediatric scald injuries.

INTRODUCTION

Scald injuries remain the most common type of burn in children. More than 250,000 children are burned each year in the United States, and 100,000 of these are scald burns.[1] These numbers reflect only children burned badly enough to need medical attention and do not include children whose caretakers do not seek help. The use of xenografting in burns was described as early as 1880,[2] followed by the report of split-thickness or intermediate-thickness skin grafts in 1929.[3] Best practices on treatment of these injuries continue to evolve as new therapies become available and as understanding of immune-mediated rejection of allografts and xenografts continues to improve.

In 2004, the authors developed a new approach to these scald burns, at their institution, based on the need to standardize a pathway for wound care. Patients with partial-thickness wounds were considered for early excision and xenografting to assist with wound closure, previously a far less common procedure done in their pediatric scald population. Xenografting has previously been shown to reduce pain, have some antibacterial action as a function of its adherence, protect against physical trauma, and provide appropriate head and moisture retention.[4]

Over the following years, the authors observed an anecdotal decrease in hospital stay and improved short-term outcomes; however, there continued to be a paucity of evidence in the literature to support these results. It was also evident

Source of Support/Funding: None.
Conflicts of Interest: None.
[a] Department of Surgery, University of North Carolina School of Medicine, Chapel Hill, NC 27599, USA;
[b] Department of Surgery, University of South Carolina School of Medicine, Columbia, SC 29209, USA;
[c] Department of Medicine, University of North Carolina School of Medicine, Chapel Hill, NC 27599, USA
* Corresponding author. 7040 Burnett-Womack, Campus Box 7195, Chapel Hill, NC 27599.
E-mail address: scott_hultman@med.unc.edu

plasticsurgery.theclinics.com

that early operative intervention for wound closure with xenografting provided the opportunity for earlier discharge to home. Decreasing hospital stay has recently been shown to directly decrease costs, reduce incidence of health care–associated infections (HAIs), and provide earlier return to activities.[5,6] The authors, therefore, hypothesized that this institutionally novel therapeutic sequence might may provide similar results in a study population.

During this time, the authors also instituted a laser practice to treat hypertrophic scars that developed from burn injuries. Although the degree of scar formation is most likely related to the depth of injury, the authors also speculated that the type of closure—xenograft, autograft, or local wound care—might also influence the development of hypertrophic scar and the subsequent need for reconstruction. With a significant amount of psychosocial development occurring during childhood and adolescence, the authors wanted to determine which of the interventions would provide the best long-term outcomes, in the shortest time frame, with the fewest interventions, to restore form and function. Children are unique compared with their adult counterparts, in that they continue to grow, and even small, initially asymptomatic scars can become problematic by not lengthening while the surrounding tissue grows.

Despite the short-term success of biologic dressings, like xenografts and allografts, in the treatment of burn wounds,[7–10] there is a paucity of information regarding long-term follow-up of children with scald injury who receive this type of wound coverage. Furthermore, long-term outcomes related to need for reconstruction, with either lasers to treat hypertrophic scars or more invasive procedures to release contracture, are not well defined. In this article, the authors report a 10-year experience with pediatric scald burns, comparing 3 different techniques of wound closure: nonoperative management, xenografting, and autografting. In addition to reporting length of stay (LOS), complications, and costs of the initial admission, reconstructive outcomes are evaluated.

METHODS

After obtaining institutional review board approval, the authors queried the institutional American Burn Association database to identify all patients under the age of 18 years who were admitted with a scald injury to the North Carolina Jaycee Burn Center. The authors identified 1867 subjects who met the inclusion criteria. The timeframe for review

was a 10-year period beginning in January 2004 and extending to December 2013. These patients were then stratified into 3 cohorts based on the wound closure method: (1) nonoperative treatment with local wound care only (although this included patients who had débridement under sedation), (2) operative débridement and xenografting of the scald injury, and (3) excisional preparation and autografting of the scald injury. Patients who underwent autografting at the primary site but also had xenografting of the donor site were assigned to the autografting category.

The data points from the American Burn Association national repository database are prospectively collected, and the initial set of variables included the following: medical record number, name, age, race, gender, county of residence, admission date, injury date, percentage total body surface area (%TBSA), *International Classification of Diseases, Ninth Revision* codes for that visit, number of operating room (OR) procedures during admission, admit status (floor, step-down, or ICU), ICU days, discharge date, LOS, hospital charges, and disposition at discharge.

After initial data receipt from the burn registrar, the authors proceed with review of individual charts, securely housed in an Epic electronic health record (Epic Systems, Verona, Wisconsin), to determine information on posthospital care, which included the following data points: length of outpatient follow-up, time to outpatient referral to a plastic surgeon, OR visits as an outpatient, time to first outpatient OR procedure, number of laser treatments, time to first laser treatment, number of outpatient skin grafts, number of outpatient tissue rearrangements (adjacent tissue rearrangement [ATRs]), and the number of outpatient nerve releases.

After obtaining these additional data points, the authors then investigated the total number of HAIs, by merging the list of patients with the institutional repository of HAIs, recorded in this same timeframe, by hospital epidemiology and infection control. This allowed comparing incidence and type of infections for the 3 different groups: autograft, xenograft, and nonoperative.

Categorical variables, such as gender, plastic surgeon referral, outpatient surgery, outpatient laser, outpatient skin grafts, and tissue rearrangements, were analyzed using 2×2 and 2×3 χ^2-square tables. Continuous/nominal variables, such as age, %TBSA, ICU days, LOS, hospital charges, length of follow-up, time to plastic surgeon consult, time to outpatient OR, time to first laser, and the number of laser treatments, were analyzed using a 2-tailed t test. Statistical significance was assigned for P values less than .05.

RESULTS

Patient demographics and in-hospital variables are shown in **Table 1**. The average age of patients in the autograft group was significantly older compared with the xenograft group (5.75 vs 3.41 years old; $P<.001$). There was no difference, however, in terms of gender ($P = .38$). %TBSA of the scald injury trended larger for the autograft group compared with the xenograft group (12.6% vs 8.1% TBSA; $P = .065$). LOS, however, was significantly longer for the autograft group compared with the xenograft group (22.9 vs 5.2 days; $<.001$). Consistent with this finding, the autograft group also had a longer stay in the ICU (7.28 vs 1.14 days; $P<.001$) compared with the xenograft cohort. Furthermore, incidence of HAIs was significantly increased for patients who required autograft (7.0% vs 0.8%; $P<.001$) compared with the xenograft cohort. Regarding the need for operative intervention, the autograft group also required statistically more visits to the OR compared with the xenograft group (1.3 vs 1.0; $P<.001$); although this is not clinically significant, this finding does reflect the need for staged excision and grafting in some of the autografted patients. The nonoperative group did require operative intervention infrequently, with an average 0.07 trips/patient, or 1 of every 14 patients, for placement of feeding tubes, superficial débridement, and dressing change under sedation.

Incidence and type of HAIs were consistent with previously published data for hospital acquired infections, [11] with pulmonary infections the most frequently encountered (**Table 2**). The autograft group had a total of 21 infections, 6 of which were pulmonary related. In descending order of frequency, the remaining HAIs were found: catheter-associated urinary tract infection (CAUTI) (6); burn cellulitis (3); and 1 each of primary blood stream infection (BSI), secondary BSI, gastroenteritis, superficial incisional infection, and urinary tract infection (UTI). The xenograft group had 4 HAIs: pulmonary (2) and 1 each for primary BSI and superficial incisional. The nonoperative group had 18 HAIs with burn cellulitis the most frequent (8), followed by pulmonary infections (2), and 1 each of the following: CAUTI, primary BSI, gastroenteritis, UTI, cholecystitis, otitis media, superficial incisional, and meningitis.

Facility charges for the initial hospitalization were significantly greater for the autograft group compared with both the xenograft and nonoperative cohorts (\$83,095 vs \$25,504 and \$17,571, respectively; $P<.001$) (**Table 3**). Length of follow-up was significantly longer in the autograft group compared with the xenograft group (286 days vs 104 days; $P<.001$); need for reconstructive surgery was significantly higher in this cohort as well (9.7% vs 3.5%; $P<.001$). The development of hypertrophic scarring was significantly higher in the autograft group compared with the xenograft and nonoperative groups (23.7% vs 8.5% vs 2.8%, respectively; all P values $<.001$).

Patients who required outpatient reconstructive surgery for hypertrophic scars, unstable wounds, and contractures were categorized into 3 groups: (1) contracture release and skin grafting, (2) ATR, and (3) laser therapy (pulsed dye laser photothermolysis and fractional CO_2 ablative resurfacing). Ten patients from the autograft cohort (2.9%) required additional outpatient skin grafting compared with 1 patient in the xenograft group (0.002%; $P<.0001$); 15 patients in the autograft cohort (4.4%) required outpatient tissue rearrangement compared with 9 patients in the xenograft group (1.7%; $P<.01$). There was no significant difference in terms of the number of

Table 1
Demographics and in-hospital variables

	Average Age	Male Gender (%)	Total Body Surface Area (%)	Average No. of Operating Room Visits	Length of Stay (d)	ICU LOS (d)	Incidence of Health Care–Associated Infections
Xenograft n = 534	3.41	55.4	8.08	1.0	5.24	1.14	0.8%
Autograft n = 339	5.75	58.4	12.56	1.3	22.86	7.28	7.0%
P	<.001	.38	.065	<.001	<.001	<.001	<.001
Nonoperative n = 994	4.15	54.7	5.75	0.07	5.09	0.72	1.8%
Total n = 1867	4.34	55.6	8.10	N/A	9.6	2.49	2.3%

Table 2
Health care–associated infections

	Autograft	Xenograft	Nonoperative	Total
Pulmonary	7	2	2	11
Burn cellulitis	3		8	11
CAUTI	6		1	7
Primary BSI	1	1	1	3
Superficial incisional	1	1	1	3
Gastroenteritis	1	—	1	2
UTI	1	—	1	2
Secondary BSI	1	—	—	1
Cholecystitis	—	—	1	1
Otitis media	—	—	1	1
Meningitis	—	—	1	1
Total	21	4	18	—

patients requiring outpatient laser therapy (18 patients in both the autograft and xenograft groups; $P = .16$), and the average number of laser treatments in each group was similar (3.3 average treatments for autograft and 3.7 for xenograft; $P = .2$). Only 1 nerve release was performed in each of the xenograft and autograft groups, with no patients from the nonoperative cohort requiring nerve decompression.

DISCUSSION

In summary, xenografting provides an attractive option for wound closure in partial-thickness scald burns, in the pediatric population. Carefully selected patients benefit from decreased ICU LOS, decreased length of hospitalization, and reduced charges. Furthermore, patients who undergo xenografting seem to have less incidence of hypertophic scarring and less need for recon structive surgery. Children with deep burns an large surface areas require autografting, and pa tients with small superficial scald burns can b managed nonoperatively with topical antimicrobia therapy, but there is clearly a cohort of severity i between these groups, who are ideal for debride ment and xenografting.

Determining the true cost of management i notoriously difficult, due to opaque cost account ing as well as adjusting for size and depth of th burn wound. Although the autograft group yielde higher inpatient charges, it also had increase LOS, ICU days, and HAIs, all of which have bee shown to increase the cost of an admission.[4] Were the authors able to decrease these variable independently of the type of wound coverage patient had, a proportional decrease in cost woul have been likely. With xenografting, however, th

Table 3
Cost and postdischarge variables

	In-Hospital Charges	Length of Follow-up (d)	Incidence of Hypertrophic Scar[a]	Need for Reconstructive Surgery
Xenograft n = 534	$25,504	104	8.5%	3.5%
Autograft n = 339	$83,095	286	23.7%	9.7%
P	<.001	<.001	<.001	<.001
Nonoperative n = 994	$17,571	74	2.8%	1.9%
Total n = 1867	$36,450	123	7.2%	3.6%

[a] Outpatient referral to plastic surgeon used as proxy (see discussion).

authors were able to effect reduced hospital charges indirectly, by decreased overall LOS. The authors' conclusion is that rapid wound closure permits earlier discharge, through reduction of post-débridement pain. Furthermore, a shorter LOS exposed patients to fewer hospital pathogens, theoretically reducing incidence of HAIs.

The autograft group had significantly increased ICU and hospital LOSs, without having an increased %TBSA, compared with the xenograft cohort. What then accounts for these differences? First, there may be selection bias, where patients who may have suffered nonaccidental scalds would be more likely to receive an autograft, because early discharge home was not an option. The authors also considered that over the past few decades, child protection services have become more robust, and, when abuse or neglect is suspected or has to be ruled out, these patients remain hospitalized longer than for accidental etiologies. This might influence clinicians to take longer before performing surgery to see where wounds demarcate, instead of trying to obtain wound coverage as early as possible for discharge home. Individual chart review from the authors' electronic health records did not provide accurate information regarding the incidence of nonaccidental scalding across the 3 treatment groups.

The pattern of autografted patients requiring more resources continued into the outpatient arena. Referral to plastic surgeon as an outpatient was used as a proxy for development of hypertrophic scarring. The authors found by individual chart review that these patients were seen by the senior author (C.S. Hultman) almost exclusively for this reason and, therefore, determined that referral would serve as an accurate proxy of this variable. The etiology and exact mechanisms for hypertrophic scarring remain elusive. Why the xenograft group had a lower incidence of hypertrophic scarring, compared with the autograft group, remains unknown, but may be due to the increased depth of injury requiring replacement of damaged dermis. In 2006, Feng and colleagues[12] compared xenografting to the exposure method, citing an experience of 535 patients over 8 years and presenting 20 individual cases. Their treatment group with xenografting had significantly decreased scar hyperplasia and improved outcomes compared with nonoperative management. The authors theorized that a single dressing would have less damage to the dermis than multiple dressing changes and that a xenograft provided the wound bed the extracellular support needed for rapid healing. This was a clinical study only and did not include histopathologic specimens or measurements of tissue growth factors to compare the 2 groups.

The histopathologic issue was partially addressed using a rat model in 2013 by Chen and colleagues.[13] This study compared xenografting to a povidone iodine cream to determine which group had better growth factors and collagen deposition. They found that the xenograft group had increased collagen, proliferating cell nuclear antigen, K10, β1 integrin, platelet-derived growth factor, epidermal growth factor, and fibroblast growth factor. The investigators hypothesized that these factors provided the xenograft group better collagen synthesis, stem cell proliferation/differentiation, and ultimately improved burn wound healing. Unfortunately, without a direct comparison to an autograft group, it is difficult to say if xenografting would have a similar expression of these cytokines as autografting.

In 2013, Hermans[9] reported their modified systematic review to determine if there was a clinical difference between xenografting and allografting. He concluded that either type of skin substitute seemed to promote rapid wound healing and re-epithelialization.[9] Barone and colleagues,[14] in 2014, evaluated xenografts vs allografts using a miniature swine knockout model where the α-1,3-galactosyltransferase enzyme was removed to prevent hyperacute rejection, due to preformed antibodies to the α-1,3-galactose carbohydrate moiety on porcine cells. They found that the knockout dermis and allograft dermis both survived 11 days without signs of hyperacute rejection. Given the ability of allografts and xenografts to permit wound closure and potentially become incorporated, at least at the level of the dermis, these biomaterials are poised to play an increasing role in resurfacing of burn wounds. Even simple modifications to xenografts, such as the manufacturing of nonmeshed grafts for use on the face to avoid imprinting, can have significant long-term cosmetic benefit.[15,16]

Close attention to the overall cosmetic outcomes by modifying operative technique continues to be of interest. In 2011 Duteille and Perrot[17] published their findings that using a Versajet for débridement in combination with xenografting in 20 patients. They claimed better cosmetic results in facial burn reconstruction, stating that the Versajet (Smith & Nephew, PLC; London, UK) was particularly adapted to facial contours compared with traditional dermatomes and Weck blades (Cadence, Staunton, VA), used for tangential excision.[17]

Finally, although the authors compared xenografting to autografting, several recent publications have proposed combining the 2 methodologies. In

2011 Sun and colleagues[18] used microskin auto-grafts under a layer of split-thickness xenografts for large surface burn coverage with good result in 31 patients with deep burn wounds. In 2013 Chen and colleagues[19] applied small portions of xenografts in their autografted wounds to test if having a combination therapy changed the wound healing process and the final results in 30 patients. They found these cografted areas tended to have healed well with no scar contracture and demonstrated a continuous basal membrane, a mature stratum corneum, rete peg formation, a uniform dermal collagen fiber structure, and fewer capillaries. They also demonstrated improved shape, and functional recovery compared with pure split-thickness autografts.

The obvious limitation of this article is that patients were not randomized into the 3 treatment groups of (1) nonoperative management, (2) débridement and xenografting, and (3) excision and autografting. Surgeons chose 1 of these 3 groups, presumably based on wound characteristics, clinical judgment of time to healing, family resources, and potentially suspicion of child abuse or neglect—which would necessarily mandate a longer LOS. Nevertheless, the data are convincing that xenografting for pediatric patients with scald injury—usually a partial-thickness burn capable of re-epithelialization—is appropriate and safe for large portion of this population. A prospective, randomized trial would help solve the additional questions that remain.

REFERENCES

1. "Pediatric Burns Fact Sheet"; The Burn Foundation. Available at: http://www.burnfoundation.org/programs/resource.cfm?c=1&a=12. Accessed February 3, 2015.
2. Lee EW. Zoografting in a burn case. Boston Med Surg 1880;103:260.
3. Diegidio P. Chapter 1: the use and uses of large split skin grafts of intermediate thickness by Blair VP, and Brown JB (1929). In: Hultman CS, editor. 50 studies every plastic surgeon should know. Boca Raton (FL): CRC Press; Taylor & Francis Group; 2014.
4. Chiu T, Burd A. "Xenograft" dressing in the treatment of burns. Clin Dermatol 2005;23(4):419–23.
5. Zimlichman E, Henderson D, Tamir O, et al. Health Care-associated infections; a meta-analysis of cost and financial impact on the US Health Care System. JAMA Intern Med 2013;173(22):2039–46.
6. Glance LG, Stone PW, Mukamel DB, et al. Increases in mortality, length of stay, and cost associated with hospital acquired infections in trauma patients. Arch Surg 2011;146(7):794–801.
7. Zajicek R, Matouskova E, Broz L, et al. New biological temporary skin cover Xe-Derma® in the treatment of superficial scald burns in children. Burns 2011;37(2):333–7.
8. Hosseini SN, Mousavinasab SN, Fallahnezhat M. Xenoderm dressing in the treatment of second degree burns. Burns 2007;33(6):776–81.
9. Hermans MHE. Porcine xenografts vs. (cryopreserved) allografts in the management of partial thickness burns: is there a clinical difference? Burns 2014;40(3):408–15.
10. Jiong C, Jiake C, Chunmao H, et al. Clinical application and long-term follow-up study of porcine acellular dermal matrix combined with autoskin grafting. J Burn Care Res 2010;31(2):280–5.
11. Weber DJ, van Duin D, Dibiase LM, et al. Health-care-associated infections among patients in a large burn intensive care unit: incidecnea nd pathogens, 2008-2012. Infect Control Hosp Epidemiol 2014;35(10):1304–6.
12. Feng X, Tan J, Pan Y, et al. Control of hypertrophic scar from inception by using xenogenic (porcine) acellular dermal matrix (ADM) to cover deep second degree burn. Burns 2006;32(3):293–8.
13. Chen X, Shi Y, Shu B, et al. The effect of porcine ADM to improve the burn wound healing. Int J Clin Exp Pathol 2013;6(11):2280–91.
14. Barone AAL, Mastroianni M, Farkash EA, et al. Genetically modified porcine split-thickness skin grafts as an alternative to allograft for provision of temporary wound coverage: preliminary characterization. Burns 2014. http://dx.doi.org/10.1016/j.burns.2014.09.003.
15. Chiu T, Shah M. Porcin Xenograft dressing for facial burns: beware of the mesh imprint. Burns 2002;28(3):279–82.
16. Hassan Z, Shah M. Porcine Xenograft dressing for facial burns: meshed versus non-meshed. Burns 2004;30(7):753.
17. Duteille F, Perrot P. Management of 2nd-degree facial burns using the Versajet(®) hydrosurgery system and xenograft: a prospective evaluation of 20 cases. Burns 2012;38(5):724–9.
18. Sun T, Han Y, Chai J, et al. Transplantation of microskin autografts with overlaid selectively decellularized plit0thickness porcine skin in the repair of deep burn wounds. J Burn Care Res 2011;32(3):e67–73.
19. Chen X, Feng X, Xie J, et al. Application of acellular dermal xenografts in full-thickness skin burns. Exp Ther Med 2013;6(1):194–8.

Chemical, Electrical, and Radiation Injuries

Jonathan Friedstat, MD[a], David A. Brown, MD, PhD[b], Benjamin Levi, MD[c],*

KEYWORDS

- Chemical injury • Ocular injury • Electrical injury • Fasciotomy • Compartment syndrome
- Radiation injury

KEY POINTS

- Chemical, radiation, and electrical injuries pose a unique challenge for burn surgeons acutely and during the reconstructive phase.
- Each chemical has unique concerns, but all benefit from immediate removal and dilution.
- Electrical injuries can cause both external flame burns and internal muscle injury.
- Compartment syndrome is an important and potentially destructive clinical sequela of electrical injury that warrants early diagnosis and treatment.
- Radiation exposure causes both short-term damage (skin, gastrointestinal tract) and long-term sequelae (increased risk of malignancy, central nervous system changes, and poor wound healing).

CHEMICAL INJURIES

Epidemiology

Chemical burns are an uncommon form of burn injury, accounting for 2.1% to 6.5% of all burn center admissions.[1] According to the 2015 National Burn Repository report of the American Burn Association, chemical injuries represented 3.4% of patients admitted to participating hospitals over the 2004 to 2015 period. The mean hospital charge for patients with chemical burns was approximately $30,000, which was significantly lower than flame, scald, or electrical injuries. More than 13 million workers in the United States are at risk for dermal chemical exposures, particularly those employed in the agricultural and industrial manufacturing industries. Skin disorders are among the most frequently reported occupational illnesses, resulting in an estimated annual cost in the United States of more than $1 billion.[2]

Overall, chemical burns in the United States occur in roughly equal proportions at work (42.9%) and at home (45.9%), with most work-related exposures occurring in an industrial setting. The highest incidence occurred in the male population between 20 and 60 year old, representing most of the industrial work force. Similarly, a 10-year retrospective study of 690 chemical burn patients admitted to a large hospital in China reported the vast majority of chemical burns occurring in the 20- to 59-year age group (95%), which were most frequently related to work. The most common burn sites were the upper extremities (32%), followed by the head and neck (28%), and lower extremities (20%).[3]

Disclosure Statement: Dr B. Levi was supported by funding from National Institutes of Health/National Institute of General Medical Sciences grant K08GM109105, American Association of Plastic Surgery Academic Scholarship, International FOP Association, Plastic Surgery Foundation Pilot Award and American College of Surgeons Clowes Award. Dr B. Levi collaborates on a project unrelated to this article with Boehringer Ingelheim on a project not examined in this study.

[a] Massachusetts General Hospital, 55 Fruit Street, Boston, MA 02114, USA; [b] Duke University School of Medicine, 8 Duke University Medical Center Greenspace, Durham, NC 27703, USA; [c] Division of Plastic Surgery, University of Michigan School of Medicine, University of Michigan, 1500 East Medical Center Drive, Ann Arbor, MI 48109, USA
* Corresponding author.
E-mail address: blevi@med.umich.edu

A vast number of hazardous chemicals are capable of damaging tissue. The Hazardous Substances Emergency Events Surveillance database of the Centers for Disease Control and Prevention published an analysis of 57,975 chemical injuries over the 1999 to 2008 time period. The chemicals most frequently associated with injury were carbon monoxide (2364), ammonia (1153), chlorine (763), hydrochloric acid (326), and sulfuric acid (318).[4] A 2004 study of military-related chemical burns treated at Brooke Army Medical Center reported 52.9% resulting from munitions (mostly white phosphorus), followed by acid exposures (9.1%), alkali exposure (6.5%), and other chemicals, such as phenol, fluorocarbon, and oven cleaner (6.2%).[1]

Beyond the initial tissue injury, sequelae of chemical burns can include wound infections, cellulitis, sepsis, and complications from scarring. Increasing age is associated with an increase in complications from chemical burns (mostly cellulitis and wound infections), with children under the age of 2 experiencing the lowest rate (2.5%). Complications in the 20- to 50-year age range plateau at 6.4% to 6.7%, which increases significantly with every decade greater than 50 to a maximum of 20.9% in patients older than 80.[5] Sepsis is the most serious complication of chemical burns, which has an overall rate of around 0.6%.[5] Mortality from chemical burns is fortunately low. In the 2014 Annual Report of the American Association of Poison Control Centers' National Poison Data System, 151,796 dermal chemical exposures reported to the agency, and only 8 proved fatal.[6]

Chemical burns are infrequent in children, afflicting 0.9% of admitted pediatric burns at the Parkland Burn Center.[7] It is also not a common form of child abuse, with only 1.4% of nonaccidental pediatric burns resulting from chemical contact.[7] Another study at Children's Hospital Michigan grouped chemical burns in a miscellaneous category of 22% of admitted pediatric patients.[8]

The following article focuses on the dermal and ocular chemical burns most frequently encountered by plastic surgeons. Although oral ingestion is a more common route of toxic chemical exposure,[6] the cause and management are beyond the scope of this article. According to the 2014 Annual Report of the American Association of Poison Control Centers' National Poison Data System, the route of exposure is usually ingestion (83.7% of cases), followed in frequency by dermal (7.0%), inhalation/nasal (6.1%), and ocular (4.3%).

Emergency Management of Chemical Burns

A general approach to the patient with chemical burns involves scene safety, protecting health care workers from exposure, removing the patien from exposure, removing any necessary clothin and jewelry, and brushing off dry chemical with a suitable instrument. Dry lime in particula should be brushed off before attempting irrigation because it contains calcium oxide that reacts wit water to form calcium hydroxide, a strong alkali. I contrast to thermal burns, many chemicals w continue to induce injury until removed, so imme diate clearance of the offending agent is para mount in the intended treatment plan.

For most chemical burn injuries, copious irriga tion with water or saline is the initial treatmen The exceptions to this are elemental metal and possibly phenols. Elemental metals produc exothermic reactions when combined with wate whereas aqueous irrigation of phenols may caus deeper infiltration into tissue. Gentle irrigation c chemical burns under low pressure is essentia because higher pressure irrigation can caus deeper infiltration of the chemical into the ski and place the patient and provider at risk fc splatter injury. Moderately warm water is ofte advised. Irrigation should be started promptl because started initial treatment in the field ha been associated with reduced severity of bur injury and a shorter length of hospitalization.[9] Irr gation should begin with the eyes and face, whic prevents further inhalation or ingestion or toxi Treatment should continue until the pH at th skin surface is neutral, which may take 2 hou or more in the case of alkali burns. Ideally, p at the skin surface should be measured 10 1 15 minutes after discontinuation of irrigatio Litmus paper, if available, is ideal for this purpos Neutralizing agents are generally not recommer ded given the potential for an exothermic read tion to occur between the 2 substances. Th delay in obtaining the neutralizing agent will als allow for deeper tissue injury if water is readi available.

Ocular injuries should be similarly irrigated wi water or saline or until neutral pH is achieve Concentrated ammonia can induce severe ant rior structural injury within 1 minute of exposur whereas lye can cause deeper injury within 3 5 minutes.[10]

The initial management of phenol injuries also somewhat controversial, with some arguir that irrigation may enhance dermal spread ar penetration of the compound. Polyethylene glyc (PEG) has both hydrophilic and hydrophobic pro erties, which may be the ideal method of phen decontamination. However, animal studies hav not shown a significant difference in phen plasma levels when burns were irrigated wi PEG or water.[11] Furthermore, because of the rari of immediate phenol availability at the burn site, irrigation with water is more often advised.[12]

Alkali Burns

Anhydrous ammonia, calcium oxide/hydroxide (lime), and sodium or potassium hydroxide (lye) are common examples of alkalis used in industrial applications or the home. Lime, found in cement and plaster, is the most common cause of alkali burns. It is also known for producing burns of limited depth owing to the precipitation of calcium soaps in fat that limit further penetration. Ammonia and lye do not produce this effect and exhibit deeper and more severe tissue injury.

Anhydrous ammonia is a pungent, colorless gas that sees use in the production of fertilizer, synthetic textiles, and methamphetamine. It is the most common injury associated with illicit methamphetamine production,[13] which has seen a resurgence in the last decade.[14] Anhydrous ammonia is typically stored in refrigerated vessels, and so leakages may cause concomitant chemical and cold injury. Tissue destruction is related to the production of ammonium hydroxide, and more specifically to the concentration of hydroxyl ions. The ensuing damage is a product of liquefactive necrosis, which results in any degree of burn from superficial to full thickness. Anhydrous ammonia is known to have a particularly high affinity for mucous membranes. Mucosa-associated injuries, such as hemoptysis, pharyngitis, pulmonary edema, and bronchiectasis, have all been associated with anhydrous ammonia exposure.[15] Inhalational exposure is extremely toxic. The report of a 2013 mass casualty in China involving anhydrous ammonia described 58 exposed employees, 10 of which died at the scene from inhalational injury, another 5 succumbed en route to the hospital, and the remainder suffered various degrees of pulmonary infection and respiratory failure.[16]

Anhydrous ammonia is soluble in water, and treatment therefore consists of immediate, copious aqueous irrigation. Because of the tendency of alkalis to linger in tissue for prolonged periods, repeat irrigation should be performed every 4 to 6 hours for the first 24 hours. Mechanical ventilation may be necessary for patients with significant facial or pharyngeal burns. Ocular exposure should be irrigated with water or saline until the conjunctival sac pH drops to less than 8.5.[17]

Hydrofluoric Acid

Organic and inorganic acids function by release of H+ and reaction with dermal proteins, which produces coagulative necrosis of the skin. Hydrofluoric acid (HF) is commonly used in the petroleum distillation industry to produce gasoline. It is also widely used in chemical and electronics manufacturing, glass etching, and smelting. Dilute solutions are found in household rust removers and metal cleaning products.[18]

HF displays a unique mechanism of action for an acid. More so than the free H+ released during dissociation, the free fluoride conjugate base ion is thought to be responsible for most tissue injury. Similar to strong alkalis, free H+ is scavenged from fatty acids, resulting in fat saponification and liquefactive necrosis. The free fluoride ion also affects calcium and magnesium cations in the serum, resulting in a systemic hypocalcemia and hypomagnesemia. Hypokalemia can also result from inhibition of the sodium-potassium ATPase and Krebs cycle enzymes.[18]

Tissue damage is progressive, which can persist for days if untreated. Pain may be immediate or delayed depending on the magnitude of exposure, and affected skin will progress from a hardened, indurated appearance to a necrotic eschar. Systemic symptoms may include nausea, abdominal pain, and muscle fasciculation. In advanced cases, QT prolongation, hypotension, and ventricular arrhythmias can occur due to the profound electrolyte disturbances.[18]

In keeping with the initial treatment of most chemical burns, immediate aqueous irrigation is indicated. Acids generally require shorter irrigation times than alkalis, which in the case of HF is approximately 15 to 30 minutes. Blisters should be debrided to allow removal of acid trapped under the desquamated epithelium. In cases of more severe HF burns, detoxification of the fluoride ion is indicated with calcium gluconate. Calcium gluconate promotes formation of an insoluble calcium salt, which can be washed from the skin surface.

Calcium gluconate can be administered by intravenous or intraarterial injection, topically with 2.5% gel, or direct subcutaneous infiltration with a 5% to 10% solution. Topical administration, although effective for superficial exposures, is incapable of neutralizing deeper burns due to the impermeability of the calcium compound. Subcutaneous infiltration may be used for localized burns, which involves injection of 0.5 mL per cubic centimeter via a 27- to 30-gauge needle. HF burns of digits have been treated with direct infiltration, although a regional nerve block is required for adequate anesthesia during the procedure. Along with the risk of digital ischemia from arterial constriction, systemic administration of calcium gluconate is recommended for digital HF burns.[19]

Intravenous or intraarterial injection with 10% calcium gluconate generally requires intensive care unit admission, telemetry, and close monitoring of serum calcium levels. Calcium chloride may also be used, although central venous access is required. The magnitude of dermal exposure need not be extensive for systemic complications to develop. An HF leakage caused by an overturned tanker truck in China in 2014 was responsible for less than 5% total body surface area (TBSA) partial- and full-thickness burns in 4 people, all of whom were treated for inhalational injury and severe hypocalcemia.[20]

White Phosphorous

White phosphorous is a nonmetallic compound that finds widespread use in munitions manufacturing, fireworks, fertilizers, and illicit methamphetamine production. It is present throughout the military arsenal as well.[21] Phosphorous will autoignite with atmospheric oxygen at temperatures greater than 30°C, forming phosphorous pentoxide that then hydrates with exposure to air to form phosphoric acid.

Tissue injury by white phosphorous is caused by both thermal and chemical burns. Phosphoric reacts exothermically with skin, liberating heat and causing thermal burns. Both phosphorous pentoxide and phosphoric acid are capable of inducing chemical burns. Metabolic derangements due to calcium binding and hypocalemia have been reported from white phosphorous absorption, such as bradycardia, QT prolongation, and ST- and T-wave abnormalities.[22] In these cases, calcium gluconate may be required to sustain plasma calcium levels.

Many have recommended the use of copper-containing solutions to neutralize white phosphorous.[22,23] Copper reacts with phosphorous to form black cupric phosphide, which is more easily removed. Copper sulfate also reduces the oxidation potential of phosphorous and consequently can limit deeper tissue injury. However, laboratory experiments have demonstrated no benefit of copper solutions over saline alone,[24] and is generally less available than water or saline. Wartime experience with white phosphorous burns suggests good efficacy with water alone.[25]

Phenol

Phenol (carbolic acid) is an aromatic hydrocarbon derived from coal tar. It has a characteristic strong, sweet odor that can be detected in burn injuries. Phenol has a notable history in surgery from the experiments by Joseph Lister in 1867 for its aseptic properties and ability to disinfect surgical instruments. Phenol is used in the production of a variety of industrial products, such as explosives, fertilizers, paints, rubber, resins, and textiles. Phenol is also used in various commercial soaps, sprays, and ointments as a germicidal antiseptic.[12] Dilute phenol solutions are also commonly used by plastic surgeons as a chemical facial peel, which are usually admixed with water, soap, and croton oil. The solution is applied topically to produce a controlled partial-thickness burn. Upon healing, the dermal collagen reorganization improves the appearance of facial rhytids, actinic keratosis, and irregular pigmentation.

Concentrated phenol and its derivatives are highly reactive with skin, which induce tissue injury by protein denaturation and coagulative necrosis. Following initial contact, coagulative necrosis of the papillary dermis may serve to delay deeper tissue penetration, highlighting the importance of immediate irrigation. Dermal phenol exposure can cause any degree of burn injury from irritation to dermatitis to full-thickness burns. Abnormal, dark pigmentation may also result from dilute phenol exposure. Because of its anesthetic properties, extensive tissue damage can occur before pain is recognized.

Phenol is poorly soluble in water, and there is some concern that inadequate irrigation will merely spread the chemical over uninjured areas of skin, resulting in a larger burn area and potentially greater systemic absorption. PEG serves as a hydrophobic solvent, which can more readily dissolve phenol. PEG is usually available in hospital pharmacies and is probably the preferred antidote for phenol burns, although this is somewhat controversial. Although the mechanism is understood, clinical studies of phenol neutralization with PEG are lacking. In a 1978 study of swine acutely exposed to phenol, plasma phenol levels were not significantly different in swine decontaminated with PEG or water.[11] Thus, as with most chemical burns, the recommended initial treatment is copious irrigation with water until PEG is available. Irrigation should continue with either PEG or water because dilute phenol solutions are more easily absorbed through the skin. Water irrigation should not be delayed while awaiting PEG availability. In a case series of 4 patients with extensive phenol burns in China, both water and PEG were used.[12]

Systemic toxicity from phenol poisoning can also result, with the cardiovascular and central nervous systems primarily affected. Neurologic symptoms include mental status changes, lethargy, seizures, or coma. Cardiovascular toxicity may present as bradycardia or tachycardia. Hypotension, hypothermia, and metabolic acidosis can

ccur with severe exposure. Treatment of sys-
emic toxicity is largely supportive with fluid resus-
tation and vasopressors as needed.

cular Injuries

hemical burns to the eye and eyelid are a
equent cause of emergency room visits, totaling
oproximately 2 million cases per year.[26] Approx-
nately 15% to 20% of facial burns involve the
ye,[27] and ocular injury stands as the second lead-
g cause of visual impairment in the United States
fter cataracts.[26] Similar to dermal chemical in-
ries, alkali exposures are more common and
enerally cause deeper and more serious tissue
amage than acid. Common offending agents in
ie household include automobile batteries, pool
eaners, detergents, ammonia, bleach, and drain
eaners.[28] Patients may present with decreased
sion, eye pain, blepharospasm, conjunctivitis,
nd photophobia. In severe cases of alkali burns,
ie globe may appear white due to ischemia of
ie conjunctiva and scleral blood vessels.

Alkali injuries such as lime and ammonia pene-
ate readily into eye, injuring stroma and endothe-
um as well as intraocular structures such as the
s, lens, and ciliary body. Acid injuries are generally
ss severe because the immediate precipitation of
oithelial proteins confers a protective barrier to
traocular penetration.[28] Periocular injuries are
ommon, where the depth of injury often correlates
ith scar formation. Debridement of devitalized
eriocular tissue is important to protect the ocular
urface from exposure keratopathy and corneal ul-
eration. Profound dermal injury may result in cica-
icial ectropion, which often requires tarsorrhaphy
' excision and full-thickness skin grafting.[26]

Ocular burns are categorized into 4 grades, with
rade IV representing the most severe. Grade I
urns are associated with hyperemia, conjunctival
cchymosis, and defects in the corneal epithelium.
rade II burns include haziness in the cornea.
rade III burns are associated with deeper pene-
ation into the cornea and present with mydriasis,
ray discoloration of the iris, early cataract forma-
on, and ischemia in less than half of the limbus.
rade IV burns appear similar to grade III but
ith ischemia involving more than half of the
nbus. They are also associated with necrosis of
ie bulbar and tarsal conjunctiva.[29]

Immediate irrigation with water is the initial ther-
by for ocular injuries, beginning at the scene and
ontinuing to the emergency department. Animal
udies have consistently demonstrated better
utcomes when the eye is rinsed early and thor-
ughly after chemical exposure,[30,31] relating to
ie progressive neutralization of pH with water

volume. Prolonged irrigation is best achieved using intravenous tubing and a polymethylmethacry-
late (Morgan) lens, although when no such device
is available, it is important to keep the eyelids
retracted to assure adequate irrigation of the conjunctiva and cornea.

ELECTRICAL INJURIES
Clinical Background

As one of the most devastating and debilitating injuries cared for in burn centers, electrical injuries
comprise 4% of all reported causes. Burn surgeons must keep in mind that electrical injuries
are unique because they may cause a flash and
external burn but also internal burns from the current, which heats up bone and burns muscle as
it invests bone. Electrical injuries occur more
frequently in adults than children because most
result from occupational exposure. Patients who
have high-voltage electrical injuries, defined as
greater than 1000 V, are at elevated risk of spine
fracture injury due to tetany and require complete
immobilization until vertebral injury is ruled out.
Providers must also evaluate patients with high-
voltage injuries for cardiac damage. Direct muscle
injury from current flow may cause gross myoglobinuria, requiring more aggressive fluid resuscitation.[32] Patients with gross myoglobinuria often
require fasciotomy of affected limbs, and a severe
electrical injury often requires monitoring in the
intensive care unit. Bone has the highest conduc-
tance, and electricity flows along the skeleton,
causing significant muscle necrosis adjacent to
the bone. TBSA is not necessarily associated
with prognosis, and TBSA does not quantify damage to deep tissues in electrical injuries. Entrance
and exit wound should be assessed when evaluating which extremities should be closely monitored for compartment syndrome.

Thermal injuries occur as electricity can
generate temperatures greater than 100°C. Elec-
troporation occurs as electrical force drives water
into lipid membrane, causing cell rupture. Tissue
resistance in decreasing order includes bone, fat,
tendon, skin, muscle, vessel, nerve. Bone heats
to a high temperature and burns surrounding
structures, such as muscle, which is the reason
muscle swelling and compartment syndrome are
common in high-voltage electrical injuries.

Alternating current causes tetanic muscle
contraction and the "no let-go" phenomenon.
This phenomenon occurs because of simultaneous contraction of (stronger) forearm flexors
and (weaker) forearm extensors. Current flow
through tissue can cause burns at entrance/exit
wounds and hidden injury to deep tissues. Current

will preferentially travel along low-resistance pathways. Current will pass through soft tissue, contact high-resistance bone, and travel along bone until it exits to the ground. Vascular injury to nutrient arteries and damage to intima and media can result in thrombosis.

Electrical exposure can cause significant injuries to other organ systems besides the skin and musculoskeletal system. From a cardiac standpoint, arrhythmias are common at the scene (any voltage) or in the hospital (high voltage ≥1000). Heart rhythm should be monitored continuously for at least 24 hours if cardiac injury is suspected at the scene or if a high-voltage injury has occurred. Ventricular fibrillation and asystole are the most common, and Advanced Cardiac Life Support should be instituted immediately. Coronary artery spasm and myocardial injury and infarction have also been described. A normal cardiac rhythm on admission, however, means dysrhythmia is unlikely, and thus, 24-hour monitoring is not needed.[33] In addition, injury to solid organs, acute bowel perforation, and gallstones after myoglobinuria have been described and should be monitored. Myoglobinuria occurs due to the disruption of muscle cells. Myoglobinuria from other causes requires increased fluid administration; however, burn resuscitation usually provides adequate fluid. Cataracts are also a long-term adverse effect of electrical injury, necessitating an ophthalmology evaluation and follow-up.

When taking the patient to the operating room for debridement and grafting of electrical injuries, the physician should perform serial debridements and allow the tissue to completely declare itself. These injuries will often evolve with progressive muscle necrosis over time, thus early grafting (within the first week) often fails to fully close the burn wound. These injuries have similarities to crush injuries, and thus, multiple trips to the operating room for debridement should not be viewed as a failure.

Pathophysiology

Electrical burns have the potential for 3 types of injury: (1) True electrical injury by current flow; (2) Arc injury from the electrical arc as it passes from the source to an object; and (3) Flame injury from ignition of clothing or surroundings. Electricity arcs occur at temperatures up to 4000°C and can create a slash injury as seen in electricians. Clinicians must keep in mind that the force of the electrical injury may throw the patient, causing additional trauma, ruptured eardrums, and internal organ contusion. Electricity flows through the tissue of greatest resistance, which

in humans is bone. In general, the severity of the injury is inversely proportional to the cross sectional area of the body part with the most severe regions seen in the wrist and ankle and decreasing proximally. Deeper tissues and region between 2 bones (tibia and fibula; ulna and radius also retain heat to a greater degree. Macroscopic and microscopic vascular injury can occur immediately and is often not reversible.[34]

Admission Criteria

All patients with high-voltage injury, electrocardiograph (ECG) changes, loss of consciousness, c concern for extremity compartment syndrom are standard indications for admission. Patients however, with low-voltage injuries and norma ECG can be discharged home if no other indication is present.[35] Although the duration of moni toring after admission is not known, most report recommend 24 hours after admission if there ar no ECG abnormalities.

Evaluation of the Extremity

Given that the entrance wound of electrical injurie often involves the upper or lower extremity and th devastating nature of compartment syndrome surgeons must be extremely vigilant when evalu ating electrical injury patients. Additional evalua tion must be performed in patients who preser with loss of consciousness or who were intubate in the field. Unlike compartment syndrome fron flame burns where the constricting tissue is th burn eschar, the constricting tissue in electrica injury patients is the fascia as the muscle swell after being heated up by the current runnin through the bone. Signs of compartment syr drome from electrical injury are similar to othe causes of compartment syndrome with pain o passive extension as the most telling sign. Add tional signs include pain out of proportion to exam ination, paresthesia, and pulselessness. The last 2 however, occur in very late stages of the process In patients who are not able to participate in an ex amination, any mechanism of concern warrant consultation by a plastic or hand surgeon an likely measurement of compartment pressure Any absolute pressure greater than 30 or diastoli pressure–compartment pressure less than 30 ind cates compartment syndrome. Fasciotomie should be performed in the presence of compar ment syndrome, making sure to decompress a compartments affected.

Fasciotomy of the Upper Extremity

There are 4 compartments in the forearm (superf cial volar, deep volar, dorsal, mobile wad) and 1 compartments in the hand (4 dorsal interossei, 3 palmar interossei, hypothenar, thenar, and adductor pollicis). When marking the incisions, the surgeon must incorporate the knowledge of this anatomy. In the hand, all compartments can be accessed through 4 separate incisions: 2 incisions along the second and fourth dorsal meta-carpal, and 1 each on glabrous-nonglabrous junc-tion of the thenar and hypothenar eminences (**Fig. 1**). In addition, a carpal tunnel release is often performed at the same time using a standard car-pal tunnel incision that is 2 to 3 cm along the inter-section of a line parallel to ulnar side of thumb (Kaplan cardinal line) and the radial part of fourth ray (**Fig. 2**). Classic descriptions of a forearm fasciotomy include a lazy S starting 1 cm proximal and 2 cm lateral to the medial epicondyle and carried out obliquely across the antecubital fossa toward the mobile wad and then curved distally and ulnarly reaching the midline at the forearm at the junction of the mid and distal one-third of the forearm and then continuing distally just ulnar to the palmaris tendon and then distally incorporating Guyon canal and the carpal tunnel. Volar release must include the pronator quadratus and deep flexor compartments as well.[36] Often a separate ulnar escharotomy is needed for elec-trical injuries with concomitant burns (**Fig. 3**). Recent studies, however, have shown that a smaller incision (**Fig. 4**) along the lazy S may be sufficient to release the volar compartments without as much morbidity or wound-healing com-plications. The dorsal compartment is released with an incision between the lateral epicondyle and ulnar styloid. To allow for improved postre-lease healing, the authors usually create a "Roman sandal" constructed of vessel loops, which apply gentle traction to the wound edges to prevent skin recoil and minimize gaping. With regards to digits, there is no true fascial compartment, and thus a fasciotomy is not indicated. However, if eschar is circumferential around the digits, the authors recommend radial and ulnar release of the eschar more dorsal to the course of the neuro-vascular bundle.

Fasciotomy of the Lower Extremity

Diagnosis of compartment syndrome in the lower extremity is similar to diagnosis in the upper ex-tremity. There are 4 compartments to the lower extremity: Superficial posterior, deep posterior, lateral, anterior. These compartments can be released through a double-incision fasciotomy with one incision centered between the fibular shaft and the crest of the tibia overlying the intra-muscular septum between the anterior and lateral compartments. After the skin is incised, subcu-taneous flaps are developed medially and laterally to expose the fascia of the intramuscular (IM)

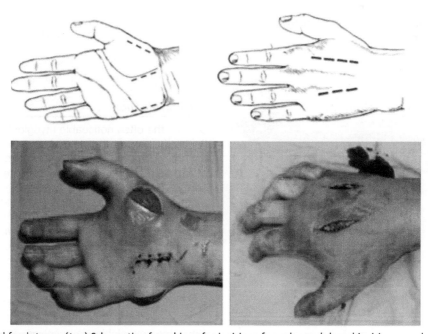

Fig. 1. Hand fasciotomy. (*top*) Schematic of markings for incisions for volar and dorsal incisions needed to release the compartments of the hand including the carpal tunnel. (*bottom*) Incisions made for release of the hand com-partments, including a carpal tunnel release.

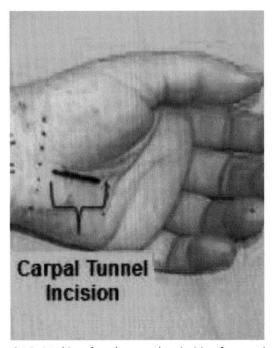

Carpal Tunnel Incision

Fig. 2. Markings for where to place incision for carpal tunnel release.

septum and fascia of the anterior and lateral compartments. Care must be taken to avoid injury to the peroneal nerves. The medial incision is placed 2 cm medial to the tibia between the anterior IM septum and tibial crest, taking care to avoid the saphenous vein and nerve. The superficial posterior compartment is decompressed by incising the gastrocnemius fascia, and the deep posterior compartment is decompressed by dividing the

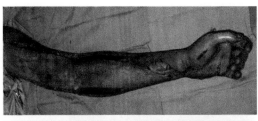

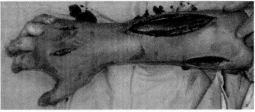

Fig. 3. Open fasciotomy incisions of the arm. (*top*) Volar incisions releasing the proximal arm and volar forearm. (*bottom*) Dorsal incisions releasing the forearm and hand.

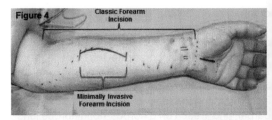

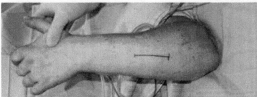

Fig. 4. Minimally invasive incision markings for forearm compartment release. (*top*) Minimally invasive volar forearm incision to release the volar forearm compartments. (*bottom*) Minimally invasive incision marked dorsally for dorsal forearm compartment release.

attachments of the soleus to the tibia, providing access to the posterior tibialis muscle.

Cardiac Evaluation

Indications for cardiac monitoring include ECG abnormality or evidence of ischemia, documented dysrhythmia before or after emergency room admission, loss of consciousness, and cardiopulmonary resuscitation in the field. Most studies recommend monitoring for 24 to 48 hours.[35] The most common arrhythmias include nonspecific ST-T changes and atrial fibrillation. Myocardial damage and dysrhythmias are seen soon after injury, and unfortunately, troponin is not always a useful diagnostic of myocardial injury.[37,38]

Renal Evaluation

Despite the often noticeable myoglobinuria in patients with severe electrical injuries, the incidence of renal failure is small. Treatment is similar to other burn patients wherein appropriate resuscitation is crucial. Historically, patients were given mannitol and sodium bicarbonate in attempts to alkalinize the urine; however, studies have failed to demonstrate improved outcomes over standard resuscitation protocols. In general, electrical injury patients with darker-colored urine should receive Lactated Ringers solution to maintain urine output double the goal rate or approximately 100 mL/h. If the urine fails to improve, the clinician should evaluate for ongoing ischemia and muscle necrosis. Once the myoglobinuria resolves, fluids should be titrated back to a urine output goal of 30 to 50 mL/h.

Secondary Complications of Electrical Injury

Cataract formation is a common complication after electrical injury and has been published to occur in 5% to 20% of electrical injury patients.[39] Early ophthalmology consultation as well as postdischarge follow-up is crucial for these patients because cataracts can arise in a delayed fashion.[40] Central and peripheral neurologic complications are also common and range from paralysis to Guillain-Barré, paresis, and transverse myelitis. Central manifestations include cognitive and emotional changes.[41,42]

Acute Burn Treatment of Electrical Injury

After stabilization and resuscitation of the electrical injury patient, general burn care principles are applied to this patient population. In general, early debridement is still a central tenant of electrical burn care. For electrical injury, however, the deeper injury to the muscle may not be evident in early debridements. Thus, serial debridements with temporary wound vacuum-assisted closure (VAC) or dressing changes help allow time for the wound to completely declare itself before autograft. The surgeon can also use a temporary coverage with human allograft as a "test" to see if the wound bed is ready. If the allograft has good take, then likely the wound is ready for autograft. Thickness of the autograft should be dictated by the location of the injury with thicker split-thickness grafts used on the hands and face (0.014- to 0.018-inch thickness).

Reconstructive Challenges of Electrical Injury

Burn injuries to the oral cavity are the most common type of serious electrical burns in young children often due to them chewing on an electrical cord, causing injury to the oral commissure. Care includes conservative management with occupational therapy and parental monitoring for bleeding from the labial artery. Subsequent reconstruction of the oral commissure is best addressed with V-Y or ventral tongue flaps.[43,44] Peripheral nerve injury is seen commonly after electrical injury. If the patient has symptoms of compressive peripheral neuropathy, a decompressive corrective surgery should be performed.[45] Late consequences of electrical injury, similar to severe thermal burns, include joint contractures and heterotopic ossification (HO). HO may be seen more commonly in electrical injury patients due to the large amount of tissue damage and the known correlation between severity of injury and HO.[46] HO is most commonly seen when the upper extremity is involved, and most frequently seen in the elbow.[47] Currently, no early

diagnostic or prophylactic strategies for this difficult complication exist.[48]

RADIATION BURNS
Clinical Background

Ever since the world was introduced to the power of nuclear weapons in 1945 with the bombings of Hiroshima and Nagasaki, the world has been forever changed. The power of nuclear weapons was seen firsthand, and the impact of radiation and its impact for injury began to be appreciated. From the bombings of Hiroshima and Nagasaki, many important lessons were learned. One was that proximity to the detonation directly impacted mortality with 86% fatality rates at 0.6 miles from ground zero, and it decreased to 27% at 0.6 to 1.6 miles, and then 2% for those 1.6 to 3.1 miles away. In addition, the mortality was highest during the first 20 days. Of the 122,338 fatalities at Hiroshima, 68,000 occurred within that timeframe. Of the 197,743 survivors, 79,130 were injured, and the remaining 118,613 were uninjured. It is estimated that those injured at Hiroshima contained 90% with burns, 83% with traumatic injuries, and 37% with radiation injuries.[49,50]

The devastation of these weapons is massive and has some understood properties. The explosion generates high-speed winds that can travel at dramatic speeds. A 20-kiloton nuclear device generates 180 mph winds 0.8 miles from the epicenter. These winds occur with a direct pressure and indirect wind drag, and the pressure wave can destroy windows and buildings and injure parts of the body that are sensitive to pressure changes, such as the lungs and ears. It results in ruptured tympanic membranes, pulmonary contusions, pneumothoraces, and hemothoraces. A fireball that results from the explosion results in thermal injuries and also sends radioactive material into the air. Near ground zero, the thermal injuries are nearly 100% fatal due to incineration from the high temperatures. Radiation is dispersed in a linear fashion and results in burns that vary in severity depending on the distance from ground zero and the time of exposure. Radiation is also dispersed into the air and follows wind patterns, ultimately settling to the ground.[49,50]

Radioactive material results in both acute injury from immediate exposure and more prolonged injury from delayed exposure to radioactive fallout or contamination. From what is known from a 10-kiloton nuclear bomb detonation, people at a distance 0.7 miles from ground zero absorb 4.5 Gy (1 Gy, Gy equals 1 Sievert, Sv). At

60 days, the radiation dose lethal dose, 50% is 3.5 Sv; with aggressive medical care, this dose might be doubled to nearly 7 Sv. To put this in context, radiation exposure from a diagnostic computed tomographic scan of the chest or abdomen is 5 mSv, and the average annual background absorbed radiation dose is 3.6 mSv. Radiation is known to impact several organ systems and result in several syndromes based on increasing exposure doses. These syndromes include the hematologic syndrome (1–8 Sv exposure), gastrointestinal syndrome (8–30 Sv exposure), and cardiovascular/neurologic systems (>30 Sv exposure), with the latter 2 being nonsurvivable.[49–51]

After initial evaluation and decontamination by removing clothing and washing radiation material from the skin, a useful way to estimate exposure is by determining the time to emesis. Patients that do not experience emesis within 4 hours of exposure are unlikely to have severe clinical effects. Emesis within 2 hours suggests a dose of at least 3 Sv, and within 1 hour is at least 4 Sv. The hematologic system follows a similar dose-dependent temporal pattern for predicting radiation exposure, mortality, and treatment. These values have been determined based on the Armed Forces Radiobiology Research Institute's Biodosimetry Assessment Tool and can be downloaded from www.afrri.usuhs.mil.

The combination of radiation exposure to burn wounds has the potential to increase mortality compared with traditional burns. Early closure of wounds before radiation depletes circulating lymphocytes may be needed for wound healing (which occurs within 48 hours). Also, in radiation injuries combined with burn or trauma, laboratory lymphocyte counts may be unreliable.[49–52] A significant difference between burn/traumatic injuries and radiation injuries is that burn/traumatic injuries can result in higher mortality when not treated within hours.

Decontamination and triage are vital to maximize the number of survivors. Initial decontamination requires removal of clothing and washing wounds with water. Irrigation fluid should be collected to prevent radiation spread into the water supply. Work by many professional organizations, including the American Burn Association has focused on nationwide triage for disaster and will be vital to save as many lives as possible. Partnerships between emergency medical services, emergency medicine, trauma surgeons, burn surgeons, medical oncology, radiation oncology, and others will be vital because their injuries will require multidisciplinary care in ways not experienced before in modern medicine. It is quite possible that expectant or comfort care could be offered to more patients than typically seen in civilian hospitals, because of resource availability after the disaster.

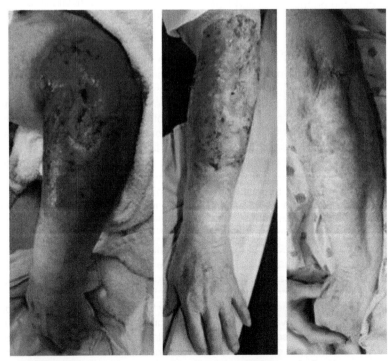

Fig. 5. Radiation burn to the arm over time as it was allowed to heal secondarily.

Iatrogenic Radiation Burns

Ionizing radiation therapy has become an important component in the treatment of many different types of cancer. It has important therapeutic treatments that include goals of curing a patient of a given malignancy as well as palliative goals, to improve their quality of life. Although there is considerable adjustment to the technique of administration, the total dose, volume, and individual variations, these are the variables considered to have the largest impact on skin changes from radiation.[53] It is also thought that in radiation-treated areas, around 85% of patients will have a moderate to severe skin reaction that can lead to blistering, ulceration, and erosion (Fig. 5).[54] When severe, it can interrupt radiation therapy, which can also have implications for their oncologic treatment and is known as acute radiation dermatitis. The other common problem patients can experience occurs months to years after treatment, whereby the skin develops progressive, permanent, irreversible changes from chronic radiation dermatitis.

Acute radiation dermatitis commonly included changes that occur within 90 days of radiation exposure.[55] There is a grading system developed by the National Cancer Institute to classify radiation dermatitis and includes 4 stages; this staging system is helpful because the clinical treatments are tied to the stage of injury. Grade 1 injuries have faint erythema or dry desquamation. Grade 2 has moderate to brisk erythema with patchy desquamation confined to creases and skin folds. Grade 3 injury contains moist desquamation outside folds with pitting edema, and bleeding from minor trauma. Grade 4 has full-thickness skin necrosis or ulceration with spontaneous bleeding. In terms of treatment, they vary based on the degree of injury. Grade 1 injuries are treated with hydrophilic moisturizers, and pruritus and irritation are treated with low-dose steroids. Grades 2 and 3 injuries focus on preventing secondary infection. Hydrogel dressing and hydrocolloids are commonly used. Grade 4 injuries are treated like full-thickness burn injuries and can require debridement with skin grafts, or flaps. Chronic wounds are watched more closely for selective debridement because they can evolve over time. They are poorly vascularized and can require more complex reconstructive procedures, including pedicled and free flaps.[53]

REFERENCES

1. Barillo DJ, Cancio LC, Goodwin CW. Treatment of white phosphorus and other chemical burn injuries at one burn center over a 51-year period. Burns 2004;30:448–52.

2. Boeniger MF, Ahlers HW. Federal government regulation of occupational skin exposure in the USA. Int Arch Occup Environ Health 2003;76:387–99.

3. Ye C, Wang X, Zhang Y, et al. Ten-year epidemiology of chemical burns in western Zhejiang Province, China. Burns 2016;42:668–74.

4. Anderson AR, Centers for Disease Control and Prevention (CDC). Top five chemicals resulting in injuries from acute chemical incidents—Hazardous Substances Emergency Events Surveillance, nine states, 1999-2008. MMWR Suppl 2015;64:39–46.

5. 2015 National Burn Repository Report of Data from 2005-2014. 2015.

6. Mowry JB, Spyker DA, Brooks DE, et al. 2014 annual report of the American Association of Poison Control Centers' National Poison Data System (NPDS): 32nd annual report. Clin Toxicol (Phila) 2015;53:962–1147.

7. Hodgman EI, Pastorek RA, Saeman MR, et al. The Parkland Burn Center experience with 297 cases of child abuse from 1974 to 2010. Burns 2016; 42(5):1121–7.

8. Shah A, Suresh S, Thomas R, et al. Epidemiology and profile of pediatric burns in a large referral center. Clin Pediatr 2011;50:391–5.

9. Leonard LG, Scheulen JJ, Munster AM. Chemical burns: effect of prompt first aid. J Trauma 1982;22: 420–3.

10. Spector J, Fernandez WG. Chemical, thermal, and biological ocular exposures. Emerg Med Clin North Am 2008;26:125–36, vii.

11. Pullin TG, Pinkerton MN, Johnston RV, et al. Decontamination of the skin of swine following phenol exposure: a comparison of the relative efficacy of water versus polyethylene glycol/industrial methylated spirits. Toxicol Appl Pharmacol 1978;43:199–206.

12. Lin T-M, Lee S-S, Lai C-S, et al. Phenol burn. Burns 2006;32:517–21.

13. Bloom GR, Suhail F, Hopkins-Price P, et al. Acute anhydrous ammonia injury from accidents during illicit methamphetamine production. Burns 2008;34: 713–8.

14. Davidson SB, Blostein PA, Walsh J, et al. Resurgence of methamphetamine related burns and injuries: a follow-up study. Burns 2013;39:119–25.

15. Amshel CE, Fealk MH, Phillips BJ, et al. Anhydrous ammonia burns case report and review of the literature. Burns 2000;26:493–7.

16. Zhang F, Zheng XF, Ma B, et al. Mass chemical casualties: treatment of 41 patients with burns by anhydrous ammonia. Burns 2015;41:1360–7.

17. White CE, Park MS, Renz EM, et al. Burn center treatment of patients with severe anhydrous ammonia injury: case reports and literature review. J Burn Care Res 2007;28:922–8.

18. Wang X, Zhang Y, Ni L, et al. A review of treatment strategies for hydrofluoric acid burns: current status and future prospects. Burns 2014;40:1447–57.

19. Yuanhai Z, Liangfang N, Xingang W, et al. Clinical arterial infusion of calcium gluconate: the preferred method for treating hydrofluoric acid burns of distal human limbs. Int J Occup Med Environ Health 2014;27:104–13.

20. Zhang Y, Wang X, Sharma K, et al. Injuries following a serious hydrofluoric acid leak: first aid and lessons. Burns 2015;41:1593–8.

21. Davis KG. Acute management of white phosphorus burn. Mil Med 2002;167:83–4.

22. Chou TD, Lee TW, Chen SL, et al. The management of white phosphorus burns. Burns 2001;27:492–7.

23. Kaufman T, Ullmann Y, Har-Shai Y. Phosphorus burns: a practical approach to local treatment. J Burn Care Rehabil 1988;9:474–5.

24. Eldad A, Wisoki M, Cohen H, et al. Phosphorous burns: evaluation of various modalities for primary treatment. J Burn Care Rehabil 1995;16:49–55.

25. Karunadasa KP, Abeywickrama Y, Perera C. White phosphorus burns managed without copper sulfate: lessons from war. J Burn Care Res 2010;31:503.

26. Pargament JM, Armenia J, Nerad JA. Physical and chemical injuries to eyes and eyelids. Clin Dermatol 2015;33:234–7.

27. Liu H, Wang K, Wang Q, et al. A modified surgical technique in the management of eyelid burns: a case series. J Med Case Rep 2011;5:373.

28. Rao NK, Goldstein MH. Acid and alkali burns. In: Yanoff M, Duker J, editors. Ophthalmology. 4th edition. Philadelphia: Saunders; 2014. p. 296–8.

29. Levine MD, Zane R. Chemical injuries. In: Marx JA, Hocksberger RS, Walls RM, editors. Rosen's emergency medicine concepts and clinical practice. 8th edition. Philadelphia: Saunders; 2014. p. 818–28.

30. Paterson CA, Pfister RR, Levinson RA. Aqueous humor pH changes after experimental alkali burns. Am J Ophthalmol 1975;79:414–9.

31. Rihawi S, Frentz M, Becker J, et al. The consequences of delayed intervention when treating chemical eye burns. Graefes Arch Clin Exp Ophthalmol 2007;245:1507–13.

32. DiVincenti F, Moncrief J, Pruitt BJ. Electrical injuries: a review of 65 cases. J Trauma 1969;9:497–507.

33. Purdue GF, Hunt JL. Electrocardiographic monitoring after electrical injury: necessity or luxury. J Trauma 1986;26:166–7.

34. Hunt JL, McManus WF, Haney WP, et al. Vascular lesions in acute electric injuries. J Trauma 1974;14:461–73.

35. Arnoldo B, Klein M, Gibran NS. Practice guidelines for the management of electrical injuries. J Burn Care Res 2006;27:439–47.

36. Leversedge FJ, Moore TJ, Peterson BC, et al. Compartment syndrome of the upper extremity. J Hand Surg Am 2011;36:544–59 [quiz: 560].

37. Kim SH, Cho GY, Kim MK, et al. Alterations in left ventricular function assessed by two-dimensional speckle tracking echocardiography and the clinical utility of cardiac troponin I in survivors of high-voltage electrical injury. Crit Care Med 2009;37:1282–7.

38. Park KH, Park WJ, Kim MK, et al. Alterations in arterial function after high-voltage electrical injury. Crit Care 2012;16:R25.

39. Boozalis GT, Purdue GF, Hunt JL, et al. Ocular changes from electrical burn injuries. A literature review and report of cases. J Burn Care Rehabil 1991;12:458–62.

40. Saffle JR, Crandall A, Warden GD. Cataracts: a long-term complication of electrical injury. J Trauma 1985;25:17–21.

41. Janus TJ, Barrash J. Neurologic and neurobehavioral effects of electric and lightning injuries. J Burn Care Rehabil 1996;17:409–15.

42. Pliskin NH, Capelli-Schellpfeffer M, Law RT, et al. Neuropsychological symptom presentation after electrical injury. J Trauma 1998;44:709–15.

43. Egeland B, More S, Buchman SR, et al. Management of difficult pediatric facial burns: reconstruction of burn-related lower eyelid ectropion and perioral contractures. J Craniofac Surg 2008;19:960–9.

44. Donelan MB. Reconstruction of electrical burns of the oral commissure with a ventral tongue flap. Plast Reconstr Surg 1995;95:1155–64.

45. Smith MA, Muehlberger T, Dellon AL. Peripheral nerve compression associated with low-voltage electrical injury without associated significant cutaneous burn. Plast Reconstr Surg 2002;109:137–44.

46. Potter BK, Burns TC, Lacap AP, et al. Heterotopic ossification following traumatic and combat-related amputations. Prevalence, risk factors, and preliminary results of excision. J Bone Jonit Surg Am 2007;89:476–86.

47. Levi B, Jayakumar P, Giladi A, et al. Risk factors for the development of heterotopic ossification in seriously burned adults: a National Institute on Disability, Independent Living and Rehabilitation Research burn model system database analysis. J Trauma acute Care Surg 2015;79:870–6.

48. Ranganathan K, Loder S, Agarwal S, et al. Heterotopic ossification: basic-science principles and clinical correlates. J Bone Jonit Surg Am 2015;97:1101–11.

49. Wolbarst AB, Wiley AL Jr, Nemhauser JB, et al. Medical response to a major radiologic emergency: a primer for medical and public health practitioners. Radiology 2010;254(3):660–77.

50. Flynn DF, Goans RE. Nuclear terrorism: triage and medical management of radiation and combined-injury casualties. Surg Clin North Am 2006;86(3):601–36.

51. DiCarlo AL, Maher C, Hick JL, et al. Radiation injury after a nuclear detonation: medical consequences

and the need for scarce resources allocation. Disaster Med Public Health Prep 2011;5(Suppl 1): S32–44.

2. Palmer JL, Deburghgraeve CR, Bird MD, et al. Development of a combined radiation and burn injury model. J Burn Care Res 2011;32(2): 317–23.

3. Bray FN, Simmons BJ, Wolfson AH, et al. Acute and chronic cutaneous reactions to ionizing radiation therapy. Dermatol Ther (Heidelb) 2016; 6(2):185–206.

54. Salvo N, Barnes E, van Draanen J, et al. Prophylaxis and management of acute radiation-induced skin reactions: a systematic review of the literature. Curr Oncol 2010;17(4):94–112.

55. Hymes SR, Strom EA, Fife C. Radiation dermatitis: clinical presentation, pathophysiology, and treatment 2006. J Am Acad Dermatol 2006;54(1):28–46.

Negative Pressure Wound Therapy for Burns

Neel A. Kantak, MD[a], Riyam Mistry, MBChB[b], David E. Varon, BA[c], Eric G. Halvorson, MD[d],*

KEYWORDS

- Negative pressure wound therapy • Burns • Skin graft • VAC

KEY POINTS

- The use of NPWT is associated with improved outcomes in a wide variety of complex wounds. Existing data support certain uses of NPWT for burn care, although studies are limited.
- Studies on the use of NPWT for acute burns suggest that NPWT may have a role in reducing edema and pain, and a positive effect on tissue perfusion and re-epithelialization.
- Of all potential applications of NPWT in burn care, using NPWT as a skin graft bolster dressing has the most supportive data. Other potential applications include management of extent of injury in acute burns, preparation of wound beds for skin grafting, and dressing skin graft donor sites. The use of modified NPWT dressings has shown promise in treating large burns.
- More scientific and clinical studies are needed to fully understand the mechanism of action, optimal method, and ideal applications for NPWT in burn patients.

INTRODUCTION

Negative pressure wound therapy (NPWT) has been used in the treatment of acute and chronic wounds for almost 20 years and is now widely used around the world. Although further research is required to specifically validate many of these treatments and to determine cost-effectiveness, existing data support the use of NPWT for certain aspects of burn care. Of all potential applications of NPWT in burn care, using NPWT as a skin graft bolster dressing has the most supportive data. Other potential applications include using NPWT to limit the extent of injury in acute burn wounds, as a bridge to skin grafting, and as a dressing for skin graft donor sites. This article reviews the literature based on application and describes our center's experience with extra-large (XL) NPWT dressings for large burns.

CLINICAL EVIDENCE ACCORDING TO INDICATION/APPLICATION
Management of Acute Burns with Negative Pressure Wound Therapy

The application of NPWT in the acute management of burn wounds was studied in hand burns by Kamolz and colleagues.[1] The goal when treating a burn acutely is to create a healing environment that protects against fluid losses, infection, and most importantly prevents further progression of the burn wound. Kamolz and colleagues[1] tested whether NPWT is better at this than conventional silver sulfadiazine cream in patients with bilateral partial-thickness hand burns who presented within 6 hours. Seven patients were used in this study with the conventional silver sulfadiazine treatment being used on the less severely burned hand. The primary outcome measure was perfusion to the

Disclosure Statement: The authors have nothing to disclose.
[a] Mid-Atlantic Permanente Medical Group, Largo Medical Center, 1221 Upper Mercantile Lane, Upper Marlboro, MD 20774, USA; [b] Department of Plastic Surgery, Royal Devon & Exeter Hospital NHS Foundation Trust, Barrack Road, Exeter EX2 5DW, UK; [c] Division of Plastic Surgery, Brigham and Women's Hospital, 75 Francis Street, Boston, MA 02115, USA; [d] Plastic Surgery Center of Asheville, 5 Livingston Street, Asheville, NC 28801, USA
* Corresponding author.
E-mail address: eric.halvorson@gmail.com

Clin Plastic Surg 44 (2017) 671–677
http://dx.doi.org/10.1016/j.cps.2017.02.023

injured skin as measured by indocyanine green angiography. The authors reported that perfusion was significantly improved on Day 3 in the burn wounds treated by NPWT. They also noted reduced edema and decreased progression of the burn wound on clinical examination of the NPWT-treated sites. Although this study was small (seven patients, 14 hands), it suggests that NPWT may have a role in preventing burn progression by improving microcirculation in the reversible zone of stasis.[1]

Beyond altering the microenvironment of the acute burn wound, NPWT may also be useful in the broader context of managing acutely ill burn patients. Banwell and Musgrave[2] have suggested that burns be treated in the acute phase with NPWT and that it is of particular benefit in clinically unstable patients for two reasons. First, full coverage of the burn (which might include complex operative procedures) may be delayed if patients are receiving treatment in intensive care. Second, it may be difficult to change dressings frequently in unstable patients, and NPWT can dramatically reduce the frequency of dressing changes. Thus, in addition to the direct benefits of limiting inflammatory injury in the microenvironment of the burn, NPWT can serve as a practical temporizing measure to achieve control of large wounds until patients become physiologically stable.

A prospective, randomized trial is needed to examine the effectiveness of NPWT in preventing progression of burn wounds, and its cost-effectiveness in management of acute burn wounds in critically ill patients.

Negative Pressure Wound Therapy as a Bridge to Skin Grafting

After the acute phase of burn injury and resuscitation, the second step is excision of devitalized tissue and coverage with skin grafts, when possible. The success of skin grafts depends on several factors, including the quality of the recipient wound bed. A well-vascularized bed with a low degree of bacterial colonization maximizes the probability of skin graft take. As such, NPWT use has been suggested as a method to prepare a wound to accept a skin graft. Although there are no good data on the use of NPWT in the preparation of burn wounds, there have been favorable studies looking at other types of open wounds. In addition to several retrospective studies,[3,4] a prospective randomized trial by Saaiq and colleagues[5] reported using NPWT versus wet-to-dry saline gauze to prepare traumatic wound sites for tie-over bolster skin

grafting 10 days after debridement. The authors found that the patients treated with NPWT had a higher skin graft take and shorter hospital stays.

Negative Pressure Wound Therapy as a Bolster Dressing for Autografts

Scherer and colleagues[6] reported the results of a retrospective study where traditional skin graft securing methods were compared with NPWT in a variety of wounds, 50% of which were burns. A subgroup analysis of the burn wounds showed a decreased graft failure rate in the NPWT group (0% vs 19%).[6]

A randomized, double-blind control trial compared the total area of skin graft loss for skin wounds (of which more than half were burns) in grafts secured with conventional methods and NPWT.[7] The authors reported a median graft loss of 0.0 cm^2 (range, 0.0–11.8 cm^2) for the NPWT group, whereas the control group median graft loss was 4.5 cm^2 (range, 0.0–5.2 cm^2; $P = .001$). The patients treated with NPWT also had significantly shorter hospital stays.

A prospective randomized control trial by Petkar and colleagues[8] of 30 burn patients compared the graft take in 21 burn wounds receiving NPWT on the split-thickness skin graft (STSG) and 19 burn wounds receiving conventional compression dressings on the STSG. They found that mean graft take was higher in the NPWT group than in the control group (96.7% vs 87.5%; $P<.001$). Most studies have not examined the use of NPWT as a bolster in exclusively burn patients. However, the previously mentioned studies all report that NPWT likely improves graft take but at a higher financial cost.

Negative Pressure Wound Therapy as a Dressing to Integrate Bilaminate Dermal Substitutes

NPWT may have a role in the integration of a bilaminate dermal substitute in a burn site, such as Integra® (Integra LifeSciences Corporation, Plainsboro, NJ). Jeschke and colleagues[9] compared the use of conventional compression dressings versus NPWT with fibrin glue changed every 4 days to secure a bilaminate dermal substitute. Once the dermal substitute had fully vascularized, an STSG was placed and the STSG take rate as a percentage of total area of dermal substitute placement was recorded. The STSG take rate was significantly higher in the NPWT plus fibrin glue group compared with conventional pressure dressings (98% vs 78%; $P<.003$) with a shorter time to definitive coverage (10 days vs 24 days;

*<.002). It is worth noting that because fibrin glue was used alongside NPWT, one cannot separate any beneficial effect of the NPWT from that of the fibrin glue.

A retrospective study by Molnar and colleagues[10] examined bilaminate dermal substitute revascularization and staged skin graft take rate with use of NPWT for securing both coverage procedures. They performed procedures on patients with exposed bone, joint, tendon, or bowel, who would have otherwise required more extensive reconstructive procedures. The authors reported 96% Integra® revascularization rate, 93% TSG take rate, and mean of 7.25 days from dermal substitute placement to skin grafting.[11–14] These studies suggest that NPWT may improve the rate of vascularization of bilaminate dermal substitutes thereby reducing the delay before skin grafting and improving eventual skin graft take.

Negative Pressure Wound Therapy as a Skin Graft Donor Site Dressing

Many burn patients require an STSG to treat their wounds. The STSG donor site is often painful and messy. Many burn surgeons still treat donor sites with some form of dry dressing; however, multiple studies suggest that a moist wound environment is preferable for donor site wound healing.[15–17] It is possible that NPWT may have a role in helping the donor site re-epithelialize faster. In our experience, the main advantage of NPWT for donor sites is that it removes wound exudate, allowing for quantification and a more stable dressing that does not move, make a mess, smell, or fall off easily. We have also found that patients seem to have less pain, perhaps because of the immobility and lack of shear associated with the dressing.

Genecov and colleagues[18] looked at the rates of skin graft re-epithelialization in 10 patients who served as their own control subjects. Two donor sites were used on each patient with one donor site being covered with occlusive dressings without negative pressure and one site being covered with NPWT. On postoperative day 7, analysis of the keratinocyte layer from punch biopsies confirmed accelerated re-epithelialization in the NPWT group in 70% of patients, equivalent rates in 20%, and delayed re-epithelialization in 10%. Statistical analysis confirmed faster re-epithelialization in the NPWT group (P<.013). The data from this experiment suggest that NPWT could help the donor site re-epithelialize faster within the first 7 days after graft harvest.

Negative Pressure Wound Therapy as an Integrated Dressing for Large Burns

Given the multiple uses for NPWT in managing a variety of burn wounds at different phases of healing, it is possible that an integrated large NPWT dressing could be useful in treating limbs and large areas of mixed burn wounds. Chong and colleagues[19] reported sandwiching limbs in large polyurethane dressings with a thin strip of sponge placed in dependent position in an approach called the "total body wrap." This technique uses the negative pressure to encourage re-epithelialization in skin graft donor sites while removing inflammatory exudate and reducing exposure to pathogens. The authors concluded that this technique could be used to promote healing and improve comfort and care in a severely burned patient, although no objective measures were recorded.

THE BRIGHAM AND WOMEN'S HOSPITAL EXPERIENCE

In the burn unit at the Brigham and Women's Hospital we have been using large NPWT dressings to treat patients with burn wounds greater than 15% total body surface area (TBSA) on a regular basis.[20] Our methods are different from those described by Chong and colleagues.[19] We apply microporous silver-impregnated foam with a silicone contact layer over donor sites and STSG recipient sites (Mepilex Ag®, Molnlycke, Gothenburg, Sweden). Both areas are then covered with similarly contoured conventional NPWT sponge (V.A.C. GranuFoam, KCI, San Antonio, TX; and/or Ioban, 3M, St. Paul, MN) and a seal is obtained using a suction pad (Sensa T.R.A.C. Pad, KCI). We have found that this combination of dressings works well on all wound types, including burned skin, open wounds, donor sites, recipient sites, and (most importantly) intact skin. Therefore, it is not necessary to tailor the dressing to each type of wound, with special bridges over intact skin. Instead, the entire extremity or body area can be covered in this two-layered dressing and covered with an occlusive dressing to obtain a seal (Fig. 1), greatly simplifying the dressing application process (and reducing operating room time).

Similar to Chong and colleagues,[19] to cover limbs we sandwich the limb between large sheets of occlusive dressing. Wall suction is applied just before the most difficult area to obtain a seal is covered, thereby assuring a seal immediately after occlusive dressing application. Areas prone to moisture or sheer forces (eg, nonexcised burn tissue, the perineum) have a double layer of occlusive dressing applied and secured in place by sutures or

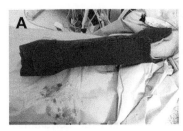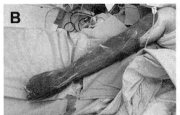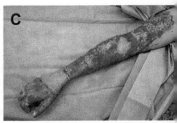

Fig. 1. Modified technique of NPWT applied to an STSG recipient site on the right arm (*A*), then covered with an occlusive dressing to obtain a seal (*B*), showing skin graft take after NPWT is removed (*C*).

staples (**Fig. 2**). Suction pads are applied in the most dependent areas, with one pump used per arm, two pumps per leg, and two pumps for the chest or back (**Fig. 3**). Pressure is applied at −125 mm Hg continuously, going down to −50 mm Hg on Day 1 to 3 for physical therapy at the discretion of the attending burn surgeon.

There is a steep but not very long learning curve to become adept in the application of large NPWT dressings and obtaining a proper seal that will hold for 5 to 7 days. Critical technical points are as follows:

1. Use a modified dressing (as described) that is effective over multiple wound types and intact

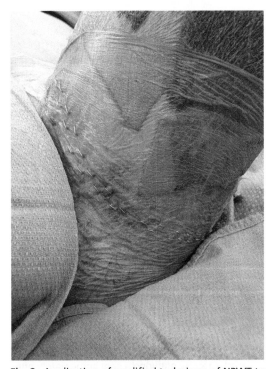

Fig. 2. Application of modified technique of NPWT to the groin area: in this case two layers of occlusive dressing and two rows of staples facilitate the maintenance of a seal to overcome shear forces and moisture.

skin, thus eliminating the need to contour dressings.
2. Wrap extremities circumferentially and obtain seal by sandwiching large occlusive dressings or using an extremity bag and proximal seal when the hands/feet are involved.
3. Save the hardest part until last. Apply wall suction before placement of the last piece of occlusive dressing, so a seal is immediately obtained.
4. Use double layers, staples, running sutures, ostomy paste, and so forth and be creative in figuring out how to obtain seal in difficult areas because you will want to use this dressing for all burns when you see the results.

A useful function of NPWT is monitoring fluid output from the wounds (which can also be predicted, as discussed later). With large NPWT dressings, fluid output is high. When it exceeds 3 L/d, we have chosen to replace it 1:1 with lactated Ringer solution. Electrolytes are checked twice daily and corrected. We prefer our technique to that of Chong and colleagues[19] because we believe graft fixation, exudate removal, and wound healing are improved by applying an NPWT sponge over the entire wound bed.

Perhaps the most important clinical benefit of using large NPWT dressings is that the surgeon and nurses in our unit have noted a dramatic decrease in pain and anxiety compared with traditional dressings that require more frequent changes. Our nurses uniformly love the dressing. Because it controls exudate, the dressings are not changed daily, which is a great reduction in tedious work and results in less patient anxiety and pain associated with such dressing changes. Many patients have little pain following surgery but increased pain after the dressing is removed at 5 to 7 days. It is possible that NPWT is modifying the inflammatory response that modulates pain perception, or that the lack of motion and sheer minimizes pain. Future studies on NPWT for burns should incorporate pain as an outcome measure.

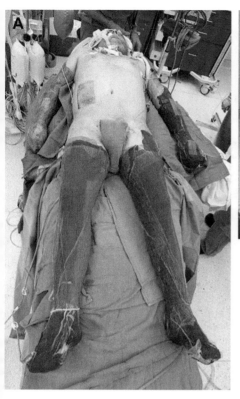
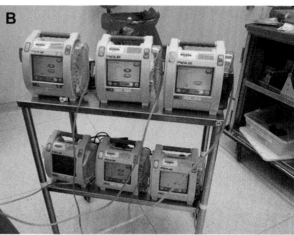

Fig. 3. Application of extra-large NPWT dressing: in this case a seal was obtained by sandwiching extremities between large sheets of occlusive dressing (*A*), then applying suction pads to the most dependent areas, with one pump used per arm, and two pumps per leg (*B*).

A recently published paper based on our early experience with XL NPWT dressings described 12 patients we treated using the aforementioned methods of XL-NPWT burn management (**Fig. 4**).[20] The mean age was 35.5 (median, 28; range, 18–63) with a mean burn size of 29.6% TBSA (median, 25%; range, 15%–60%). Half of the patients we studied had also suffered an inhalation injury, and 11 of the 12 patients required mechanical ventilation for an average of 16.5 days (median, 15; range, 2–40 days). The mean time from injury to grafting was 7.75 days (median, 7.5; range, 2–17 days) and the mean TBSA covered with STSG and NPWT was 35.1% (median, 32%; range, 17%–44%).

The average graft take was 97% (median, 100%; range, 85%–100%) with the STSG donor sites re-epithelializing after an average of 11.25 days (median, 11; range, 10–14 days), although this later information was only from 4 patients. Two patients developed acute kidney injury (AKI) that resolved and one developed a hematoma within 12 hours of surgery. The hematoma was evacuated and the NPWT dressing resealed with no further complications. The length of stay (LOS) for our patients averaged 37.9 days (median, 32.5; range, 19–66) and all 12 of our patients survived without any wound infections. Of interest, two patients had TBSA burns greater than 35% and their LOS were shorter than the ABA Burn Respiratory national averages (39 vs 62 days and 50 vs 68 days, respectively). Patients with smaller burns had variable LOS, chiefly because of social issues. Our sample size is too small to make any conclusions regarding the effect of XL-NPWT on LOS.

Fluid output from the wounds during the first 5 days of grafting averaged 101 ± 66 mL/% TBSA covered per day. Average output for the donor sites was double that of the recipient site at 132 ± 83 mL/%TBSA versus 61 ± 37 mL/%TBSA, respectively. These numbers are used to predict fluid loss from burn wounds covered with NPWT dressings, although measuring actual output is obviously more accurate. Nevertheless, predictions can make the intensive care unit team more prepared to resuscitate such patients in the postoperative period.

Lamke and Liljedahl[21] studied the evaporative water losses from burn wounds and skin graft donor sites reporting that water loss was three times higher from donor sites compared with grafted sites (1.2 vs 0.36 mL/cm^2/d, respectively).

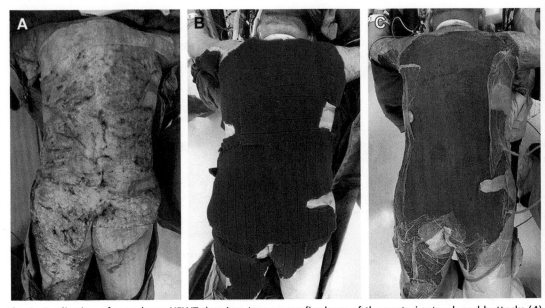

Fig. 4. Application of extra-large NPWT dressing. Large campfire burn of the posterior trunk and buttocks (*A*), covered with xenografts and autografts followed by a microporous nonadherent foam with a silicone contact layer followed by conventional NPWT sponge (*B*). Proximal thighs were then circumferentially wrapped and sealed using an occlusive dressing sandwich technique (*C*) and staples/sutures were used in the perineum. This seal held for 6 days.

The results from our patients followed a similar trend with fluid loss from the donor site being double that of the recipient site. Two of our patients developed AKI; this may have been caused by a lack of experience in using XL-NPWT and an underestimation of fluid loss. On the other end of the fluid resuscitation spectrum, however, none of our patients developed lung edema from overresuscitation and they were able to discontinue manual ventilation earlier than burn patients in other studies, although our study is too small to perform meaningful statistical analysis.[22]

We have found that our modified NPWT dressing is a safe and effective dressing for treating large burn wounds, and a technology-based improvement for patients, nurses, and surgeons alike. Our results regarding graft take are similar to those achieved by Petkar and colleagues[8] with the difference being our burn wounds were much greater than the 10% TBSA burns in their study. Our average healing time of 11.25 days for STSG donor sites corroborates the study by Genecov and colleagues,[18] which showed that NPWT enhanced donor site re-epithelialization.

SUMMARY

Although the literature supporting NPWT for burns is not robust, there is good evidence to support its use as a bolster dressing for skin grafts. Other studies suggest that it may reduce conversion in the zone of stasis, it may improve integration of bilaminate dermal substitutes, and it may improve donor site re-epithelialization. Based on our early experience we have found that a modified NPWT dressing is a safe and effective dressing for large burn wounds because it provides an integrated dressing for management of various wound types in a single burn patient. Our modified NPWT dressing is much easier to apply than traditional NPWT dressings. In addition, accurate measurement of wound exudate helps guide fluid resuscitation and achieve appropriate fluid balance, reducing the risk of pulmonary edema and AKI. Exudate management is a chief advantage of NPWT for burns, resulting in greater ease of use and a stable dressing that requires less work to realize superior outcomes. We also believe that NPWT promotes re-epithelialization, protects against infection, and reduces anxiety and pain. The multiple potential advantages of NPWT for burns converge to make it a compelling dressing.

Having less frequent dressing changes helps reduce the burden on the nursing staff, reduces bacterial colonization, and reduces narcotic requirements. Decreased narcotic requirements and more precise fluid management, with avoidance of fluid overload and subsequent pulmonary edema, may lead to decreased ventilatory support nd intensive care unit LOS. Decreased wound olonization may lead to decreased wound infections and decreased infections at other sites that re prone to infection from colonizing bacteria eg, pneumonia, central line infections). Some disdvantages include cost, time for dressing appliation, a learning curve for dressing application, nd the requirement of an extra trip to the operting room for removal of the dressings. Attention to maintenance of a negative pressure seal before emoval of the dressings also requires vigilance nd a well-trained nursing staff. On occasion, all-suction is required.

In balance, we believe that the advantages of PWT outweigh the disadvantages, and that the otential for improved outcomes and decreased OS could make it a highly cost-effective dressing.

EFERENCES

1. Kamolz LP, Andel H, Haslik W, et al. Use of sub-atmospheric pressure therapy to prevent burn wound progression in human: first experiences. Burns 2004;30(3):253–8.
2. Banwell PE, Musgrave M. Topical negative pressure therapy: mechanisms and indications. Int Wound J 2004;1(2):95–106.
3. Dunn RM, Ignotz R, Mole T, et al. Assessment of gauze-based negative pressure wound therapy in the split-thickness skin graft clinical pathway-an observational study. Eplasty 2011;11:e14.
4. Campbell PE, Smith GS, Smith JM. Retrospective clinical evaluation of gauze-based negative pressure wound therapy. Int Wound J 2008;5(2):280–6.
5. Saaiq M, Hameed-Ud-Din, Khan MI, et al. Vacuum-assisted closure therapy as a pretreatment for split thickness skin grafts. J Coll Physicians Surg Pak 2010;20(10):675–9.
6. Scherer LA, Shiver S, Chang M, et al. The Vacuum Assisted Closure Device: a method of securing skin grafts and improving graft survival. Arch Surg 2002;137:930–4.
7. Llanos S, Danilla S, Barraza C, et al. Effectiveness of negative pressure closure in the integration of split thickness skin grafts: a randomized, double-masked, controlled trial. Ann Surg 2006;244(5):700–5.
8. Petkar KS, Dhanraj P, Kingsly PM, et al. A prospective randomized controlled trial comparing negative pressure dressing and conventional dressing methods on split-thickness skin grafts in burned patients. Burns 2011;37(6):925–9.
9. Jeschke MG, Rose C, Angele P, et al. Development of new reconstructive techniques: use of Integra in combination with fibrin glue and negative-pressure therapy for reconstruction of acute and chronic wounds. Plast Reconstr Surg 2004;113(2):525–30.
10. Molnar JA, DeFranzo AJ, Hadaegh A, et al. Acceleration of Integra incorporation in complex tissue defects with subatmospheric pressure. Plast Reconstr Surg 2004;113:1339–46.
11. Heimbach D, Luterman A, Burke J, et al. Artificial dermis for major burns. A multi-center randomized clinical trial. Ann Surg 1988;208:313–20.
12. Machens HG, Berger AC, Mailaender P. Bioartificial skin. Cells Tissues Organs 2000;167:88–94.
13. Sheridan RL, Hegarty M, Tompkins RG, et al. Artificial skin in massive burns: result to ten years. Eur J Plast Surg 1994;17:91.
14. Honari S, Gibran NS, Engrav LH, et al. Three years' experience with 52 Integra (artificial skin) patients since FDA approval. J Burn Care Rehabil 2000;21:190.
15. Voineskos SH, Ayeni OA, McKnight L, et al. Systematic review of skin graft donor-site dressings. Plast Reconstr Surg 2009;124(1):298–306.
16. Wiechula R. The use of moist wound-healing dressings in the management of split-thickness skin graft donor sites: a systematic review. Int J Nurs Pract 2003;9(2):S9.
17. Rakel BA, Bermel MA, Abbott LI, et al. Split-thickness skin graft donor site care: a quantitative synthesis of the research. Appl Nurs Res 1998;11(4):174–82.
18. Genecov DG, Schneider AM, Morykwas MJ, et al. A controlled subatmospheric pressure dressing increases the rate of skin graft donor site reepithelialization. Ann Plast Surg 1998;40:219–25.
19. Chong SJ, Liang WH, Tan BK. Use of multiple VAC devices in the management of extensive burns: the total body wrap concept. Burns 2010;36(7):e127–9.
20. Lund C, Browder N. The estimation of area of burns. Surg Gynec Onst 1944;79:352–8.
21. Lamke LO, Liljedahl SO. Evaporative water loss from burns, grafts and donor sites. Scand J Plast Reconstr Surg 1971;5:17–22.
22. Mackie DP, Spoelder EJ, Paauw RJ, et al. Mechanical ventilation and fluid retention in burn patients. J Trauma 2009;67:1233–8 [discussion: 8].

Management of the Chronic Burn Wound

Stephen Tyler Elkins-Williams, MD[a], William A. Marston, MD[b],
Charles Scott Hultman, MD, MBA[a],*

KEYWORDS

• Chronic wound • Hyperbaric oxygen therapy • Marjolin ulcer • Topical growth factor

KEY POINTS

- There exists little evidence to promote or refute the use of hyperbaric oxygen therapy (HBOT) in acute burn wounds.
- Diabetic foot burns could be separately considered, given the body of evidence in chronic diabetic foot wounds. Further research is necessary to prove the efficacy of HBOT in this setting.
- Marjolin ulcers are malignant degeneration of chronic wounds and occur most commonly in unexcised full-thickness burns.
- Average time from the initial injury to development of a Marjolin ulcer is 30 years. Cancers from Marjolin ulcers tend to be more aggressive than common skin cancers.
- There are many cytokine growth factors available for use on burn wounds. Some promising studies have been performed; additional research will help determine optimum patient selection and treatment regimens.

INTRODUCTION

Perhaps one of the most challenging problems in burn care is obtaining stable, definitive closure of the chronic wound that has failed to heal, using conventional techniques. Although most of the burn literature focuses on management of acute wounds, including timing, depth, and type of excision, as well as method of skin grafting, obtaining permanent closure of chronic wounds can be elusive. This article reviews specific considerations in the workup and management of chronic burn wounds, realizing that resurfacing is not complete until the burn surgeon obtains complete closure of the integument.

Critical to restoring integrity of the skin is obtaining a detailed history about the wound, which helps build a differential diagnosis as to why the wound has failed to close, either secondarily or through surgical intervention. How and when did the burn occur? What previous attempts

have been used to facilitate wound healing? Have physical therapy and occupational therapy been involved in executing a plan? Are there environmental or patient-related issues that have prevented the wound from closing? This history, combined with serial physical examination of the wound, will help build a list of possible causes:

- Mechanical: location over tendon or extensor joint
- Metabolic: diabetes, hypothyroidism, autoimmune disorders
- Infectious: acute or chronic
- Vascular: inflow (arterial) and outflow (venous), especially in extremities
- Lymphatic: destruction of regional network causing lymphedema
- Radiation: progressive microvascular fibrosis
- Neoplastic: possible Marjolin ulcer or cutaneous metastasis

[a] Division of Plastic and Reconstructive Surgery, Department of Surgery, University of North Carolina Medical Center, University of North Carolina at Chapel Hill, Chapel Hill, NC 27599, USA; [b] Division of Vascular Surgery, Department of Surgery, University of North Carolina Medical Center, University of North Carolina at Chapel Hill, Chapel Hill, NC 27599, USA
* Corresponding author.
E-mail address: Scott_Hultman@med.unc.edu

Clin Plastic Surg 44 (2017) 679–687
http://dx.doi.org/10.1016/j.cps.2017.02.024

- Personal: smoking, not compliant with splinting or garments, poor wound hygiene
- Social: limited resources and poor access to care (transportation, wound care supplies, caregiver)
- Psychiatric: substance abuse, Munchausen syndrome

This article reviews 3 issues pertinent to management of the chronic burn wound: (1) use of hyperbaric oxygen to facilitate wound closure, (2) application of topical growth factors, (3) and diagnosis and treatment of Marjolin ulcers.

HYPERBARIC OXYGEN THERAPY
Introduction

The Undersea and Hyperbaric Medical Society defines hyperbaric oxygen therapy (HBOT) as "an intervention in which an individual breathes near 100% oxygen intermittently while inside a hyperbaric chamber that is pressurized to greater than sea level pressure."[1] In clinical practice, this pressure typically exceeds 1.4 atm.[1]

The concept of using hyperbaric pressure to treat patients dates back to 1662; a British clergyman named Henshaw thought that hyperbaric pressures could speed healing in acute medical conditions. He created a sealed chamber that he named the Domicilium, using organ bellows to control changes in pressure. Henshaw could not use isolated elemental oxygen in his treatments, however, as it would not be discovered until more than a hundred years later.[2]

Over the course of the late nineteenth and early twentieth centuries, progress was made with the use of oxygen for treatment of decompression sickness, first in normobaric settings and later with the additional of hyperbaric pressures. But it was not until 1955 that Churchill-Davidson and colleagues[3] published "High-Pressure Oxygen and Radiotherapy," using HBOT to potentiate the effects of radiation therapy in patients with cancer, in *The Lancet*. Thus began the era of modern HBOT in medicine.

Current Uses

The use of HBOT quickly expanded to a be used in a wide variety of medical conditions, most of which initially lacked evidence or standard protocols. The Undersea and Hyperbaric Medical Society was founded in 1967 and maintains a current list of accepted medical indications for HBOT use, one of which is acute thermal burn injury (**Box 1**).[4]

Hyperbaric Oxygen and Burns

The theory behind use of HBOT in burn injuries is sound. Animal models have demonstrated that

---

Box 1
2014 Undersea and Hyperbaric Medical Society's indications for hyperbaric oxygen therapy

- Air or gas embolism
- Carbon monoxide poisoning
- Clostridial myositis and myonecrosis (gas gangrene)
- Crush injury, compartment syndrome, and other acute traumatic ischemias
- Decompression sickness
- Arterial insufficiencies
- Severe anemia
- Intracranial abscess
- Necrotizing soft tissue infections
- Osteomyelitis (refractory)
- Delayed radiation injury (soft tissue and bony necrosis)
- Compromised grafts and flaps
- Acute thermal burn injury
- Idiopathic sudden sensorineural hearing loss

HBOT can increase the partial pressure of oxygen in end organ tissues. This elevation is achieved by increasing the Pa_{O_2} of the blood to 10 to 15 times normal, which creates a steep gradient down which oxygen may diffuse into hypoxic tissues.[5] Theoretically, increasing oxygen tension in burn patients could decrease leukocyte activation, reduce so-called secondary injury, and even reduce tissue edema through an oxygen osmotic effect.

Evidence in Burns

Despite this, very little quality research has been done on the effectiveness of HBOT on patients with burn injuries. In the 2004 Cochrane review, Villanueva and colleagues[6] found only 2 quality randomized controlled trials (RCTs) evaluating the effectiveness of HBOT in patients with acute thermal injuries.[6]

1. Hart and colleagues,[7] 1974: 16 patients, 10% to 50% total body surface area (TBSA) burns, randomized to routine burn management and HBOT or routine burn management with sham HBOT
   a. Intervention: 100% oxygen at 2 atmosphere absolute (ATA) for 90 minutes every 8 hours for 24 hours, then every 12 hours until healed
   b. Mean healing times shorter in the intervention group (19.7 days vs 43.8 days, $P<.001$).

c. Method criticisms: did not describe allocation concealment methods; no definition of healing given, and no description of the wound size and depth at presentation given
d. Questionable applicability: skin grafts in less than half of the patients enrolled, calls into question relevance in the early excision and grafting era

Brannen and colleagues,[8] 1997: 125 patients randomized to routine burn management or routine burn management plus HBOT
a. Intervention: 100% oxygen at 2 ATA for 90 minutes twice a day for a minimum of 10 treatments, maximum of one treatment per percent TBSA
b. Primary outcome: length of stay
c. Secondary end points: mortality, acute fluid requirements, number of operations required
d. No statistically significant difference in any of these outcomes

There have been several nonrandomized comparative studies performed over the years that have suggested improvements with HBOT in survival, hospital length of stay, and speed of reepithelization.[5] However, multiple investigators have concluded that there is currently insufficient evidence to either support or refute the use of HBOT in the setting of acute thermal burns.[5,6]

Any future studies seeking to clinically investigate HBOT in acute burn patients will need to seek to understand the degree, type, and size of burn that will see the most benefit. Additionally, the optimal frequency, duration per session, and overall length of therapy need to be explored.

Diabetic Foot Burns

The data for use of HBOT in chronic wounds are more established. A recent Cochrane review of the literature determined that HBOT improved healing for diabetes-related foot ulcers and likely reduced the rate of major amputation in this same population.[9] The evidence was not as strong for venous stasis ulcers, but there was evidence that HBOT may help to reduce the size of these wounds.

Given the success of HBOT in diabetic foot wounds, there has been a recent investigation by Jones and colleagues[10] into developing a protocol for management of foot burns in diabetic patients. Their protocol for determining which patients would benefit from HBOT is summarized (Fig. 1):

The patients who are then determined to benefit from HBOT undergo 14 treatments; if the transcutaneous partial pressure of tissue oxygen measurements is improving, patients receive 6 additional treatments. Those patients who are to be skin grafted are treated both preoperatively and postoperatively. Unfortunately, this protocol has only ever been compared against a group of historic controls from the 1970s and 1980s. There are no data currently available that compares HBOT with standard treatment in patients with diabetic foot burns.

Challenges

There are practical challenges of administration of HBOT in burn patients that must be considered. The most severely injured acute burn patients, those who would stand the most to gain from the potential benefits of HBOT, are typically intubated and critically ill. The risks of leaving the burn intensive-care-unit setting and being transported to an HBOT chamber 2 to 3 times daily are not trivial. Additionally, these types of patients would require the use of multi-place HBOT chambers to accommodate nursing and support staff. Multiplace chambers are not likely to be as available as the cheaper and smaller mono-place chambers more commonly in use.

Summary/Recommendations

The theory behind application of HBOT in burn wounds seems sound, and some early trials have shown promise. However, to date there is inadequate evidence to make judgment on its efficacy. There are some practical challenges in administration of HBOT in acute burn patients. Future study, likely across multiple centers, will be necessary to determine the optimum patient selection and treatment protocol for HBOT use.

TOPICAL GROWTH FACTORS
Introduction

Cytokine growth factors have been found to promote wound healing in a variety of ways:

- Encourage chemotaxis of inflammatory cells
- Stimulate endothelial cells
- Affect the migration of various cells
- Stimulate angiogenesis
- Inhibit apoptosis
- Mediate the synthesis of other cytokines.[11]

Mechanism of Action

In order for wounds to heal, they undergo a standard progression through various stages of wound healing (Fig. 2):

At each stage, different humoral factors and cells interact in specific ways. Changing these interactions, or the timing of the interactions, can alter wound healing and lead to hypertrophic scars

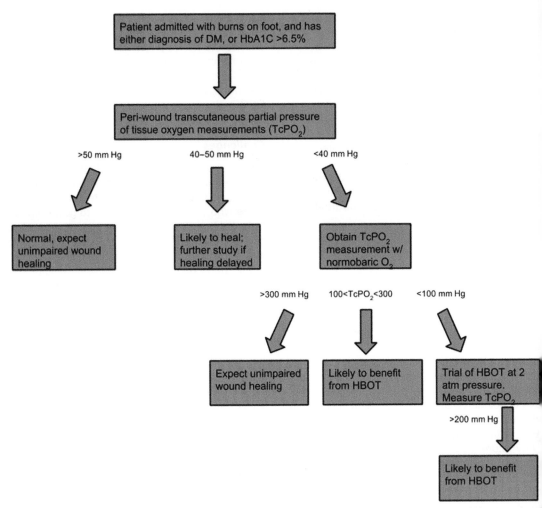

Fig. 1. Algorithm for use of HBOT in diabetic foot burns. DM, diabetes mellitus; HbA$_{1c}$, hemoglobin A$_{1c}$. (*Data from* Jones LM, Rubadue C, Brown NV, et al. Evaluation of TCOM/HBOT practice guideline for the treatment of foot burns occurring in diabetic patients. Burns 2015;41(3):536–41.)

or nonhealing wounds. The key to successfully using cytokine growth factors in burn wounds is to choose the proper growth factors that can speed wound healing without causing adverse effects.

Types of Growth Factor

There have been a wide variety of types of cytokine growth factors that have been investigated for burn wounds. These growth factors include platelet-derived growth factor (PDGF), fibroblast growth factors (FGFs), epidermal growth factors (EGFs), transforming growth factor (TGF) alpha, vascular endothelial growth factor, insulinlike growth factor I, nerve growth factor, TGF beta, granulocyte-macrophage colony-stimulating factor (GM-CSF), and amnion-derived cellular cytokine solution.[12] Although the heterogeneity of the types of available growth factors gives clinicians

and investigators a diverse toolbox, the diversity can also make it difficult to compare and pool studies.

Types of Burn Wounds

Further complicating matters are the different types of wounds with which one might wish to use a cytokine growth factor. They could be applied to partial-thickness burns, full-thickness burns, the interstices of meshed skin grafts, or even skin graft donor sites. Ching and colleagues[12] performed a very thorough review of available studies, in both animal and human models, investigating the use of the full spectrum of cytokine growth factors. Although their use in partial-thickness burns comprised most of the data, studies have been performed in full thickness burns as well as over skin grafts and

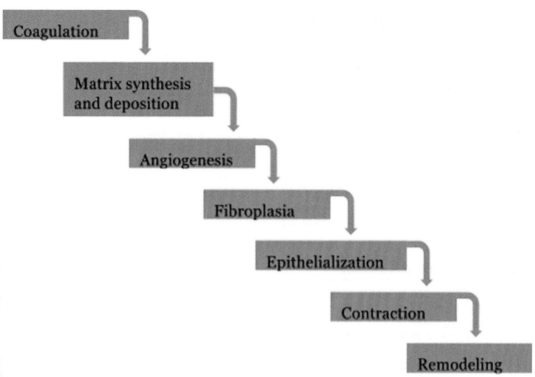

Fig. 2. Phases of wound healing.

even to donor sites. There is encouraging evidence for all types of cytokine growth factors in speeding wound healing. They do note, however, further study to generate high-quality human data is warranted.

Current Evidence

There have been several recent high-quality RCTs demonstrating the effectiveness of EGF and PDGF in simulated partial-thickness burns in animal models.[13,14] In addition, as Zhang and colleagues[15] demonstrated, at least 13 RCTs have been performed in human subjects. All of these studies were performed in Asia (China and Japan), and many of them were never published in English. Although the investigators expressed concern over various methodological flaws in the studies, they did note a consistent positive improvement in speed and quality of wound healing seen with FGF, EGF, and GM-CSF in partial-thickness burns.

These particular cytokines are likely suited to partial-thickness burns. By definition, the depth of a partial-thickness burn is limited to the papillary dermis (grade IIa) or reticular dermis (grade IIb). FGF and EGF are mitogens for endothelial cells and dermal fibroblasts, whereas GM-CSF works directly on the keratinocyte and endothelial cell. Because deeper structures, such as subcutaneous fat, muscle, and blood vessels, are spared, growth factors targeting these additional tissue types are likely unnecessary.[16]

Future Challenges

There is certainly a theoretic concern for cytokine growth factors to stimulate oncogenesis. The mechanisms by which growth factors promote tissue repair are also those implicated in malignant degeneration. Fortunately, tumor development has not yet been seen in clinical or experimental studies.[16] Given our knowledge of the latency time for Marjolin ulcers, however, the typical follow-up time seen in human studies of GFs is inadequate to detect future chronic malignant changes as an adverse effect.

Summary

Overall, the use of cytokine growth factors, particularly FGF, EGF, and GM-CSF, has shown promise in speeding the healing of partial-thickness burns. Additional large trials attempting to determine the optimum dosage regimen and delivery method of GFs will be useful in the future to maximize patient benefit.

MARJOLIN ULCERS
Introduction

Jean-Nicolas Marjolin was born in 1780. At a young age, he rose to become the Chair of Surgical Pathology at the University of Paris by 1819. He was a contemporary of Dupuytren, who served concurrently as the Chair of Operative Medicine. In 1828, Marjolin published an article describing "cancer-like ulcers."[17] Later, in 1850, Dr Robert Smith described neoplastic changes in a chronic ulcerating scar tissue and labeled this "Warty ulcers of Marjolin."[17] De Costa again described malignant degeneration of burn scars in 1903 as Marjolin ulcers, and the name stuck.[17] Today, the term generally refers to any long-term malignant changes in chronic scars.

Pathophysiology and Epidemiology

It is thought that any chronic inflammatory condition, not just burn scars, can lead to Marjolin ulcers. Other inciting conditions are seen in **Box 2**:

Incidence is difficult to determine, but numbers cited in the literature range from 0.77% to 2.0% of deep burns that have been allowed to heal by secondary intention.[11] By far the primary histologic type of Marjolin ulcer is squamous cell carcinoma (SCC), with Marjolin ulcer accounting for up to 2% of diagnosed SCCs. The second most common histologic type is basal cell carcinoma (BCC) of the skin; Marjolin ulcers contribute to 0.03% of these overall. Rare cases of melanoma, sarcoma, squamo-BCC, dermatofibrosarcoma protuberans, and mesenchymal tumors have been reported as well.[11]

The exact pathogenesis of Marjolin ulcers is unknown, though several mechanisms have been proposed. Lymphatic obliteration is thought to diminish the body's ability to detect cellular mutations, allowing atypia to persist longer and transform into carcinoma. Additional potential causes include

- Chronic irritation
- The avascular nature of the scar
- Release of toxins from damaged tissues
- Immunologic factors
- Repeated trauma

Another theory, the 2-hit hypothesis, states that the burn causes some baseline mutations in the cell. These mutations leave them more susceptible to future DNA damage (for instance, from UV radiation) leading to malignant changes.[11,17]

Marjolin ulcers can develop in any anatomic location, though the most common site is the lower extremities, followed by the upper extremities.[18] They are more common in men, though this may be a result of the increased incidence of burns in men as well. All age groups can acquire Marjolin ulcers; the latency period inversely relates to patients' age at time of injury. That is, children typically have a very long latency time, whereas the elderly have a much shorter latency interval.[11]

There are 2 type of Marjolin ulcers:

- Acute: much rarer; malignant degenerations within 1 year
- Chronic: more common; any Marjolin ulcer taking place more than 12 months after injury

The latency period for chronic ulcers can vary widely (ranging from 11–75 years), but the average is thought to be 30 years.[19] When considering classifying a new diagnosis of malignancy as a Marjolin ulcer, it is useful to keep in mind the criteria proposed by Giblin and colleagues[20] as seen in **Box 3**.

Clinical Presentation

Any nonhealing or ulcerative wound that appears in a chronic scar should raise suspicion for a Marjolin

---

Box 2
Other conditions potentially leading to Marjolin ulcer
Vaccinations
Snake bites
Osteomyelitis
Pressure sores
Spinal Cord Injury
Pilonidal abscess
Dermatitis artefacta
Venous stasis ulcers

Box 3
Establishing relation of cancer to burn scar
1. Incontrovertible evidence of the burn (by wound or scar)
2. Cancer origin within the boundaries of the burn scar
3. Absence of precursory or similar neoplasm on the site before the burn
4. Histologic type of cancer compatible with the type of tissue that was burned (ie, SCC, BCC, and so forth, in burned skin)
5. Appropriate interval of time between burn injury and development of cancer

cer. The clinical appearance is most commonly a at, ulcerative lesion with elevated margins and urrounding induration. They can also appear as n exophytic lesion resembling granulation tisue.[11,17,19] There should be a low threshold to obtain a biopsy in the appropriate clinical scenario.

Workup and Treatment

Once a biopsy confirms the diagnosis, patients hould be worked up with staging in accordance with usual oncologic principles.

- There is no TMN staging specific to Marjolin ulcers.
  - The staging system for the histologic type of tumor should be used.
- Marjolin ulcers tend to be more aggressive than common skin cancers.
  - Metastasis rate of 27.5%[14]
- A thorough lymph node examination should be performed.
- Consider imaging to look for distant metastases.
  - Chest radiography
  - Brain computed tomography
  - Abdominal ultrasound or cross-sectional imaging

Surgery remains the primary treatment of Marjolin ulcers. A wide excision of the primary lesion should be performed. Most investigators advocate for at least 2-cm margins,[11,17,19] with a split-thickness skin graft or flap coverage of the wound. Occasionally, amputation is needed. Most agree that a prophylactic lymph node dissection is not indicated. Clinically positive nodes warrant biopsy and/or lymph node dissection. Some investigators advocate for a sentinel node biopsy to be performed if nodes are clinically negative. There is no standard agreed on protocol for the addition of adjuvant therapies after adequate surgical excision. Those described include radiotherapy; chemotherapy with agents, such as topical 5-fluorouracil, methotrexate, and L-phenylalanine mustard; and intra-arterial limb isolation perfusion therapy.[17] Poor prognosis when compared with other types of skin cancer is to be expected.

Prevention

Prevention is perhaps the best strategy in treatment of Marjolin ulcers. Allowing burn wounds to go unexcised and heal by secondary intention places patients at much high risk for development of Marjolin ulcers in the future. Patients with resultant fragile burn scars should have these re-excised, or at the minimum closely monitored, to ensure that they do not undergo malignant transformation.

In developed nations, early excision and grafting is standard. The patients most at risk for development of Marjolin ulcers are those with poor access to health care. In a recent large series from Bangladesh, Das and colleagues[21] included 140 patients with burn scar ulcers over a 10-year period, of which 46 (33%) were found to have malignant changes. Of the patients with malignancy, 77% had a primary-level education or less. Appropriate treatment of deep burns with excision and grafting at the time of injury minimizes the future risk of malignant transformation of resultant scars to Marjolin ulcers.

Case Report

The authors present a 75-year-old woman who had sustained a more than 50% TBSA burn from a house fire when she was 4 years old. Over the course of 11 months, she developed a nonhealing ulcer in the right upper quadrant of her abdominal wall, managed initially by a wound care center, with topical growth factors and biological dressings. Punch biopsy was eventually obtained, revealing a diagnosis of SCC, arising from her burn scar. Physical examination by the senior author was positive for an ulcerative, 5 × 8-cm skin lesion (**Fig. 3**), which was fixed to the underlying fascia but negative for axillary or

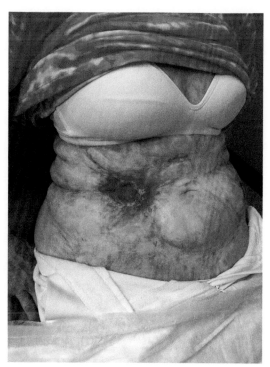

Fig. 3. A 75-year-old woman with a Marjolin ulcer in right upper abdominal wall.

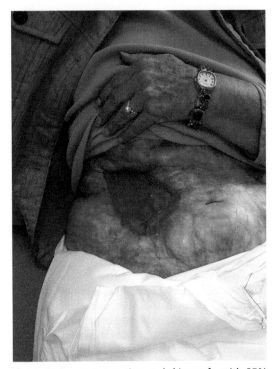

Fig. 4. Status post resection and skin graft, with 85% take, secondary to zoster infection in dermatome.

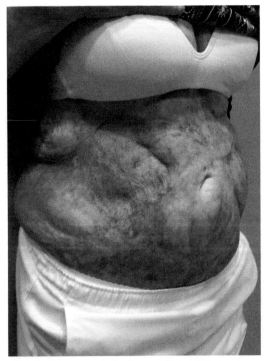

Fig. 5. Three years following wide local excision, no evidence of recurrent disease.

inguinal adenopathy. Computed tomography scan demonstrated extension to, but not through the anterior rectus abdominis fascia, with no evidence of nodal involvement. At the time of surgical resection, 1 month later, the lesion had grown to 7 × 9 cm and was excised with a 2- to 3-cm margin, leaving a 13 × 14-cm defect that was skin grafted. Sentinel lymph node biopsy was also performed with lymphoscintigraphy and lymphazurin blue dye, localizing the basin to the right groin, where 2 sentinel lymph nodes were removed. Frozen-section biopsies were obtained from all 4 quadrants, as well as the deep margin, all of which were negative for tumor, as were the lymph nodes from the right groin. Her postoperative course was complicated by a herpes zoster wound infection, which resulted in an initial 85% take of her skin graft (**Fig. 4**). Three years later, she remains free of disease (**Fig. 5**). Tumor surveillance is performed by semiannual physical examination.

REFERENCES

1. Indications for hyperbaric oxygen therapy. 2014 Available at: https://www.uhms.org/resources/hbo indications.html. Accessed July 11, 2016.
2. Dauwe PB, Pulikkottil BJ, Lavery L, et al. Does hyperbaric oxygen therapy work in facilitating acute wound healing: a systematic review. Plast Reconstr Surg 2014;133(2):208e–15e.
3. Churchill-Davidson I, Sanger C, Thomlinson RH. High-pressure oxygen and radiotherapy. Lancet 1955;268(6874):1091–5.
4. Undersea and Hyperbaric Medical Society (UHMS). In: Weaver LK, editor. Hyperbaric oxygen therapy indications: the hyperbaric oxygen therapy committee report. 13th edition. North Palm Beach (FL): Best Publishing Company; 2014.
5. Wasiak J, Bennett M, Cleland HJ. Hyperbaric oxygen as adjuvant therapy in the management of burns: can evidence guide clinical practice? Burns 2006;32(5):650–2.
6. Villanueva E, Bennett MH, Wasiak J, et al. Hyperbaric oxygen therapy for thermal burns. Cochrane Database Syst Rev 2004;(3):CD004727.
7. Hart G, O'Reilly R, Broussard N, et al. Treatment of burns with hyperbaric oxygen. Surg Gynecol Obstet 1974;139(5):693–6.
8. Brannen AL, Still J, Haynes M. A randomized prospective trial of hyperbaric oxygen in a referral burn center population. Am Surg 1997;63:205–8.
9. Kranke P, Bennett MH, Martyn-St James M, et al. Hyperbaric oxygen therapy for chronic wounds [review]. Cochrane Database Syst Rev 2015;(6):CD004123.
10. Jones LM, Rubadue C, Brown NV, et al. Evaluation of TCOM/HBOT practice guideline for the treatment of

foot burns occurring in diabetic patients. Burns 2015;41(3):536–41.

11. Saaiq M, Ashraf B. Marjolin's ulcers in the post-burned lesions and scars. World J Clin Cases 2014;2(10):507–14.

12. Ching YH, Sutton TL, Pierpont YN, et al. The use of growth factors and other humoral agents to accelerate and enhance burn wound healing. Eplasty 2011;11:e41.

13. Alemdaroğlu C, Değim Z, Celebi N, et al. An investigation on burn wound healing in rats with chitosan gel formulation containing epidermal growth factor. Burns 2006;32(3):319–27.

14. Travis TE, Mauskar NA, Mino MJ, et al. Commercially available topical platelet-derived growth factor as a novel agent to accelerate burn-related wound healing. J Burn Care Res 2014;35(5):e321–9.

15. Zhang Y, Wang T, He J, et al. Growth factor therapy in patients with partial-thickness burns: a systematic review and meta-analysis. Int Wound J 2016;13(3):354–66.

16. Lee KC, Joory K, Moiemen NS. History of burns: the past, present and the future. Burns Trauma 2014; 2(4):169–80.

17. Copcu E. Marjolin's ulcer: a preventable complication of burns? Plast Reconstr Surg 2009;124(1): 156e–64e.

18. Kerr-Valentic MA, Samimi K, Rohlen BH, et al. Marjolin's ulcer: modern analysis of an ancient problem. Plast Reconstr Surg 2009;123(1):184–91.

19. Pekarek B, Buck S, Osher L. A comprehensive review on Marjolin's ulcers: diagnosis and treatment. J Am Col Certif Wound Spec 2011;3(3):60–4.

20. Giblin T, Pickrell K, Pitts W, et al. Malignant degeneration in burn scars: Marjolin's ulcer. Ann Surg 1965; 162:291–7.

21. Das KK, Chakaraborty A, Rahman A, et al. Incidences of malignancy in chronic burn scar ulcers: experience from Bangladesh. Burns 2015;41(6): 1315–21.

Index

Note: Page numbers of article titles are in **boldface** type.

Clin Plastic Surg 44 (2017) 689–693
http://dx.doi.org/10.1016/S0094-1298(17)30077-9
0094-1298/17

Moving?

Make sure your subscription moves with you!

To notify us of your new address, find your **Clinics Account Number** (located on your mailing label above your name), and contact customer service at:

Email: journalscustomerservice-usa@elsevier.com

800-654-2452 (subscribers in the U.S. & Canada)
314-447-8871 (subscribers outside of the U.S. & Canada)

Fax number: 314-447-8029

Elsevier Health Sciences Division
Subscription Customer Service
3251 Riverport Lane
Maryland Heights, MO 63043

*To ensure uninterrupted delivery of your subscription, please notify us at least 4 weeks in advance of move.

Printed and bound by CPI Group (UK) Ltd, Croydon, CR0 4YY

08/05/2025

01864699-0014